Review & Study Guide

PSYCHIATRIC NURSING
PROMOTING MENTAL HEALTH

Elaine R. Zimbler
Educational Consultant and Associate
Center for Nursing Education and Testing
Martinsville, New Jersey

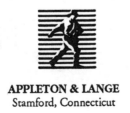

APPLETON & LANGE
Stamford, Connecticut

Copyright © 1997 by Appleton & Lange
A Simon & Schuster Company

97 98 99 00 01 / 10 9 8 7 6 5 4 3 2 1

Prentice Hall International (UK) Limited, London
Prentice Hall of Australia Pty. Limited, Sydney
Prentice Hall Canada, Inc., Toronto
Prentice Hall Hispanoamericana, S.A., Mexico
Prentice Hall of India Private Limited, New Delhi
Prentice Hall of Japan, Inc., Tokyo
Simon & Schuster Asia Pte. Ltd., Singapore
Editora Prentice Hall do Brasil Ltda., Rio de Janeiro
Prentice Hall, Upper Saddle River, New Jersey

Editor-in-Chief: Sally J. Barhydt
Development Editor: Barbara Severs
Production Editor: Maria T. Vlasak
Typography: Thomas M. O'Brien
Cover Design: Libby Schmitz

PRINTED IN THE UNITED STATES OF AMERICA

ISBN 0-8385-8121-8

90000

9 780838 581216

TABLE OF CONTENTS

TABLE OF CONTENTS

PREFACE

REVIEW AND STUDY GUIDE FOR PSYCHI-ATRIC NURSING: PROMOTING MENTAL HEALTH has been developed to help students learn the important concepts in mental health nursing. The textbook *Psychiatric Nursing: Promoting Mental Health* by Ann Wolbert Burgess and 33 contributors is the basis for the material presented in this Review; the text's organization is followed here, chapter by chapter.

REVIEW AND STUDY GUIDE FOR PSYCHI-ATRIC NURSING: PROMOTING MENTAL HEALTH can be helpful to learners with many different needs. For students who are having their first experience in psychiatric nursing, it can be used as a tool to assist them in conceptualizing what they have read in their textbook. In some cases, the *Review and Study Guide* may be used itself as a text. For students who are preparing for the NCLEX-RN examination, this book is a review of vital issues in psychiatric nursing. In addition, multiple-choice questions, similar to those used for the computerized NCLEX-RN, appear at the end of the book. Moreover, this publication is a useful review of basic concepts for nurses who, after an absence of some time from practicing psychiatric nursing, are returning to that work. Similarly, those who are beginning their psychi-atric nursing work experience will find the book a helpful study guide.

Each chapter in *REVIEW AND STUDY GUIDE FOR PSYCHIATRIC NURSING: PROMOTING MENTAL HEALTH* begins with Terms to Define. You may find that you are familiar with some of the vocabulary; some terms, however, may be new to you. Depending on your learning style, you may choose to define these terms before read-ing the chapter, or you may prefer to read the chapter to discover definitions.

To assist you in focusing your thinking as you read through each chapter, Gaining A Perspec-tive has been developed. It presents issues or prob-lems that you should consider as you read the chapter's Key Concepts that follow. The Key Con-cepts address the most salient ideas addressed in the chapter.

After you have read the Key Concepts, you are asked, in Taking Another Look, to answer, per-haps in writing, the questions posed in Gaining a Perspective. The intention is that you spend time thinking about the application of the conceptual material presented in the Key Concepts.

You will note that at the end of each chapter you are referred to the section Suggested Re-sponses. Those responses are intended to give you some ideas about how you might have ad-dressed the problems raised in Gaining A Per-spective. Because the goal is for you to think crit-ically, the quality of your responses cannot be stressed enough.

The last section of this book contains 100 mul-tiple-choice questions with content similar to that which may be on the NCLEX-RN examina-tion. Correct answers and rationales are provid-ed for each of these questions in the last section of the book.

— Elaine R. Zimbler

ACKNOWLEDGEMENTS

It has indeed been a privilege for me to develop this *Review and Study Guide*. My thanks to Ann Wolbert Burgess and her colleagues for providing me with *Psychiatric Nursing: Promoting Mental Health*, a wonderful source of material. It is a pleasure to see a text that addresses the issues that are so pressing in today's psychiatric mental health environments. Barbara Severs, Senior Development Editor in Nursing at Appleton & Lange, took my raw materials and, because of her expertise, made this book a product to be proud of. Barbara is so knowledgeable, but it is her support, patience, and calmness that I appreciate most. Lastly, I would like to thank my family, Shari, Ray, Rebecca, and Andy, for providing me with an environment that allows me to continue to develop and grow.

SECTION I
ENTERING THE 21ST CENTURY

1 BEGINNING THE PSYCHIATRIC NURSING EXPERIENCE

TERMS TO DEFINE

TERMS TO DEFINE

patient reactions, demands

routes toward self-awareness

self-inventory

social networks

GAINING A PERSPECTIVE

After you have read the Key Concepts for this chapter, describe your feelings or intentions in regard to the following two questions.

1. What type of feelings are you and other students likely to have prior to beginning a psychiatric nursing experience?

2. How do you intend to prepare for the beginning experience?

Key Concepts

- **SELF-INVENTORY** is a way for an individual to reflect as objectively as possible on one's own thoughts, feelings, and behaviors. The inventory is a way to distinguish between **self** and **others**, enabling a nurse to understand what is unique about the patient without projecting one's own misconceptions and emotions to the patient. Self-appraisal is emphasized in psychiatric nursing because the primary tool for intervention is the therapeutic relationship and alliance.

- **INTERVIEWING ONESELF** is helpful by asking questions that relate to beginning and practicing psychiatric nursing. Following are examples of questions that might be asked.

  Do you have strong feelings or emotions when you think of walking into a psychiatric hosptial or unit? What are they?

  Are you afraid of being hurt?

  What has been your experience with mentally ill individuals?

- **FEELINGS OF BEING FRIGHTENED OR IN-ADEQUATE** are not uncommon for students before beginning a new venture. To manage fear and anxiety, factual information must be sought. For example,

  Mental illness is not contagious.

  Most mentally ill patients are not violent.

- **RECOGNIZING THAT A SITUATION IS STRANGE AND ACKNOWLEDGING FEEL-INGS OF ANXIETY** are helpful responses in the initial stage of one's experience in psychiatric nursing. As time goes on, you will find that you are more comfortable addressing the behaviors that upset you and communicating them to the patient.

- **IN BEGINNING THE CLINICAL EXPERIENCE,** students describe feeling awkward, useless, and appearing like a novice. They believe they have no understanding of how people behave or what psychological problems are. Students are beginners, but in psychiatric nursing they have a good start, as they have spent years talking with people and listening to them.

- **PSYCHIATRIC PATIENTS, LIKE ALL PEOPLE, HAVE THEIR OWN THOUGHTS AND FEELINGS, AS WELL AS LIFE.** Students need to learn about them. Although it is important to learn about a patient from reading a chart or talking with others who know the patient, too much emphasis on these activities may be a clue that a student is afraid or blocked in some way from moving forward.

- **SUPERVISION IS A PROCESS** whereby student and supervisor review the student's clinical work; it is not to analyze the student, but to help with the self-inventory assessment.

- **IDENTIFYING WITH PATIENTS** or thinking that you have symptoms or emotions similar to those of your patient happens to students in any rotation. Strong emotions similar to the patient's are often the initial underdeveloped capacities for empathy—an initial phase of identification. An awareness should develop that you are a separate individual and that you need not to feel guilt or responsibility for the other (patient). This is a part of developing a capacity of self-awareness.

- **A STUDENT'S STRONG EMOTIONS CAN BE INSIGHTS** into the patient's defensive behaviors, as well as your own defensive behaviors and prejudices. As part of self-inventory you might ask:
  Are strong emotions coming from expectations

that you have of what is appropriate behavior? Do you believe that persons who demand much, or keep repeating how depressed they are, are self-centered and indulging themselves? The demanding patient can be interesting, complicated, and exasperating.

- **PATIENTS MAKE STATEMENTS THAT ELICIT EMBARRASSMENT, GUILT, AND EXCESSIVE SELF-CONSCIOUSNESS FROM STUDENTS.** Patients seem to put staff "on the spot." Through supervision and after being "put on the spot," the student learns how to separate himself or herself and personal reactions from the patient.

- **IF YOU SAY THE WRONG THING,** you may be in the best position to learn something.

- **WHILE ASSESSING PATIENTS, STUDENTS OFTEN BECOME CONCERNED ABOUT OFFENDING PATIENTS WITH PARTICULAR QUESTIONS.** The fear of hurting the patient arises for some students in asking questions about impulse control, including suicidal and violent behavior; orientation to reality; sexual behavior; or interpersonal traumatic events. The nurse must be comfortable in realizing that these events are possibilities in any person's life.

- **OUR COMMUNICATION AND RELATIONSHIPS WITH OTHERS ARE IMPORTANT MEANS FOR LEARNING ABOUT OURSELVES.** Family relations, the first of our social networks, provide some of the most enduring lessons in self-awareness. School provides additional lessons through relationships with teachers and peers. In nursing, the student-supervisor relationship can be an influential avenue of self-awareness. Another influential relationship is with a mentor. A mentor is a guide who supports, facilitates, and promotes the intellectual and career development of another person. Lessons learned in these relationships are modified by life experiences, which usually include other deep and lasting relationships. Counseling and therapy are additional ways to learn about oneself.

- **READING IS A ROUTE TO SELF-AWARENESS.** Through the formal study of psychiatric mental health nursing, students are exposed to written ideas about clinical practice. Reading fiction and nonfiction (especially autobiographies) helps one learn about human nature and oneself.

- **WRITING IN A DIARY**, journal, or log also enhances self-awareness. The notes can be unstructured and written sporadically or regularly. In addition, process recordings — a more formal method of writing — help students deal more effectively with clients. Process recordings usually include verbatim accounts of nurse-client communication, and are helpful in clinical supervision. Over time, at regular intervals, the recordings can be reviewed and summarized to document major patterns or themes and the overall progress of the nurse-client interaction.

TAKING ANOTHER LOOK

You are now ready to respond to the issues raised in Gaining a Perspective at the beginning of this chapter. After you have written or thought about your responses, you may want to look at the Suggested Responses on page 317.

2 PSYCHIATRIC NURSING

TERMS TO DEFINE

advanced level psychiatric nursing

ANA Statement on Psychiatric Mental Health Clinical Nursing

basic level functions

Coalition of Psychiatric Nursing Organizations (COPNO)

phenomena of concern

primary mental health care

subspecialization

GAINING A PERSPECTIVE

Consider the three questions listed below, and respond to them in more depth after you have read the Key Concepts in this chapter.

1. What are your purposes and expectations in learning about psychiatric nursing?

2. Where do you think the focus of psychiatric nursing will be in the future?

3. What type of qualifications do you need to practice in the psychiatric mental health area?

Key Concepts

• **THE RE-INTEGRATION OF PHYSICAL AND PSYCHOSOCIAL CARE** for persons with mental illness is an area that psychiatric nurses are in an advantageous position to pursue. Psychiatric nursing is revitalized when the emphasis is on the connections among brain, spirit, mind, and body.

• **THE ANA STATEMENT ON PSYCHIATRIC MENTAL HEALTH CLINICAL NURSING PRACTICE** defines psychiatric mental health nursing as the diagnosis and treatment of human responses to actual or potential mental health problems. Psychiatric nursing is a specialized area of nursing practice that employs neurobiological principles and theories of human behavior as its science and the purposeful use of self as its art.

Psychiatric nursing focuses on 12 phenomena of concern:

Maintenance of optimal health and well-being and prevention of psychobiological illness.

Self-care limitations or impaired functioning related to mental and emotional distress.

Deficits in the functioning of significant biological, emotional, and cognitive systems.

Emotional stress or crisis components of illness, pain, and disability.

Self-concept changes, developmental issues, and life-process changes.

Problems related to emotions such as anxiety, anger, sadness, loneliness, and grief.

Physical symptoms that occur along with altered psychological functioning.

Alterations in thinking, perceiving, symbolizing, communicating, and decision making.

Difficulties in relating to others.

Behaviors and mental states that indicate the patient is a danger to self or others or has a severe disability.

Interpersonal systems, sociocultural, spiritual, or environmental circumstances or events that affect the mental and emotional well-being of the individual, family, or community.

Symptoms, side effects/toxicity associated with psychopharmacological intervention and other aspects of the treatment regimen.

• THE EARLIEST KNOWN METHOD OF TREATING MENTALLY ILL INDIVIDUALS may be described as the supernatural, or mystical, model of healing. For centuries the behavior of the mentally ill was interpreted as being caused by demons, malevolent gods, witches, werewolves, vampires, planet movement, and atmospheric changes. Inhuman conditions existed throughout the ages and knowing about them should help the student appreciate the significance of reforms in the mental health field.

• THE CUSTODIAL METHOD was the model of healing the mentally ill that replaced the mystical model. Demonology declined when the Greek physician Hippocrates suggested that mental disorders probably had their origins in some brain dysfunction, but this philosophy was only temporary.

Two major trends emerged: vigorous use of the supernatural to account for mental disturbances and increased inhumane treatment for the mentally ill. In response to some of the cruel aspects of treatment, moral management emerged through the efforts of Philippe Pinel (1745-1826), William Tuke (1732-1822), and Dorothea Dix (1802-1887). Moral management was humane treatment for the mentally disturbed while they were in mental institutions (asylums).

• DETENTION RATHER THAN TREATMENT was employed in mental institutions during the 19th century. The stigma of mental illness was communicated to the patient. When organized nursing was introduced into hospital settings, however, major changes occurred in the care of the

mentally ill. The Nightingale model of training was brought to America in 1873.

• LINDA RICHARDS (one of the first trained nurses) believed that mentally ill persons needed nursing care, which led to the creation of schools of nursing in state hospitals and training programs in other institutions. Yet, by the end of the 19th century the vast majority of professional nurses who worked in psychiatric hospitals had little or no training in psychiatry. In the early 1900s there was little demand for "asylum" nurses, as the mental hospitals employed attendants at very low wages. The goal of establishing psychiatric affiliations for students in all schools of nursing was not reached until later in the 20th century.

• THE MENTAL HEALTH ACT OF 1946 marked the beginning of psychiatric nursing as a nursing specialty and mental health profession. It provided federal funds for the support of psychiatric nursing at both the graduate and undergraduate levels. In 1949, the National Institute of Mental Health was established to identify and promote goals and priorities for the mental health field. Public concern for poor treatment in state mental hospitals spurred signing into law in 1955 the Mental Health Study Act. In 1961, a report (Action for Mental Health) strongly emphasized community-based services and a reduction in inpatient facilities. In 1963, the Community Mental Health Centers Act was signed into law, and over time it provided assistance to communities for construction and operation of community mental health centers.

In 1978 the Report to the President from the Commission on Mental Health recommended development of mental health centers throughout the country that would respond to changing circumstances and to the diverse cultural and racial backgrounds of people. The report clearly identified nurses as members of the interdisciplinary mental health team and made nurses eligible for third-party reimbursement. These recommendations were to be implemented through the law passed in 1978, but because of changes in political attitudes and decentralization of funds from the federal to state level, the recommendations were never fully implemented. Consequently, the trend toward block grants to states continues.

- **THE SECOND WORLD WAR RENEWED INTEREST IN PSYCHIATRIC CARE** and profoundly affected psychiatric nursing. The passage and funding of the National Mental Health Act of 1946 influenced the scope and direction of psychiatric nursing and psychiatric nursing education because it encouraged nurses to fill a wide variety of roles. In addition, a study by the National League for Nursing (1950) concluded that special training was required for psychiatric nurses.

  Doctoral education in nursing gained momentum in 1955 when the United States Public Health Service (USPHS) initiated the Special Pre-doctoral Research Fellowships (direct grants to students to finance doctoral education) and the Nurse Scientist Training Programs, which provided grants to schools of nursing.

- **THE PSYCHIATRIC NURSE IS A CLINICIAN ACTIVELY INVOLVED IN:**

  Primary preventive interventions to educate about mental health risks before illness occurs.

  Secondary preventive interventions to treat mental illness as quickly as it is diagnosed

  Tertiary preventive interventions to minimize the effects of long-term or chronic psychiatric illness.

- **DISSEMINATING GOOD SCIENTIFIC RESEARCH** will, it is believed, continue to improve the quality of patient care. The psychiatric nurse has a history of involvement in practice-based research and theory development. In 1952, Gwen Tudor's research indicated that the social milieu of the psychiatric ward operated to maintain deviant patient behavior and emphasized the critical role of the nurse in managing that milieu. In 1954, Schwing's "The Way to the Soul of the Mentally Ill" and Sechehaye's "Symbolic Realization" focused on nurses' therapeutic potential

with patients, as did Hildegard Peplau's work. **Hildegard Peplau, June Mellow, and Ida Jean Orlando were probably most influential** in developing a conceptual base for psychiatric nursing. Peplau's framework provides a system within which the nurse helps the patient to examine situational factors, with the focus on improving interpersonal competencies that have been lost or never learned. Within the system the patient's behavior is observed. Together the nurse and patient describe and analyze behaviors, and connections are noted. New patient behaviors are tested and integrated, while the nurse assesses his or her own interpersonal behavior.

Mellow's nursing therapy gives the patient an opportunity to participate in a corrective emotional experience in order to facilitate integration of the ego. The nurse must be able to cope with intense patient feelings and manage his or her own feelings during the relationship (skills similar to those needed for psychoanalytic psychotherapy).

Orlando's theory concerns the dynamic nurse-patient relationship.

- **EFFORTS ARE COALESCING TO MAKE PSYCHIATRIC NURSING STRONGER.** The Coalition of Psychiatric Nursing Organizations (COPNO) is composed of two representatives from each of the following: the ANA Council on Psychiatric and Mental Health Nursing, the American Psychiatric Nursing Society, the Society for Education and Research in Psychiatric Nursing, and Advocates for Child Psychiatric Nursing. The group formulated a task force to revise the Statement on Psychiatric Mental Health Nursing Practice and the Standards of Psychiatric Mental Health Nursing Clinical Practice. The report addressed primary mental health care and the scope and levels of psychiatric mental health clinical practice.

- **PRIMARY MENTAL HEALTH CARE IS DEFINED AS** the continuous and comprehensive services necessary to promote mental health, prevent mental illness, maintain health, manage and/or refer mental and physical problems, diagnose and treat mental disorders and their sequelae, and facilitate rehabilitation. In diagnosing human responses to actual or potential mental health problems, theory is applied to human phenomena through the process of assessment, diagnosis, planning, intervention or treatment, and evaluation. To help develop a treatment plan based on assessment data and theoretical premises, the psychiatric mental health nurse uses nursing diagnoses and standard classifications of mental disorders, such as those found in the Diagnostic and Statistical Manual (DSM) of Mental Disorders of the American Psychiatric Association and the International Classification of Diseases.

- **PSYCHIATRIC NURSES ARE SPECIALIZED REGISTERED NURSES (RNs)** educated in nursing and licensed to practice in their individual state. Currently, RNs are qualified for specialty practice at the basic and advanced levels, which are differentiated by educational preparation, experience, type of practice (i.e., clinician, administrator, educator, or researcher), and certification.

  At the basic level of specialization the psychiatric nurse is licensed, has a baccalaureate degree, demonstrates clinical skills, and is certified. Certification is a formal process that validates the nurse's competency and permits the use of "C" after RN (RN,C).

  At the advanced level, the nurse has a master's degree and is nationally certified as a clinical nurse specialist (RN,CS).

  Doctoral programs in nursing may focus on either advanced development of the clinician role with a research component related to specific clinical problems (Doctor of Nursing Science — DNSc) or research and theory development in the science of psychiatric mental health nursing (Doctor of Philosophy—PhD). Subspecialization in a specific area of practice may be categorized according to a develop-

mental period (e.g., child and adolescent, geriatric), a specific mental/emotional disorder (e.g., addiction, depression), a particular practice focus (e.g., family, community), and/or a specific role or function (e.g., forensic nursing, psychiatric liaison).

- **PSYCHIATRIC NURSING HAS CLINICAL PRACTICE FUNCTIONS.** At the basic level, interventions promote and foster health, assess dysfunction, assist clients to regain or improve their coping abilities, and prevent further disability. The interventions focus on psychiatric patients and include health promotion and maintenance, intake screening and evaluation, case management, provision of a therapeutic environment (i.e., milieu therapy), tracking clients and assisting them with self-care activities, administering and monitoring psychobiological treatment regimens, (including prescribed psychopharmacological agents), health teaching, crisis intervention and counseling, and outreach activities such as home visits, community action, and advocacy.

- **PSYCHIATRIC NURSING HAS PROGRESSED** from a custodial function; it has improved the care of psychiatrically ill and emotionally distressed individuals, and advocated for an optimal level of mental health for all people.

TAKING ANOTHER LOOK

You are now ready to respond to the questions raised by Gaining a Perspective at the beginning of this chapter. After you have written or thought about your responses, you may look at the Suggested Responses on page 317.

3 PATTERNS OF PSYCHIATRIC NURSING PRACTICE: INTEGRATING THE ARTS WITH THE SCIENCE

TERMS TO DEFINE

empirics

esthetics

ethics

personal knowledge

syntactical learning

GAINING A PERSPECTIVE

1. Consider what might be the best way to learn about psychiatric nursing. Think about such things as the experiences you would need, how much time it would take you, and what type of facilities would be required. Then, after you have read the following Key Concepts, describe more concretely what is required in your psychiatric nursing education.

Key Concepts

- **FOR SYNTACTICAL LEARNING,** students are encouraged to think by viewing wholes — whole patients within whole communities.

- **BARBARA CARPER'S FRAMEWORK (1978) IS FOUNDED ON FOUR PATTERNS OF KNOWING.** It includes the idea that nursing knowledge comes from formal instruction and common everyday forms of knowing. The four patterns are:
  - Empirics. Traditional ideas of science using such methods as observation, experimentation, description, and prediction.
  - Personal knowledge. Knowing ourselves, our values, and how we can be helped to interact with another human.
  - Ethics. Moral knowledge, for example, respect for human dignity.
  - Esthetics. The art of nursing—its beauty and the understanding of what is possible in the practice of nursing.

  The four patterns are interrelated and dynamic.

- **THE CORE CONTENT (CURRICULUM) OF PSYCHIATRIC NURSING** is presented in Study Guide Table 3-1.

  In keeping with current trends, the curriculum is community oriented; the clinical portion includes a significant community practicum. The key assumption underlying the core content (curriculum) is that mental health practice is fundamental to everything that happens to the patient, whether in a psychiatric hospital, critical care unit, or any treatment environment.

Table 3-1

Core Content	PMHN Course Content	Competencies
Growth and development	Appropriate care for psychiatric clients	Plan and implement age appropriate care
Neuroanatomy, neurophysiology, neuroendocrinology, neuroimmunology	Nuerocognitive alterations in mental illness, and neurobiological alterations in mental illness, stress management	Demonstrate basic assessment skills to include: a. sensory perception, cognitive deficits b. information processing resulting in alterations of behavior and social functioning and bio-psychoneuroimmunological changes
Diagnostic thinking Inductive, deductive, and reproductive reasoning Syntactical thinking	Major psychiatric diagnostic classifications per DSM; mental health alterations and nursing diagnosis; client in context	Identify symptoms of each category. Desribe what data is present and demonstrate how conclusions are reached.
Basic management principles Case management Psychiatric treatment	Referral processes Expected outcomes of psychiatric treatment Behavior change Supportive relationship Insight	Ability to participate in case management and management of psychiatric care. Plan for a continuum of care. Mobilize resources to provide, safety, structure, and support for the mentally ill. Refer patients for counseling and therapy.
Critical pathways Interdisciplinary roles	Critical pathways related to major mental illness Roles of various mental health care providers, including roles of psychiatric nurses with various levels of education	Implement critical pathways related to patients with major mental illnesses. Demonstrate ability to work with various members of the interdisciplinary team.
Health care promotion and illness prevention	Smoking cessation; exercise, endorphin, enkephelina, nutritional aspects of mental health; principles of sobriety	Plan and facilitate a mental health promotion plan for a client with serious mental illness.
Community health	Community mental health; community support initiative; at-risk populations; social policy regarding care of mentally ill	Participate in delegating care and making appropriate referrals for psychiatric patients. Identify at-risk populations and major policy governing mentally ill.
Conceptual nursing models	Psychiatric nursing models of care	Determine model of care and articulate its fit within PMHN context.

Table 3-1 continued

Core Content	PMHN Course Content	Competencies
Ethical and legal principles, values, clarification	1. Nurse Practice Acts 2. Standards of practice or PMHN 3. Confidentiality 4. Least restrictive treatment	Clarify personal values continuously re mental illness. Facilitate others to clarify values and attitudes related to self and mental illness.
Person as consumer, person with family and context, family/significant other Person with family and context	Principles of collaborative relationships with individuals, and families, consumer, and advocacy groups Systems theory	Demonstrate ability to assist with individuals and families in developing and implementing context-sensitive care plans for psychiatric patients.
Basic pharmacology	Major psychotropic agents for identified psychiatric illness that includes: a. action and expected effects b. side effects and toxicity c. potential interactions with other medications	Evaluate effects of medication on patients, including symptoms, side effects, toxicity, and potential interactions with other medications/substances. Teach patients and families medication management. Evaluate outcomes of medications.
Principles of learning and learning theories	Psychoeducational approaches to working with individuals, families, and consumers	Demonstrate ability to develop and implement a teaching project related to mental health-illness issues.
Communication theory and skills	Therapeutic use of self: a. understanding, using, and controlling effective responses b. integrating effective and cognitive responses with appropriate interventions c. continuing clarification and maintenance of professional boundaries d. evaluating interventions with psychiatric clients	Demonstrate therapeutic use of self: Self-assessment Self-observation
Crisis intervention Violence Stress-crisis continuum	Concept of anxiety, coping Principles of anger and aggression Crisis intervention with psychiatric clients by level of stress	Assess potential violence; intervene in acute agitation.
Cultural and ethical differences Spiritual needs	Compare and contrast psychiatric symptoms and cultural and spiritual self expression	Provide culturally and spiritually competent care that meets client needs.
Child/adolescent development	Recognition of major child/adolescent disorders; contrast with adult disorders	Articulate interventions that might be used with children/adolescents who have behavioral deviations.

continued

Table 3-1 continued

Core Content	PMHN Course Content	Competencies
Chronic illness	Symptoms management in seriously and persistently mentally ill Relapse care/prevention	Establish therapeutic relationship with seriously and persistently mentally ill patients.
Advocacy	Consumer advocacy groups	Observe functioning of advocacy groups. Become acquainted with and support these groups, and articulate their roles.
Concepts of risk and screening for psychiatric emergencies	Risk factors, screening, and referral related to psychiatric illness and social problems: a. suicide/homicide b. substance abuse c. violence/abuse	Screen for substance use/abuse. Screen for victim violence/abuse. Screen for suicide and homicide.
Group process	Therapeutic factors in group intervention	Demonstrate beginning group participation/leadership skills. Trace the nature and scope of thinking about psychopathology.
History (from demonology to biology) Development of the psychosocial and sociocultural points of view	Mental illness through the ages. Ideas carried over through history; ideas carried over through the arts Normal and abnormal behavioral through the eyes of the scientist	Trace the progress that has been made in the understanding of human behavior.
Human sexuality	Impaired sexual expression/sexual dysfunction	Trace the sexual farce continuum. Differentiate between "normal" sexuality and sexual dysfunction. Refer for treatment of STDs

- **TO ACHIEVE THE ASSESSMENT AND DIAGNOSTIC SKILLS NEEDED** in psychiatric practice, it is necessary to have a broad knowledge base. Neuroanatomy, neurophysiology, neuroendocrinology, neuroimmunology, and recent findings in human growth and development are content that is necessary for the student to understand the rationale behind nursing interventions.

- **CONTENT STRESSES ETHICS AND HEALTH CARE'S MORAL CODE.** The structural practice of nursing includes the following elements:
  Tasks of caring.
  Recognition of patients' rights and responsibilities, including legal status, right to treatment, right to refuse treatment, and right to be treated in the least restrictive environment possible.
  Nurses' rights and responsibilities, guided by the Standards of Nursing Practice and the Code of Ethics.
  Ethical issues are of particular concern as health care becomes increasingly profit driven.

- **NURSES ARE ENABLED TO TALK WITH PATIENTS AND THEIR FAMILIES, AS WELL AS LISTEN TO THEM,** by using communication theory and skills, personal knowledge, and intuition. This is key to *all* nursing practice.

- **CENTRAL TO NURSING IS UNDERSTANDING CERTAIN HUMAN EXPERIENCES,** such as the nature of self, anguish, guilt, and love. Interacting with individuals as well as reading their literature and viewing their artistic creations can help to explain or illustrate how patients experience feelings and thoughts that sometimes they cannot express.

TAKING ANOTHER LOOK

You are now ready to respond to the question raised in Gaining a Perspective at the beginning of this chapter. After you have written or thought about your response, you may want to look at the Suggested Responses on page 318.

SECTION II
BASIC PROFESSIONAL CONCEPTS

4 BRAIN AND BEHAVIOR

GAINING A PERSPECTIVE

Consider the questions listed below. After you
have read the Key Concepts of this chapter,
describe in more detail your thoughts about these
subjects.

1. How does learning about brain function assist
   with learning about psychiatric illness?

2. How will your nursing practice be affected by
   knowing that some drugs used therapeutically
   can cause psychiatric problems?

Key Concepts

• **PSYCHOLOGY AND BIOLOGY ARE NOT
  MUTUALLY EXCLUSIVE** aspects of mental illness. Scientists are exploring the relationships
  between physiological functions and anatomical structures and their associations with mental processes including consciousness, memory, and emotions.

• **NEURONS,** the nerve cells that are the fundamental units of the nervous system, send and
  receive impulses (messages) within and outside
  the brain, helping to regulate such behaviors
  as breathing, eating, movement, and emotional status. Neurons are composed of some of the
  common structural components found in other types of cells (see Study Guide Figure 4-1).

Figure 4-1
Cell Structure

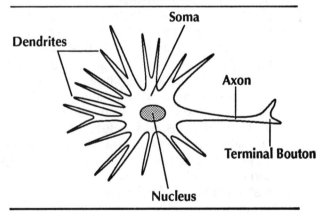

A single axon extends from the cell body of
each neuron and relays information away from
the cell body. Some axons have a protective
covering, or sheath, called myelin, which has
an insulating effect and assists in the rate of
transmission. Clinical degenerative demyelination leads to slowed conduction and subse-

quent behavioral impairments, such as in multiple sclerosis. The terminal bouton at the end of the axon contains thousand of vesicles that store chemicals (neurotransmitters), which are released into the synaptic cleft when the cell is excited, or stimulated. Axons, cell bodies, and dendrites form an ongoing system to transmit impulses in the nervous system.

Neurons are classified in several ways.

Structurally
- Number of processes from cell body, i.e., unipolar, bipolar, or multipolar
- Axonal length, i.e., long — Golgi type I; short (majority) — Golgi type II

Functionally
- Motor: transmit signals to muscles, glands, and blood vessels
- Sensory: receive stimuli from internal and external environments
- Interneuron: interconnect other neurons (generally Golgi type II)

Specificity for Neurotransmitter Release
- Cholinergic: release acetylcholine
- Serotonergic or dopaminergic: release serotonin or dopamine

The body's environment, such as oxygenation, nutrition, external toxins, internal structural changes, and stress, influences neuronal functioning. Lack of oxygen leaves nerve cells vulnerable to damage or death, potentially impairing associated behavioral functions. Poor nutrition, including vitamin deficiencies, results in behavioral manifestations of clinical significance, e.g., depressed mood, or neuritis. External toxins, such as lead, can cause encephalopathy. Internal changes, such as tumors, can cause behavioral impairment. Stress can cause a chain of physiological responses that lead to altered behavior.

- **NEURONAL FIRING** permits the transmission of impulses from one cell to another. At the synapse, the terminal bouton of one neuron is within close contact to the axon, dendrites, or cell body of another. The actual synapse involves the membrane of the presynaptic cell (the sender), the synaptic cleft, and the membrane of the postsynaptic cell (the receiver).

- **THE NERVOUS SYSTEM** is composed of two main interactive organizations: the central and peripheral systems.

Central Nervous System (CNS): structure and function

- **Brain**

Weighs approximately 1350 grams; made of nerve cells that form gray and white matter; has three lining membranes (meninges) — the pia mater (inner), arachnoid (middle), and dura mater (outer). Subdivisions of the brain are as follows:

CEREBRUM. Has two cerebral hemispheres with six lobes—frontal, parietal, temporal, occipital, insular, and limbic. (See Study Guide Figure 4-2. NOTE: The insular and limbic lobes are not shown because they are tucked underneath the frontal and temporal lobes.) The cerebrum is the center for intellectual functions; plays a primary role in processing emotion and sensory input and impulses from the voluntary muscles of the body. The cortex forms the outer layer of the cerebral lobes and has a major role in processing sensory information.

THALAMUS. Primary function is to receive and relay sensory impulses such as pain, or visual (excluding olfactory) from the body; integrates sensory and motor stimuli; plays a role in regulating mood and memory.

EPITHALAMUS. Contains the pineal gland which produces melatonin.

HYPOTHALAMUS. Plays a primary role in maintaining bodily homeostasis (e.g., regulates body temperature, water balance, circadi-

Figure 4-2
Four of Six Lobes of Cerebral Hemispheres

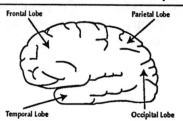

an rhythms); involved in expression of moods (limbic system); stimulates autonomic nervous system and release of a variety of hormones. (see Study Guide Table 4-1).

PITUITARY GLAND (HYPOPHYSIS). Has two lobes; controlled by the hypothalamus; key in hormone synthesis (see Study Guide Table 4-1).

LIMBIC SYSTEM. Includes several components: the hippocampal formation (including the hippocampus), which is concerned with memory and learning; the amygdala, involved in feeding, sexual, and aggressive behaviors; the thalamus, hypothalamus, and cingulate gyrus, which if damaged can cause such problems as mutism and akinesia; and the limbic midbrain nuclei (origin of noradrenergic, dopamine, and serotonin transmitter pathways).

CEREBELLUM. Functions to maintain balance and muscle tone and to coordinate voluntary muscles; impairment produces such problems as loss of balance, muscle incoordination, and hypotonia.

BRAINSTEM. Includes the pons and medulla oblongata. Controls sleep and wakefulness; directs visual and auditory reflexes; medulla controls respiration, gastrointestinal motility, and circulation; contains pathways relaying information to other areas of the CNS and from the CNS to peripheral tissues; has nuclei that play a role in neurotransmitter functioning; 10 of the 12 cranial nerves (III-XII) emerge from the brainstem; the spinal cord, which includes 31 pairs of nerves, extends down from the brainstem.

VENTRICLES. The choroid plexus within the ventricles produces cerebrospinal fluid (CSF) at the rate of 500ml/day and a steady-state volume of 100-140ml in an adult. The four fluid-containing ventricles (cavities) are interconnecting. CSF cushions the brain, delivers hormones, and transports waste products.

Peripheral Nervous System (PNS): structure and function

• Spinal nerves

Afferent spinal nerves relay information to the central nervous system, and efferent nerves away from the CNS; visceral afferent

Table 4-1
HYPOTHALAMIC AND PITUITARY HORMONES

Hypothalamus
Corticotropin-releasing hormone..........................CRH
Gonadotropin-releasing hormone.....................GnRH
Growth hormone-inhibiting hormone (somatostatin)
Growth hormone-releasing hormone................GHRH
Prolactin-inhibiting factor (dopamine)....................PIF
Prolactin-stimulating factor......................................PSF
Thyrotropin-releasing hormone............................TRH

Pituitary (anterior)
Adrenocorticotropic hormone............................ACTH
ß-lipotropin
Follicle-stimulating hormone ....FSH
Growth hormone ....GH
Lutenizing hormone..LH
Melanocyte-stimulating hormone.........................MSH
Prolactin
Thyroid-stimulating Hormone ....TSH

Pituitary (posterior)
Antidiuretic hormone (vasopressin)......................ADH
Oxytocin...OT

neurons send stimuli to the CNS; somatic afferent neurons send signals from the voluntary muscles and skin to the CNS. A transverse cross section of the spinal cord shows gray matter surrounded by white matter. The gray matter consists of three regions: dorsal horn, lateral horn, and ventral horn. The dorsal and lateral horns are associated with the afferent neurons, the ventral horn with efferent signaling.

• Efferent division of the PNS

SOMATIC NERVOUS SYSTEM. Responsible for voluntary movement or innovation of skeletal muscles

AUTONOMIC NERVOUS SYSTEM. Frequently involved in symptoms of psychiatric disorders; responsible for a wide spectrum of involuntary, automatic functions (e.g., peristalsis, heart beat); has three divisions: sympathetic, parasympathetic, and enteric. (See Study Guide Figure 4-3.)

– Sympathetic division. Involves preganglionic neurons that arise from the thoracic

Figure 4-3
Peripheral Nervous System

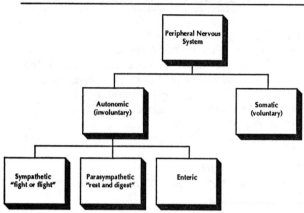

and lumbar areas of the spinal cord; referred to as adrenergic system or "fight or flight" stress response system. Stress can be physical, emotional, or both; secretes two neurotransmitters—acetylcholine (released from the preganglionic sympathetic neurons) and norepinephrine (released from the postganglionic sympathetic neurons); norepinephrine and epinephrine increase tissue response in organs with receptors specific for these adrenergic hormones.

– Parasympathetic division. Involves preganglionic neurons that originate from cranial and sacral regions; referred to as the "rest and digest" response or cholinergic system; fosters a normal hemostatic state and functions to conserve energy.

– Enteric division. Primarily concerned with regulating gastrointestinal motility.

• **PSYCHIATRIC DISORDERS ARE THOUGHT TO BE INFLUENCED** by abnormal patterns of interaction between the neurochemical messenger systems in the brain. This is in contrast to neurological disorders, which are often associated with structural lesions in the CNS. How the major neurotransmitter systems influence behavior, emotion, and cognition is summarized below.

Neurotransmitters are often secreted following a circadian rhythm; classification is based on chem-

ical structure (see Study Guide Figure 4-4). **Neurotransmitter receptor** subtypes differ in their bonding affinity for neurotransmitters and for the drugs related to the particular neurotransmitter; subtypes are located in different function areas and mediate different behavioral and therapeutic effects; major receptor types include cholinergic, dopaminergic, noradrenergic, and serotonergic systems; stimulation or inhibition of receptors results in desired and unwanted behavioral responses.

• **PSYCHIATRIC ILLNESSES ARE ASSOCIATED WITH ALTERATIONS IN SEVERAL NEUROTRANSMITTERS.** Research suggests that increased dopamine, increased norepinephrine, and the balance between dopamine and serotonin in the CNS may play a role in schizophrenia. Excessive CNS concentrations of excitatory amino acid glutamate may also contribute to psychotic symptomatology. Major depression has been associated with reduced CNS norepinephrine function and with reduced levels of serotonin metabolite 5-HIAA (5-hydroxyindoleacetic acid) in the cerebrospinal fluid. Anxiety has been linked to increased norepinephrine CNS concentrations.

Figure 4-4

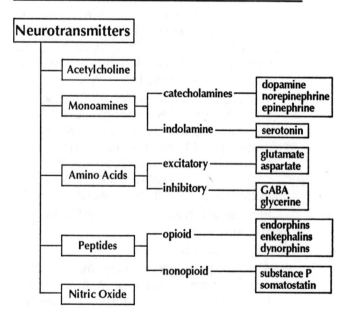

Serotonin may influence eating behavior, particularly regulating satiety. Reduced serotonin levels may be implicated in impulsive and aggressive behaviors. Other disorders such as impaired memory (including Alzheimer's disease) involve a number of neurotransmitters. Abnormalities in neurotransmitter functioning are believed to be involved in conditions such as migraine headaches, Huntington's chorea, and Parkinson's disease.

- **LABORATORY TECHNIQUES** include brain imaging and electrophysiology.

  Computed tomography (CT) is imaging that produces a series of cross-sectional x-rays to construct a three-dimensional image of the brain; used to assess bone structure and suspected organic brain disorders.

  Positron emission tomography (PET) involves administering a radioactive compound prior to obtaining cross-sectional images, which are transformed to three-dimensional images; examines brain glucose utilization, blood flow, and neurotransmitter activity.

  Single photon emission computed tomography (SPECT) is similar to PET but uses a longer acting radioactive compound; permits computer detectors to rotate around the head and make additional planar images.

  Magnetic resonance imaging (MRI) uses a magnetic field projected onto the brain; energy from brain activity is detected by sensors to produce an image; distinguishes between white and gray matter; can identify areas of demyelination.

  Electroencephalogram (EEG) measures electrical activity in the brain and is used to differentiate between organic and functional disorders.

  Polysomnography uses an EEG to obtain electrophysiological measurements of brain activity during sleep; also records eye movements (REM and non-REM); abnormal REM sleep is associated with depression.

  Evoked potentials (EP) are EEG measurements recorded in response to an external stimulus; timing of peaks in wave recording provides an index of cognitive processing.

TAKING ANOTHER LOOK

You are now ready to respond to the questions raised in Gaining a Perspective at the beginning of this chapter. After you have written your responses or thought more about them, you may want to look at the Suggested Responses on page 318.

5 MENTAL HEALTH LEARNING AND TEACHING

GAINING A PERSPECTIVE

Think about the questions that follow and after you have read the Key Concepts of this chapter, respond specifically to the two situations described below.

1. What would you, as a nurse, need to know about learning theory to effectively teach patients and their significant others?

2. How would you deal with a situation in which you, the nurse, are asked to prepare a program to teach teenagers about mental illness?

Key Concepts

- **MOTIVATION IS A CRITICAL ISSUE IN HEALTH TEACHING.** How to motivate people is outlined in two approaches (See Study Guide Table 5-1).

The content approach to motivation concerns what within people motivates them to behave in a certain way. The implications of need hierarchy theory (Maslow's theory) for patient teaching are:

Multiple needs generally determine motivation.

A patient's need for satisfaction can be linked to desired outcome.

What motivates one person may not motivate another.

The process approach to motivation focuses on the direction or choice of pattern behaviors. Learning is a change in behavior that results from reinforced practice, whether practice reflects encoded neural pathways or a strengthening of certain responses. The change in behavior is assumed to be long-term and different from the changes induced by such factors as fatigue and maturation.

Reinforcement is basic to much of learning theory and includes two kinds of conditioning:

Classical (Pavlovian). A conditioned reflex; the reflex (behavior) occurs given certain conditions.

Instrumental (operant). The consequences of the behavior determine the frequency of the behavior.

Table 5-1
MAJOR APPROACHES TO MOTIVATION

Approach	Theories	Primary Concern
Content	Need hierarchy theory	Concerned with what motivates people
Process	Reinforcement theory	Concerned with *how* people are motivated

The implications of learning theory are the basic concepts behind behavior modification. Health behaviors that lead to desirable consequences are likely to be repeated. Health behaviors that lead to undesirable consequences are less likely to be repeated. This reasoning involves three components:

Stimulus. An event that leads to a response

Response. A unit of behavior that follows a response

Reinforcement. A consequence of a response

The consequences of a person's behavior are dependent upon his or her response to a stimulus. At least four types of reinforcement modify patient behavior (see Study Guide Table 5-2).

- **LEARNED EXPERIENCES ARE THE BASIS OF MUCH HUMAN AND ANIMAL BEHAVIOR.** Experiences, stored as memory, determine much of current perception and performance. The notion that memory affects behavior in the presence and/or absence of conscious awareness appears in theories of implicit (procedural) and explicit (declarative) memory (see Study Guide Table 5-3).

Implicit memory (patterns) is essential to survival and growth and development, and important to advanced levels of memory and learning (imprinting). Explicit memory is the major domain of learning: working memory.

One is not born with a memory. The neural

Table 5-2
TYPES OF REINFORCEMENT

POSITIVE REINFORCEMENT: Strengthens behavior by providing a desirable consequence when a desirable behavior occurs.

AVOIDANCE LEARNING: Strengthens behavior by teaching individuals to respond in ways that avoid undesirable consequences.

EXTINCTION: Weakens behavior by withholding a desirable consequence when an undesirable behavior occurs.

PUNISHMENT: Weakens behavior by providing an undesirable consequence when an undesirable behavior occurs.

Table 5-3
IMPLICIT AND EXPLICIT MEMORY NETWORKS

Procedural (Implicit)	Declarative (Explicit)
Gentically based neural system	Developmental neural system
Located in brainstem/hippocampus	Rooted in brainstem/neocortex
Patterns of learning and memory	Associative earning
Priming and imprinting	Working memory
Simple classical conditioning	Operant memory
Out of awareness	Remembering events
No spontaneous recall	Spontaneous recall possible
Skills	Domain of learning
Observed through behavior and symptoms	Language and meaning networking
Hard to alter or change	Linked to associative stimuli

pathways of implicit and explicit memory need to develop and mature (see Study Guide Table 5-4).

Memory process begins early; children can remember events. Perception and encoding of events occur early in the life of attentive children, but children do have difficulty with conceptualizing complex events, identifying relationships such as cause and effect, recognizing feelings, and attributing intent. Ability to order and interpret perceptions, an acquired skill, is not really reliable until a person is about 12 years old. Storage of information does not change with age. Children's ability to retrieve through recall and reporting events is compromised by other domains of development that may not be sufficiently sophisticated to communicate the memory.

The three types of memory include:

- RECOGNITION. Simplest form; within the capacity of an infant.

- RECONSTRUCTION. Involves reinstating the context in which the original memory occurred; match between encoding a situation and retrieval of environmental factors.

- FREE RECALL. Most complex; retrieval of previously observed events from storage with few or no prompts; strongly age related; develops gradually; depends on development of language and higher levels of organizing thoughts.

Table 5-4
MEMORY DEVELOPMENT

Memory Process	Definition
Acquisition	Perception of information
Storage	Encoded data/event
Retrieval	Recall
Types of memory	
Recognition	Sensory system cue
Reconstruction	Restating context
Free recall	No cues or prompts
Strategies for remembering	
Rehearsal	Repeat/memorize
Categories	Organize data
Associative cues	Conduct memory search

Strategies for remembering use internal processes, such as visualization and rehearsal, organization of memories according to themes, categories, and common elements, as well as the use of external and internal cues to conduct searches. The use of these strategies begins in childhood and improves as use and age increase.

- **INFORMATION MUST BE PROCESSED TO LEARN.** Human information processing occurs in stages.

  Sensory registration. Sensory impulses (e.g., sounds) are transmitted to the cortical level where they are perceived as a simple sensory message; not necessarily categorized — may remain at the sensory state without an informational signal or symbol value.

  Pattern recognition. Perceptual; accomplished by a process of comparing the stimulus pattern to be identified with patterns previously stored as part of long-term or short-term memories.

  Short-term memory. Cognitive process; stimuli must last long enough for individual to remember; rehearsal (or repeating the stimulus to be remembered) facilitates memorization.

In the information processing experience, the only elements that can be directly observed and measured are the initial stimulus and the resulting end response. The intervening processes are hypothetical constructs that may be inferred and that can be analyzed in terms of general questions, such as those that follow:

What is being processed? The three domains of processing are sensory, perceptual, and cognitive; is the primary influence of the stimulus physical energy or information? Relative emphasis given to energy and information differs: energy stimuli are defined with reference to their physical characteristics (e.g., light intensity); information stimuli are more complicated.

Where is it being processed? Two physiological approaches are considered:

Is the processing more peripheral or central in the CNS?

In which hemisphere of the brain is the processing?

When does processing occur? Stages are generally described as:

Input. When energy and information components of the stimuli are incorporated

Classification of components

Organization of the classified components

Interpretation of what has been processed

Output, which culminates in a response

The mental codification of experience (schema) is made possible by three levels of information processing:

Sensory. Processed within the peripheral nervous system, brain stem, basal ganglia, and amygdala; conditioned learning is first noted in this processing stage; number and types of processing may differ depending on type of stimuli, task, and the person's phase of practice or experience.

Perceptual. Processing involves the neurological ability to retain aspects of perceptual experience as memory; as human development proceeds ability to retain sensory experience as perceptual representations occurs— remembered sights (iconic memory) or sounds (echoic memory).

Cognitive. Processing requires development of the neural system that permits response and retention, cognitive interpretation, and description of internal and external perceptions, using language for symbols of experience. **Research suggests** that information processing in psychiatric patients may differ from that of mentally healthy individuals.

- **THE HEALTH TEACHING PROCESS HAS SEVERAL COMPONENTS**

  Assessment of the patient. Variables, for example, occupation, sex, age, sociocultural background, influence the style and technique of teaching; variables such as patient cognitive and psychological levels (including memory capacity, perception of illness, level of stress) influence level of teaching.

  Plan for teaching and implementation. After patient needs are identified, information to be taught is planned; motivation and learning pace are considered; an environment conducive to learning is prepared; content is made relevant and organized.

  A nurse's teaching skill will be enhanced by:
  - using an organized plan
  - presenting content in small segments
  - using language free of jargon
  - routinely asking questions and seeking feedback
  - maintaining eye contact
  - using audiovisual aids when possible
  - requesting a return demonstration from the patient when appropriate
  - offering positive reinforcement (praise) when learning occurs

  Teaching style involves:
  - knowing content to be taught
  - being aware of one's own security in teaching
  - being flexible in approach
  - listening carefully to the patient
  - presenting content calmly, unhurriedly, and in an interesting way.

  Evaluation. To determine if learning has occurred; changes in patient's behavior are assessed.

TAKING ANOTHER LOOK

You are now ready to respond to the questions raised in Gaining a Perspective at the beginning of this chapter. After you have written or thought about your responses, you may want to look at the Suggested Responses on page 319.

6

STRESS, COPING, AND DEFENSIVE FUNCTIONING

GAINING A PERSPECTIVE

Think about the two questions presented below. Then, after you have read the Key Concepts, respond in more detail to the queries.

1. What are some of the stressors that you have had in your life and the defense mechanisms that you use to cope with them effectively?

2. How would you, a nurse, deal with a patient whom you may not be treating especially well, but who constantly says to you, "You are so good to me. I feel like you are my guardian angel."?

Key Concepts

• **STRESS AND ITS POSSIBLE EFFECT ON MENTAL HEALTH** have become increasingly important in nursing, psychiatric nursing in particular. Two related definitions of stress are pertinent: stress is a stimulus that upsets an individual's balance, or homeostasis; it is also an individual's response to that stimulus. The focus in psychiatric nursing is the individual's biological, psychological, social, and/or cultural reactions to a stressor (or activator) and the consequences of those reactions with respect to psychiatric illness. Stress is global and includes emotions such as fear, anger, anxiety, depression, or a combination of these, as well as the wide range of human responses (see Study Guide Figure 6-1).

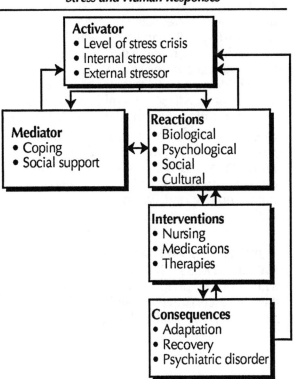

Figure 6-1
Stress and Human Responses

- **NORMALITY, IN THE BROADEST DEFINITION OF MENTAL HEALTH,** may be conceptualized as an individual's ability to successfully cope with stress and conflict, permitting optimal functional ability. Mental health is on a continuum and permits varying levels of stability throughout the life span.

- **WHAT CONSTITUTES "ABNORMAL" BEHAVIOR** is an understanding that nurses must develop. "Normalcy" is generally defined as behavior that falls within a recognized "standard" of a given culture. Abnormal thoughts, feelings, and behaviors are often difficult to specify, however. What distinguishes eccentric behavior from psychiatric illness is that in psychiatric illness an individual's thoughts, feelings, and behaviors have impaired his or her functioning. The person's inability to adaptively cope with psychological conflict weakens self-esteem and eventually interferes with the ability to effectively accomplish the necessities of daily living.

  The percentage of the population who are mentally ill or require treatment for maintaining mental health or for substance abuse has risen significantly—in any one year 20% of adults in the United States suffer from an active mental disorder; 32% can be expected to have a mental illness sometime during their life. Disorders vary according to age—12% of 63 million children and adolescents suffer from some form of mental disorder; 4 million older Americans are suffering from Alzheimer's disease.

  Mental disorders are clinically significant behavioral or psychological syndromes or patterns that are associated with an individual's current distress or disability, with a significantly increased risk of death, pain, or disability, or with an important loss of freedom.

- **COPING, THE MEDIATING BEHAVIOR BETWEEN STRESS AND ANXIETY,** influences whether the individual will maintain homeostatic balance. Coping activities modify the negative effects of social and psychological strain.

- **ANXIETY RESULTS WHEN A STRESSOR OVERWHELMS** a person's ability to resolve or cope with the stressor. Anxiety is a ubiquitous emotional state. It is experienced when the self-identity or essential values of a person are threatened, but has no specific object. The feeling state in anxiety is characterized by

  A subjective sense of dread, apprehension, threat, failure, helplessness, or impending disaster

  A sense of losing control, being disoriented, or committing a dangerous act

  A fear of sudden death

  Common physical or somatic alterations in body systems are listed below.

  Circulatory system. Perspiration, clammy hands, flushing, blushing, feeling hot or cold.

  Respiratory system. Heavy breathing, sighing respirations, hyperventilation, dizziness.

  Gastrointestinal system. Abdominal pain, anorexia, nausea, dry mouth, diarrhea, constipation, "butterflies" in the stomach.

  Genitourinary system. Urinary frequency, various interferences with sexual function.

  Cognitive functioning. Impaired attention span, poor concentration, impaired memory, changes in outlook and future planning.

  Anxiety occupies a focal point in the dynamics of all human adjustment and is a driving force for most of our adjustments in life. Peplau's classical levels of anxiety are described below.

  Mild. Can motivate learning, stimulate growth and creativity; sensory field increases; individual more alert to the environment.

  Moderate. Tends to narrow perceptual field; individual unable to attend to the factors operating in the environment, but can focus if directed to do so.

  Severe. Drastically reduces perceptual field; goal of individual is to get relief; individual needs a great deal of direction to attend to a specific area; self-awareness is diminished.

  Panic. Loss of control; individual disorganized and needs another human being to function; perceptual field blocked; self-awareness almost absent; feelings are dread, terror, awe, and danger.

Figure 6-2
Functions of the Ego

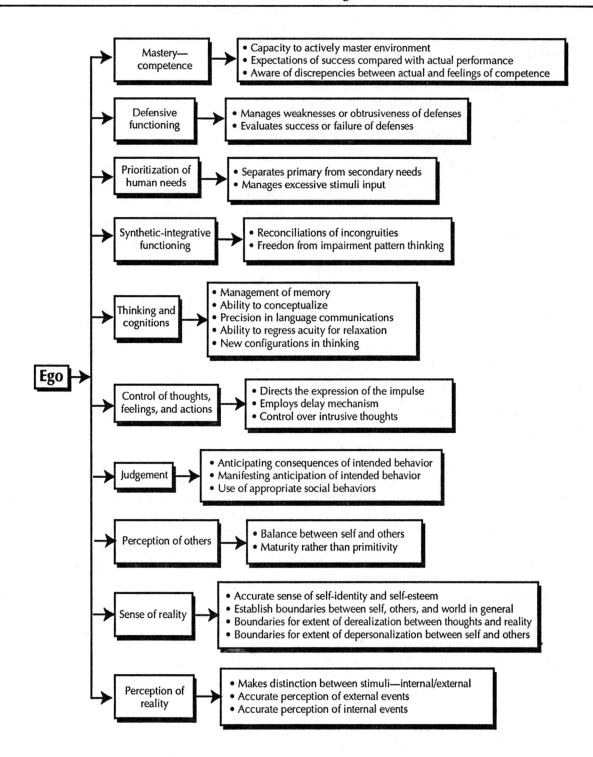

- **A PERSON'S DEFENSIVE FUNCTIONING AND STRUCTURE** may be studied by observing his or her use of defense mechanisms. Personality style may be understood in this way. Defensive functioning is part of the coping process. Studies about ego development and defense mechanisms have taken two major directions: first, studies of various ego functions (including defensive functioning) that are primarily conflict-free and result from maturational aspects of intellectual functioning; second, studies of the major mechanisms of ego defense.

  According to Freud, the ego is the reality balance; it mediates pressures of the environment and instinctual satisfaction and preserves the integrity of an individual. A study on the role of the ego describes 10 major functions of the ego (see Study Guide Figure 6-2).

  In examining a patient's mental status, psychiatric nurses may benefit from being able to assess ego function as it relates to defense mechanisms. Ego development is involved in individual coping and adaptation.

  The hypothesis underlying the psychodynamic model of the human mind is that all human behavior makes sense. The model, with the goal to make sense of behavior, places the psyche (ego, self, mind, soul) in the active consciousness. Without ego the individual is under control of instinctual drives; ego gives personality its boundaries and its direction. The psychodynamic view of mental health posits that mental symptoms arise when conflicting emotions, such as love or hate and assertiveness or passivity, produce unmanageable distress.

  Defense mechanisms, then, are adaptive functions of the personality and specific intrapsychic processes that operate unconsciously. They are employed to seek relief from emotional conflict.

- **A PERSON'S DEFENSE LEVEL, RANGING FROM MATURE AND HEALTHY TO PSYCHOTIC,** is an indication to the psychiatric nurse of the potential of the patient to recover from an illness. Assessing what that level is assists the nurse to determine interventions (see Study Guide Table 6-1).

  Defenses in the high adaptive level, associat-

Table 6-1

DEFENSE LEVELS WITH EXAMPLES OF DEFENSE MECHANISMS

High-Adaptive Level	*Disavowal Level*
• Anticipation	• Denial
• Affiliation	• Projection
• Altruism	• Rationalization
• Humor	*Major Image-Distortion Level*
• Self-assertion	
• Self-observation	• Autistic Fantasy
• Sublimation	• Projective Identification
• Suppression	• Splitting
Mental Inhibitions Level	*Action Level*
• Displacement	• Acting Out
• Dissociation	• Apathetic Withdrawal
• Identification	• Help-Rejecting Complaint
• Intellectualization	• Passive Aggression
• Isolation of Affect	• Regression
• Reaction Formation	*Defensive-Dysregulation Level*
• Repression • Undoing	
Minor Image-Distortion Level	• Delusional Projection
	• Psychotic Denial
• Devaluation	• Psychotic Distortion
• Idealization	
• Omnipotence	

ed with good coping skills, result in optimal adaptation in handling stressors, usually maximize gratification, and allow conscious awareness of feelings, ideas, and their consequences. Eight high adaptive defenses are listed below.

- ANTICIPATION. Emotional reactions are thought about and experienced in advance.
- AFFILIATION. Individual deals with emotional conflict by turning to others for help or support; problems are shared, but affiliation does not imply making someone else responsible for the problem.
- ALTRUISM. Individual deals with emotional conflict by meeting the needs of others; receives gratification either vicariously or from responses of others.
- HUMOR. Amusing or ironic aspects of a stres-

sor or conflict are emphasized.

- SELF-ASSERTION. Feelings are addressed directly in a way that is not coercive or manipulative.
- SELF-OBSERVATION. One's own thoughts, feelings, motivation, and behavior are reflected on, and the response is appropriate.
- SUBLIMATION. Unacceptable instinctual drives are diverted into socially and personally accepted channels.
- SUPPRESSION. Unacceptable ideas or impulses are voluntarily relegated from the conscious mind.

Defensive functioning at the mental inhibitions level (self-sacrificing defenses) keeps potentially threatening ideas, feelings, memories, wishes, or fears out of the awareness. These eight defenses are listed below.

- DISPLACEMENT. Redirection of an emotion from one idea, object, or person to another.
- DISSOCIATION. Detachment of emotional significance from an idea, situation, object, or relationship.
- IDENTIFICATION. Unconscious adoption or patterning of the personality characteristics of an admired other.
- INTELLECTUALIZATION. Excessive use of abstract thinking or making generalizations to control or minimize disturbing feelings.
- ISOLATION OF AFFECT. Separation of ideas from the feelings originally associated with them.
- REACTION FORMATION. Direction of overt behavior or attitudes in the opposite direction of the individual's underlying motives, feelings, or wishes.
- REPRESSION. Involuntary banishment of unacceptable or painful thoughts, feelings, and impulses into the unconscious.
- UNDOING. An endeavor to actually or symbolically erase a previously consciously intolerable experience.

Defense mechanisms at the minor image-disturbing level, employed to regulate self-esteem, can interfere with interpersonal relationships, but not necessarily with achievement and accomplishment. Defense mechanisms at this level are listed below.

- COMPENSATION. Conscious or unconscious attempt to overcome real or imagined inferiority or inadequacies.
- DEVALUATION. Attributing exaggerated negative qualities to self or others.
- IDEALIZATION. Attributing exaggerated positive qualities to others.
- INTROJECTION. Symbolic assimilation (taking into self) of loved or hated attitudes, wishes, ideals, or persons.
- OMNIPOTENCE. Acting or feeling as though one possesses special powers or abilities and is superior to others.
- SUBSTITUTION. Replacement of an unattainable or unacceptable need, emotion, drive, or goal with one that is attainable and acceptable.
- SYMBOLISM. Mechanism by which an external object is used to represent an internal idea, belief, attitude, wish, or feeling.

The disavowal level of defense mechanisms is characterized by keeping unpleasant or unacceptable stressors, impulses, ideas, affects, or responsibility out of awareness with or without their misattribution to external causes. Nursing intervention seeks to help the person deal with reality. Three defense mechanisms at this level are listed below.

- DENIAL. Unconscious disavowal of thoughts, feelings, wishes, needs, or external reality factors that are consciously unacceptable.
- PROJECTION. Attributing to another person or object thoughts, feelings, motives, or ideas that are unacceptable to self.
- RATIONALIZATION. An attempt to modify unacceptable motives, feelings, needs, or impulses into those that are acceptable.

Major image-distortion level defenses are characterized by gross distortion or misattribution of the image of self or others. The defenses are habitually used and their use guarantees problems in interpersonal relationships. Three defenses at this level are listed below.

- AUTISTIC FANTASY. Emotional conflicts dealt with by excessive daydreaming as a substitute for human relationships, more effective action, or problem solving.

- PROJECTIVE IDENTIFICATION. Falsely attributes to others his or her own unacceptable feelings, impulses, or thoughts.
- SPLITTING. Compartmentalizes opposite affect states and fails to integrate positive and negative qualities of self into cohesive images; self and images tend to alternate between polar opposites (e.g., exclusively good or exclusively bad).

Action-level defensive functioning deals with internal or external stressors by using action or withdrawal. The common feature at this level is that all behaviors indicate the person's inability to deal with his or her impulses by taking action on his or her behalf. Action-level defenses are described below.

- ACTING OUT. Individual deals with emotional conflict through actions rather than reflection or feelings.
- CONVERSION. Elements of intrapsychic conflict are disguised and expressed symbolically through physical symptoms.
- APATHETIC WITHDRAWAL. Behavior is avoidant and lacks energy, suggestive of a depressed mood.
- HELP-REJECTING COMPLAINING. Repeated requests for help, which disguise overt feelings of hostility or reproach toward others, and then rejection of suggestions, advice, or help that others offer.
- PASSIVE AGGRESSION. Indirect expression of aggression toward others.
- REGRESSION. Return to an earlier and subjectively more comfortable level of emotional adjustment.

Level of defensive dysregulation is characterized by failure of defense regulation to contain reactions to stressor, leading to a pronounced break with objective reality. Defensive dysregulation is defined below.

- DELUSIONAL PROJECTION. Projected thoughts are false, fixed ideas.
- PSYCHOTIC DENIAL. An assertion that something obviously true is neither true nor part of reality.
- PSYCHOTIC DISTORTION. A belief that has no grounding in reality.

TAKING ANOTHER LOOK

You are now ready to respond to the questions posed in Gaining a Perspective at the beginning of this chapter. After you have written or thought about your responses, you may want to look at the Suggested Responses on page 319.

7 HUMAN GROWTH AND DEVELOPMENTAL TASKS

TERMS TO DEFINE

attachment

consolidation

developmental framework

life-cycle stage

midlife transition

normative crisis

regression

transition

GAINING A PERSPECTIVE

Think about the two situations described below, and after you have read the Key Concepts of this chapter discuss your ideas in more depth.

1. What factors, including developmental tasks, would you, as a nurse, consider when helping a 15-year-old deal with the loss of a parent?

2. What are likely to be the effects of an infant's successfully forming a secure attachment with his or her parent(s)?

Key Concepts

• **UNDERSTANDING HUMAN DEVELOPMENT AND THE EMOTIONAL REACTIONS EXPECTED AT VARIOUS STAGES OF THE LIFE CYCLE** helps in supporting ill individuals and their families. The life-cycle stages are defined by specific tasks, conflicts, and viewpoints occurring during relatively stable periods. Some stages are universal; some are influenced by culture. Each developmental line proceeds at its own pace. A person may advance rapidly in some areas and remain the same or regress in other areas, according his or her own unique biological (including gender), psychological, and social (including culture) condition.

• **CARL JUNG**, the first mental health researcher to focus on the life cycle, believed that personality had developed by adolescence, which facilitated individuals assuming family, work, and community responsibilities at that time. The next major opportunity for personal growth, Jung believed, was around 40 years, a midlife stage.

• **LIFE CHANGE GENERALLY OCCURS THROUGH A SEQUENCE OF PREPARATION** (transition), rapid change (normal development or normative crisis, such as childbirth or marital crisis), and finally, consolidation (achievement of a new stage or plateau). Transitions involve repetitious acts or regression to reexperience the past while planning for the future. The primary characteristic of normative crisis is turmoil. Some regression, revival of earlier more childlike behavior in response to stress, tends to be experienced during the developmental process.

• **IN A DEVELOPMENTAL FRAMEWORK,** the focus is on evolving communication skills, as well as physical growth and affective development.

Table 7-1

DEVELOPMENTAL TASKS

Infancy	Attachment. Assistance in the regulation of bodily states, emotion.
Toddlerhood	Development of symbolic representation and further self-other differentiation. Problem-solving, pride, mastery motivation.
Preschool	Development of self-control; the use of language to regulate impulses, emotions; store information; predict and make sense out of the world. Development of verbally mediated and semantic memory. Gender identity. Development of social relationships beyond immediate family and generalization of expectations about relationships. Moral reasoning.
Latency age	Peer relationships. Adaptation to school environment. Moral reasoning
Adolescence	Renegotiation of family roles. Identity issues (sexuality, future orientation, peer acceptance, ethnicity). Moral reasoning.
Young Adult	Continued differentiation from family. Refinement and integration of identity with particular focus on occupational choice and ultimate partners. Moral reasoning.

Source: National Psychological Maltreatment Consortium, 1995, Office for the Study of the Psychological Rights of the Child, School of Education, Indiana University-Purdue University at Indianapolis. Reprinted with permission.

Variability that is characteristic of these developmental skills may be based on culture and gender differences. (See Study Guide Table 7-1. NOTE: This framework is not helpful for tracking adult behavior, therefore it is not detailed in this table.)

- **INFANCY TASKS** 0 to 12 months of age
  Regulation of bodily states and emotions
  - Apgar score is first formal assessment; assessment at one and five minutes after birth.
  - Newborns have remarkable sensory (visual, smell, etc.) ability.
  - Gross motor abilities
    —Primitive at birth
    —By 16 weeks—holds head up
    —By 28 weeks—sits with support
    —By 40 weeks—creeps
    —By 1 year of age—walks
  - Rapid physical growth; weight triples.

- Cries to communicate fatigue, pain, hunger, fear, discomfort, anger, or wish for contact. Other communication is smiling, reaching, looking away, and speaking (one to two words by 1 year).

Attachment
- Emotional/affectional tie formed between one person and another; lasts over time; leads to seeking physical closeness to the caregiver; describes infant's thoughts, feelings, and behaviors towards caregiver(s).
  —Begins in the first hours of life
  —Interaction produces a strong affective response, enhanced by looking, crying, clinging, and vocalizing
  —May not occur if abuse or neglect occurs
  —Attachment critical in the first year or may cause developmental problems
- Four types of attachment
  —Secure attachment. Child has separation anxiety in a new situation or when afraid;

wants to be close to parent.

—Insecure attachment. Parent does not respond; negative implication for development of trust and healthy relationships.

— Anxious resistant attachment. Brought on by parental inconsistency, frequent separations; manifests itself in excessive separation anxiety.

— Anxious avoidance attachment. Parent rebuffs infant when child seeks comfort; extreme case of abuse or neglect.

- **TODDLERHOOD TASKS** 1 to 3 years old
  Physical
  - Running by 30 months
  - Sleeping about 12 hours per day
  - Slower growth and decrease in appetite
  - Desire to feed self
  - Sense and control of bladder/sphincter muscles—prerequisites for toilet training (18-30 months)

  Other landmarks
  - At 18 months recognizes self in mirror; maintains and uses mental symbols; has gaps between understanding of consequences and wanting to explore
  - Social referencing in first half of second year looks to parent for emotional clues about a new event (exploring environment)
  - By 3 years of age speaks about 300 words and in short sentences
  - From 16 to 24 months the rapprochement subphase begins; the child realizes separateness and feels ambivalence about attachment and dependency needs; by last half of third year child becomes comfortable with brief separation as he or she struggles with psychological autonomy and separateness
  - From 24 to 36 months understands emotions and can verbally identify them; identifies with a gender role
  - Piaget's preoperational stage of intellectual development from 2 to 7 years of age; can classify and problem solve by trial and error; egocentric; symbolic play

- **PRESCHOOL** 3 to 6 years old
  - Aware of sex differences
  - Parallel play (playing side by side) becomes associative play (pairs or small groups)
  - Moral reasoning begins with belief that all events can be explained by the action of a force that wills it to happen
  - Moral development involves justice, punishment, and the belief that guilt is determined by amount of damage done
  - Improved communication ability by 5 years of age; more articulate with language; development running ahead of the ability to understand concepts
  - Children begin to show signs of romantic behavior toward parent of opposite sex and rivalry toward same-sex parent

- **LATENCY – MIDDLE CHILDHOOD** 6 to 12 years old
  - Cognitive and motor capacities develop to allow gradual independence from family
  - Can perceive and understand more complex sensory stimuli; handedness is determined
  - Balance, equilibrium, large muscle control, and timing improve; 7- to 10-year-olds play sports
  - Signs of puberty are evident, usually from age 10 to 12 years
  - Piaget's intellectual stage of concrete operations begins; can consider more than one dimension simultaneously
  - Morality is subjective
  - More able to control drives and inhibit certain behaviors to postpone gratification
  - Peer relationships develop; single-sex groupings for play; subculture not involving adult influence develops; peer acceptance sought

- **ADOLESCENCE**
  - Neurologic development is mature
  - Attain reproductive capacity; hormonal changes plus social and cultural factors tend to increase interest in sexuality and sexual experimentation
  - Piaget's stage of formal operations is attained;

Table 7-2
ADULT LIFE CYCLE: STAGES, TASKS AND ISSUES

STAGE	TRANSITIONAL ISSUES	RITE OF PASSAGE	SYMPTOMS OF CRISIS	PATHOLOGIC OUTCOME
Pre-adulthood	Novice, student	Matriculation	School/work phobia	Agoraphobia
Adulthood Consolidation	New title	Graduation	Repeated career changes	Pseudoadult
Courtship	Experimentation	Dating "trial marriage"	Premature or delayed commitment	Schizoid character, precocious adult
Marriage Transition	Contract with spouse	Marriage ceremony	Boredom or constant warfare	Separation or divorce
Pregnancy	Physical change	Baby shower, childbirth education	Hypochondriasm, detachment	Denial
Childbirth	Pregnancy	Labor and delivery	Excessive anxiety prepartum and during labor	Postpartum depression
Parenting	Primary maternal preoccupation	Naming ceremony	Marital unrest, developmental delay in child	Parental deprivation or overstimulation of child
Midlife	Mourning loss of youth	Midlife crisis	Withdrawal, sudden life change	Depression, substance abuse
Transition to Old Age	Repository of cultural values	Retirement, illness, death of spouse/friends	Regression	Depression, pseudodementia

abstract thought used to consider theories, devise and test hypotheses

- Renegotiation of family roles; more independent; increased arguing with parents
- Intense peer friendships develop
- Temporary increase in less mature defense mechanisms
- Belief of omnipotence may lead to dangerous risk-taking
- Fluctuations in self-esteem, moods, images of self
- For teens with gay/lesbian identity, problems with self-acceptance arise; peers and parents may be nonsupportive

- **TRANSITION TO ADULTHOOD** (see Study Guide Table 7-2)
  - Transition to an occupation; trying different roles, styles, and techniques
  - Experimentation with intimate relationships
  - Problems may occur from inability to fully separate from parents
    Pseudoadult: a "child" who never grows up
    Precocious adult: detaches early; self-parenting; seems competent but stilted and lifeless

- **CONSOLIDATION OF ADULTHOOD** approximately 30 years of age
  - **Fixity of adulthood**; commitments and loss of options

Marriage is a transition to a committed partnership; ideally between two mature individuals; see other person as a whole separate individual. Marital crisis can occur in the following situations:

- If a couple marry before they have consolidated their own adult identities
- During life-cycle stages

CHILDBIRTH — making room for a new person and adjustment in relationship; parenting skills are influenced by strength of parental partnership and experience each has had with his or her own parents

PARENTING — reexperiencing, reworking of one's own childhood

CHILDLESSNESS — can cause feelings of guilt; can cause divorce if both parents do not come to a compromise

MIDLIFE — "empty-nest"

Single parenting presents many challenges; need to meet own needs without negatively impacting needs of children

- **MIDLIFE TRANSITION** between 35 and 55 years of age

Introspection and reassessment in light of mortality

Begin a process of individuation and personality flowering or a process of spiritual and psychological decay

Launching children into the world

Differences between men and women:

WOMEN Biological functioning changes (menopause); conflict in roles of mother and woman (working); time for self-expression (childbearing completed); changes may be more symbolic (more health conscious, more family oriented); some feel "second chance" at life

A universal human life cycle was proposed by Daniel Levinson and colleagues from their studies of men between the ages of 35 and 45; consisting of specific eras and periods in a set sequence, a psychosocial theory of adult development

- BEREAVEMENT

Loss plays a necessary role in every life transition.

Coming to terms with ambivalence about the deceased is necessary.

- TRANSITION TO LATER LIFE

Task to enhance and maintain a sense of inner emotional integrity in face of increasing external threats

RETIREMENT is an experience of loss of authority and power; need to find new sources of productivity and creativity.

ISOLATION, which is a threat to integrity, requires construction of a new social network.

- DEATH AND DYING

Idea of one's own impending death is emotionally traumatic.

Kubler-Ross describes acceptance of death-related tasks; denial and isolation, anger, bargaining, and acceptance are roughly analogous to the stages of bereavement.

Relationship with death has new meaning as one develops.

TAKING ANOTHER LOOK

You are now ready to respond to the questions that are raised in Gaining a Perspective at the beginning of this chapter. After you have written or thought about your responses, you may want to look at the Suggested Responses on page 320.

8 SYSTEMS THEORY AS A MODEL FOR UNDERSTANDING FAMILIES

TERMS TO DEFINE

bargaining mode of transaction

coercion mode of transaction

gemeinschaft mode of transaction

genogram

legal/bureaucratic mode of transaction

modes of transaction

social exchange paradigm

systems theory

team-cooperative mode of transaction

GAINING A PERSPECTIVE

Think about the following questions, and after you have read the Key Concepts of this chapter you will be able to reply in more depth.

1. What verbal interactions might take place if members of a family (subsystems) were using coercion as a mode of transaction?

2. What would your family look like on a genogram?

3. What could happen when nurses who see their own families as departing from normal begin to work with families similar to their own?

4. What are some societal trends that have an effect on family and what questions do these issues raise?

Key Concepts

• **THE FAMILY IS AN ELUSIVE CONCEPT;** its shape, character, and functions have been interpreted very differently by historians, sociologists, psychologists, and anthropologists. Nurses must be knowledgeable about families, because no matter what the area of their practice, they will encounter families as context or supporters of the individual patients for whom they are caring. Indeed, at times they will deliver care for the entire family. At other times nurses will experience families as barriers to care. These barriers may not always be obvious, but discovered when plans of care are disrupted.

• **PRIVACY ABOUT FAMILY LIFE** has produced what sociologists call pluralistic ignorance. Systematic, rigorous research on the intimacies of family life is in its infancy, although scholars have been interested in studying marriage and the family for several centuries.

• **"FAMILY" IMPLIES THAT SEVERAL UNIVERSALS ARE OPERATING**

Sexual relations between close relatives are forbidden. (Note: Husbands and wives are not relatives; they are strangers who marry.)

Men and women cooperate through a division of labor based on gender.

Marriage is a durable, although not necessarily lifelong, arrangement.

Culture, not biology, determines the rules of family organization, such as gender relationships. In this modern world, family patterns are so fluid that the United State Census Bureau has difficulty measuring trends. Today's family, however, is:

• most likely to have two or fewer children.

• likely to have the mother employed outside the home.

- has members marrying at an older age than previously.
- less permanent.

Although some Americans choose not to marry, 90% do.

- **INTRAPSYCHIC AND INTERPERSONAL THE-ORIES** preceded family systems theory.

In early 1900, families were kept apart from psychiatric patients (who were housed in large state hospitals); patients were thought to need some distance and respite from their relatives to abate whatever noxious forces had been operative; families were implicated as the cause of the current problem(s) in historical ways.

World War II, when men were treated for the stress of war, provided impetus for interpersonal strategies, such as group therapy; sources of psychic distress or mental illness shifted from the far past (historical) to the here and now.

The National Institute of Mental Health was created in 1946; work of scientists on schizophrenia and other severe mental illness focused on interpersonal theories (Harry Stack Sullivan's work).

- **Mothers were implicated** as cause of illness and operated in the here and now, not in the past, to maintain the illness.
- **Professional's behaviors** were also examined.
- **Professionals engaged in therapeutic interactions** with patients.
- **Focus not on the family as a system but on dyads**—the patient and one significant other examined in sequence.

- **SYSTEMS THINKING, IN TAKING IN MORE OF THE PROBLEM'S SURROUNDING CONTEXT,** expanded intrapsychic or interpersonal dynamics considerably. The system is viewed as the patient. A system is defined as sets of elements standing in interaction. The theory is a logical-mathematical field that deals with scientific doctrines of wholeness, dynamic interaction, and organization. By 1950, psychiatrists began to involve total family systems in their treatment plans. A spirit of openness and col-

legiality replaced the close, private ambience of psychoanalytic approaches.

- **SYSTEMS THEORY PRINCIPLES**

The whole is greater than the sum of its parts. An entity, a quality, or an abstract essence in a system cannot be understood as simply an additive, mechanistic operation; parts of anything without organization remain just parts, becoming only an identifiable system when they are organized.

Rules of organization are not directly visible, nor are they written down; however, they are easily detected by asking or observing. A family's rules of organization are determined by their culture, embodying ethnic, religious, and social factors. Tradition is a ritualized, remembered, and enacted set of rules of organization (places people in roles). Each human social system, e.g., work system and nation, takes on its own identity from the rules of organization.

Janus effect and hierarchical order, another principle of systems theory, states that a system is a set of interacting parts organized by rules. The boundaries, or parameters, of these systems vary in size and complexity. The system may be as small as a cell nucleus, or may have thousands of parts, as does a nation. Holon is the term used to capture the essence of the system under analysis; it means the interacting parts and their boundary. A system or holon has subsystem parts, arranged hierarchically. Subsystems are seen as inferior (beneath, in complexity) to systems and suprasystems (above the system level). For example, a nuclear family might be considered the system, and the marital dyads and siblings the subsystems. The nuclear family system would have the large extended family as the suprasystem.

Depth and breadth of hierarchies — the arrangements of systems — yield a clue to complexity.

Adaptation in this context is two units or subsystems interacting with each other by exchanging matter, energy, or information. Maladaptation occurs when one or several desired exchanges do not occur or are blocked, or a transaction is attempted which is not desired by either subsystem.

When the system is maladapted or confronted with a new or different situation, decision-making functions are called into play. In human systems, decision making is closely related to power issues. Cultural norms are also a guide to understanding the types of power in given social situations.

• **THE SOCIAL EXCHANGE PARADIGM** (Study Guide Figure 8-1) is a framework for analyzing the substance (the what) of exchanges between subsystems.

Figure 8-1 SOCIAL EXCHANGE PARADIGM

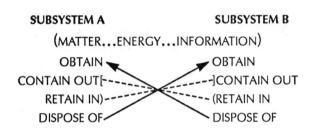

• **THE MODES OF TRANSACTION PARADIGM** focus on the ways (the hows) that exchanges might be handled. Interacting subsystems try to persuade others to comply with their wishes, needs, requests, etc., using strategies — modes of interaction.

Bargaining mode, applied in home environment and workplaces.

Legal-bureaucratic mode, formalistic, relying on two interacting subsystems valuing the notions of rules, duties, and job descriptions.

Gemeinschaft mode, a familistic stance in which warmth, affection, and interpersonal bonding are relied on.

Team-cooperative mode in which interacting members are part of a group or team effort that would not be completed unless the members pull together to get the work done.

Coercion mode operates when two subsystems do not belong to a larger system that has an available, operative set of rules for interacting

short of force, fraud, deception, and violence. It is a default category.

Families tend to prefer one of the modes more than others. Subsystems within the family may not be using the same mode; however, subsystems within families have probably been socialized to the same set of values and norms, including the appropriateness of the rules for conducting their interchanges. Conflicts do occur, but the normative order is maintained more often than not.

• **IN THE ASSESSMENT AND TREATMENT PHASES** of working with clients (in the context of family, school, or work systems) the Social Exchange Paradigm and the Modes of Transaction Paradigm are useful tools for clinicians.

• **USING SYSTEMS THEORY AS A FRAMEWORK FOR UNDERSTANDING** what, why, and how people do what they do provides a rich, nonjudgmental approach to clinical work. Symptoms used as diagnostic signs in psychiatric diagnoses are not viewed as "owned" by the individual, but rather are statements about system maladaptation or signals of distress for the system.

• **USING A PICTURE, OR GENOGRAM,** to diagram all family members makes the systems framework easier to implement when working with families. Rather then record data about significant family-member relationships in the usual paragraph or sentence notation pattern, a genogram can be used. The genogram provides a succinct picture of family structure and relationships, including all members. It can be drawn quickly using plain paper and a pencil. The family can watch what is being drawn.

Construction of a genogram follows several rules.
  • Males (men and boys) are indicated in boxes, females (women and girls) in circles.
  • Marriages are indicated by straight horizontal lines, connecting male (left) to female (right). (Dotted lines indicate cohabitation without marriage, or for some,

same-sex couples.)

- Children are indicated on a sibling line (horizontal line below the parents, connected by a vertical line), eldest to the left. Pregnancies are indicated by triangles; adoptions are shown by dotted lines.
- Divorces are noted by "//" on a marriage line.
- Death is noted by "/" through a box or circle.
- People who are not family members may be indicated by using dotted lines.
- Other data that may be included are:
  —Birth date (b).
  —Education or occupation.
  —Ethnicity/religion.
  —Health/illness (may use color coding to track illness), risk factors.
  —Geographic location.

(See the example of the Flanagan Family genogram in Study Guide Figure 8-2.)

- **WHAT IS NORMAL AND WHAT IS NOT NORMAL IN FAMILY LIFE** is not always clear to clinicians. If nurses feel uncomfortable exploring the psychological aspects of their patients' families, they miss opportunities to suggest repairs and to get the families rethinking their animosities and cutoffs. Systems analysis allows nonjudgmental discussions to take place, and encourages the development of better solutions to very troublesome situations.

A theme emerging is that no single pattern distinguishes well-functioning families from pathological families. No single family structure is healthier than other arrangements. Families are tremendously complex and an array of variables is operative at any one moment. Faulty conclusions can be avoided by forming tentative hypotheses and then engaging the family to mutually explore them.

- **COUNSELING AND TEACHING ABOUT PARENTING** are part of many professionals' work — today there are specialists in every dimension of individual and family function. Children do not become well-adjusted adults unless nurtured in some type of close, continuing social

Figure 8-2
The Flanagan Family

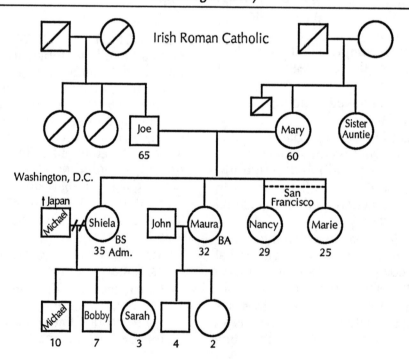

unit, where norms are clearly set, self-esteem is fostered, and issues of separateness and connectedness are worked on openly and directly.

- **THE FUTURE OF THE FAMILY** cannot be predicted without placing it squarely in its social context. According to recent trends, it seems likely that the following future directions for families are possible.

  Human potential, tenderness and warmth, and psychosocial needs will have increasing value as a primary focus of families, rather than material pursuits.

  The trend toward decreasing numbers of children per family will continue. Consequently, greater attention will be paid to parent-child relationships and an increased use of professionals as parenting advisers.

  Neighborhoods will be reinvented, along with community support centers.

  Extended families will gain the attention of researchers, as will grandparent-grandchild relationships.

  A new ideal — strength without domination — will gain impetus and influence in family socialization patterns.

  The challenge will be to keep abreast of changes in family patterns and dynamics and to use this knowledge to provide humanistic and enlightened patient care. Thinking "systems" should prove to be an asset.

TAKING ANOTHER LOOK

You are now ready to respond to the questions that were raised in Gaining a Perspective at the beginning of the chapter. After you have written or thought about your responses, you may want to look at the Suggested Responses on page 320.

9 CULTURE, ETHNICITY, AND RACE IN MENTAL HEALTH AND ILLNESS

TERMS TO DEFINE

Chrisman Culture-Sensitive Case Model

culture

ethnicity

race

racism

stereotyping

GAINING A PERSPECTIVE

Think generally about the situation outlined below, and after you have read the Key Concepts for this chapter respond in greater detail to the query.

1. What advice would you, a nurse, give a co-worker about working with the mostly black-American population that is on the inpatient psychiatric unit where both of you will work?

Key Concepts

- **TO HAVE KNOWLEDGE ABOUT THE RELATIONSHIP BETWEEN PSYCHIATRIC SERVICES AND CULTURE, RACE, ETHNICITY, AND SOCIOECONOMIC STATUS IS NECESSARY** for health care providers in order to help ensure sensitive competent care for diverse patient populations. In nursing, the formal area of study is called "Transcultural Nursing"; many individuals involved in this area of study are nurse anthropologists.

- **CURRENT MIGRATORY PATTERNS AND INCREASED BIRTH RATES AMONG PARTICULAR RACIAL AND ETHNIC GROUPS** are rapidly changing the demographics of the United States and, therefore, the characteristics of many patients currently seen by health care providers. Nurses will be called upon with increasing frequency to care for patients who are very different from themselves culturally, racially, and ethnically.

- **THE TERMS THAT ADDRESS CULTURAL DIVERSITY ARE NOT CLEARLY DEFINED** and are seldom used consistently.

- **CULTURE IS A LEARNED, SHARED, AND SYMBOLICALLY TRANSMITTED DESIGN FOR LIVING.** It is socially acquired and socially transmitted by symbols including customs, techniques, beliefs, institutions, and material objects. "Vertical transmission" is the passing on of a culture from one generation to another (e.g., teaching children values and beliefs). "Horizontal transmission" occurs when individuals learn from their peer group. "Oblique transmission" takes place when cultural norms are learned from other adults/institutions that are part of the individual's original culture. Individuals are then enculturated and socialized. In contrast to enculturation and socialization, acculturation and resocialization refer to cultural and psychological changes brought about by contact with persons who belong to a different culture and exhibit different behaviors.

Cultural orientation must be determined by careful assessment and should not be assumed simply on the basis of an individual's race or ethnicity.

- **ETHNICITY IS DEFINED AS A CONSCIOUSNESS OF GROUP BELONGING**—a group that is differentiated from others by symbolic markers (culture, biology, territory), that is rooted in bonds of a shared past, and that has a perceived ethnic interest. Racial groups may be comprised of a number of ethnic groups who have among themselves relatively distinct cultures. Ethnic groups are socially distinguishable by virtue of their cultural orientation, heritage, and distinct sense of difference.

- **RACE IS POPULARLY DEFINED BY USING SKIN COLOR AS THE MARKER OF DIFFERENCE;** "white," "black," "yellow," and "red" commonly describe divergent groups of people. Race, in its broadest sense, is primarily biologically determined. To provide culturally competent care, nurses need to be cognizant that myriad ethnic and cultural differences can exist among members of groups who are considered as comprising the "same race."

- **COOKBOOK APPROACHES BASED ON THE STRUCTURAL FUNCTIONALISM OF ANTHROPOLOGY CAN SERVE TO STEREOTYPE** a group and cause the caregiver to think about the ethnically, racially, and culturally diverse patient in fixed generalizations that are too often reductionist and negative. It is important to know that cultural bias based on unfamiliarity can be eliminated in part by learning about the customs, beliefs, and values of the divergent group. A critical task facing nursing is the development of methods to eliminate racism, racial prejudice, and insidious discrimination from nursing practice.

- **SUBTLE STEREOTYPING OR NEGATIVE**

RACIAL INFLUENCES AFFECT DIAGNOSIS AND TREATMENT. Negative racial countertransference feelings are influenced by exposure of psychiatric nurses and other health care providers to newspapers, television, and other media where a disproportionate number of stories report negative events, especially about black Americans.

- **GENERALIZATIONS ABOUT ETHNIC, RACIAL, AND CULTURAL PATTERNS MAY HELP FAMILIARIZE THE NURSE WITH DIVERSE GROUPS.** Generalizations should be used as guidelines in organizing one's thoughts about people with diverse backgrounds. Generalizations become stereotypes when they are inappropriately used as fixed truths. Equally counterproductive to treatment is the nurse's failure to understand the importance of race, ethnicity, and culture on the individual's or family's understanding of an illness and their response to it. The concepts of race, ethnicity, culture, and the mitigating concept of socioeconomic status have to be understood systematically; their relationships are very complex.

- **RACISM IS AN ONGOING CONSTANT STRESSOR IN THE LIVES OF BLACK PATIENTS.** Nurses who are racially, culturally, ethnically, or socioeconomically different from the black patients they are working with must accept this fact. Psychiatric nurses who are arguably more focused than other nurses on establishing a therapeutic relationship with patients must learn to discuss racial difference with a patient if the nurse is white and the patient black. It is part of forming a therapeutic bond.

Race is the most obvious determinant of how one is viewed in this society. The psychiatric nurse must move beyond broad guidelines about race, ethnicity, and culture and assess what is reality for the patient.

- **THE CHRISMAN (1991) CULTURE-SENSITIVE CARE MODEL** is a conceptual framework that takes into account racial, ethnic, and cultural diversity. It is based on three principles: knowledge, mutual respect, and negotiation. The nurse with crucial knowledge about cultural diversity will be able to assess cultural factors related to a patient, and then promote those factors that are helpful and encourage the patient to accept some modification. Nurses can use this and other models for gathering knowledge about culturally and ethnically diverse groups with whom they frequently come in contact in their clinical work.

Gaining knowledge

- Reading books and articles.
- Talking and listening to patients and families. Nurses may have to identify why the information is being sought.
- Knowing beliefs, particularly religious ones helps in assessment and treatment. Spirituality may be a coping mechanism, particularly among black patients.

Establishing mutual respect

- Knowledge can be the basis for developing mutual respect.
- Listen to what the patient is describing as his or her experience — do not minimize it or try to identify by claiming to understand and citing a similar experience.
- Maintain a role of respect. Do not assume that calling patients by their first names is acceptable. Avoid patronizing and/or insulting behaviors.
- Clinicians' knowledge of their own ethnocentric beliefs will help them develop insight into how the beliefs influence their responses.

Negotiating treatment

- Broad knowledge and respect for the patient's cultural and racial identity and ethnicity can be used by the clinician to make care delivery more culturally sensitive and competent.

TAKING ANOTHER LOOK

You are ready to respond to the question that was raised in Gaining a Perspective at the beginning of this chapter. After you have written or thought more about your response, you may want to look at the Suggested Responses on page 321.

10 SPIRITUALITY AND PATIENT CARE

GAINING A PERSPECTIVE

Think about the situation presented below, and after you have read the Key Concepts for this chapter describe your response in more depth.

1. How would you, a nurse, handle the following situation?

   A patient tells you that he feels his life has no meaning. He says that he used to have deep faith in God, but that things have gone badly for him and that he thinks that there is no use in believing.

Key Concepts

- **THE PURPOSE OF LIFE** has traditionally been debated and philosophized by humankind. Persons suffering from psychological tragedies or psychiatric disorders generally struggle with the meaning of life events.

- **SPIRITUALITY** is the umbrella under which religion and religiosity stand. Spirituality, for the purposes of this book, encompasses a personal relationship with a higher being. It involves transcendent values, such as beauty and love, and a commitment to spiritual principles for one's life, for example, being truthful and caring. Spiritual qualities include gentleness, tolerance, patience, and forgiveness. Religiosity encompasses a chosen religious belief system.

- **SPIRITUAL WELL-BEING** can be defined as the affirmation of life in a relationship with God, self, community, and environment — a relationship that nurtures and celebrates wholeness. Spiritual well-being implies spiritual and psychological health, expressed through the experience of feeling alive, purposeful, and fulfilled.

- **A DISPARITY HAS DEVELOPED BETWEEN THE IMPORTANCE PLACED ON SPIRITUALITY AND RELIGIOSITY BY PATIENTS AND BY PROVIDERS OF MENTAL HEALTH CARE.** Sometimes issues of spirituality and religious belief are dismissed as irrelevant in the care of an individual who is struggling with a psychiatric illness. Holistic care deals with more than broken minds; it addresses broken bodies, hearts, and souls.

- **THE STANDARDS OF PSYCHIATRIC MENTAL HEALTH CLINICAL PRACTICE (ANA 1994)** state the importance of spiritual care: "...interpersonal, systematic, sociocultural,

CHAPTER 10

Figure 10-1

Assessment of Spiritual Awareness

1. **THE INDIVIDUAL'S NEED FOR A MEANINGFUL PHILOSOPHY OF LIFE** (a challenging object of self-investment is being met)
   a. What is important to you in life right now?

If the person responds with nothing...
   Ask. What was important to you?
   b. What does "being old" mean to you? Do you consider yourself old?

2. **SOURCE OF HOPE**
   a. Do you think your life has become better or worse as you have gown older?
   b. Do you foresee your life as better in the future?
   c. When you're discouraged or feeling hopeless, what keeps you going? Where have you found strength in the past?

3. **TRUSTING RELATIONSHIPS WITH GOD, PEOPLE, AND NATURE** (Your relationship with God, people, and nature—how do you keep that together?) What is the person's image of God?
   a. Do you believe in a power greater than yourself? Can you tell me about that power, i. e., who or what it is?
   b. Do you feel more like being alone or with other people right now?

4. **SELF-ACTUALIZATION**
   a. How much control do you believe you have over what happens to you in life?
   b. To what extent do you believe other forces play a role in what happens to you in life?
   c. Do you have a personal means for meeting your inner spiritual needs? Describe it.
   d. What do you believe about death?
   e. What are your special creative abilities?
   f. Tell me what beauty means to you. What is there in the world that you consider beautiful?

---

spiritual, or environmental circumstances or events which affect the mental and emotional well-being of the individual, family, or community...."

Spiritual issues are mentioned in the ANA Code for Nurses (1985) in regard to respecting human dignity, recognizing everyone's equal right to health care regardless of national, ethnic, religious, racial, cultural, political, economic, developmental, role, and sexual differences. Nurses enable the patient to live with as much physical, emotional, and spiritual comfort as possible, and they support the values the patient has treasured in life.

NANDA lists two diagnoses: Spiritual Distress and Potential for Enhanced Spiritual Well-Being.

- **ONE OBSTACLE TO EFFECTIVELY DEALING WITH SPIRITUAL NEEDS** is that exploration and resolution of such needs require a person to confront his or her limitations. A prerequisite for effectively managing one's own spiritual needs and those of others is to acknowledge the legitimacy and universality of these needs for all persons. Self-assessment, the process of getting in touch with one's own spiritual beliefs and values, is thus essential to clarify and integrate such beliefs and values into one's own life. Self-assessment is also important for the mental health care worker in order to resolve underlying dormant conflicts that might otherwise become manifest within the context of a therapeutic relationship.

  To assist patients with spiritual care, it is critical that nurses be willing to discuss spirituality with the patient and a person's relationship with God.

- **THE NURSING ADMISSION HISTORY CAN SYSTEMATICALLY ASSESS** the nature of a patient's spiritual and religious beliefs, as well as the reciprocal relationship between those beliefs and the current illness or life situation. Such assessments include inquiry into more than the patient's religious group affiliation.

- **A SPIRITUAL AWARENESS TOOL** is based on work that recognizes that people construct meaning from their experiences. The tool is developmental in that it recognizes that people change over time and that the criteria used to construct meaning change also. This developmental approach helps to understand patients' spiritual awareness in a way that respects their evolving dignity (see Study Guide Figure 10-1).

TAKING ANOTHER LOOK

You are now ready to respond to the question posed by the situation described in Gaining a Perspective at the beginning of this chapter. After you have written or thought about your response, you may want to look at the Suggested Responses on page 321.

11 LEGAL AND ETHICAL ISSUES IN PSYCHIATRIC NURSING

GAINING A PERSPECTIVE

Think about the issues presented below, and after you have read the Key Concepts in this chapter address the questions more fully.

1. How would you, the nurse, explain to Mrs. Jones, who is a patient in need of inpatient psychiatric care, what it would mean if she decided to seek voluntary admission to the psychiatric unit?

2. How would you, the nurse, handle a situation in which Mrs. Lawton, a competent patient, tells you that she is refusing to have the electroconvulsive therapy (ECT) that the psychiatrist is suggesting?

3. What are your concerns about the concept of privilege and patients treated in the community who have a potential to do harm? For example, suppose a patient told a nurse that she intended to harm a member of her family.

Key Concepts

- **LEGAL ISSUES RELATED TO THE CARE OF MENTALLY ILL PATIENTS** have become, in the last 30 years, a consideration in providing therapeutic interventions. Nurses should be familiar with current legal and ethical problems to ensure adequate care for patients.

- **BEFORE THE MIDDLE OF THE 19th CENTURY,** the decision to admit a patient to a psychiatric facility was wholly within the discretion of the hospital administrator. From 1840 to 1880, Dorothea Lynde Dix conducted a personal crusade to expose the conditions existing in poorhouses and local jails where many mentally ill persons were ultimately placed. She effectively lobbied in many states for the creation of public psychiatric institutions. The increase in the availability of institutions focused attention on the need for rational, fair procedures, particularly for persons in need who refused to voluntarily admit themselves to psychiatric hospitals.

    The efforts of Dix and other activists also instigated statutes requiring that no one could involuntarily be committed without a jury trial by peers. By the end of the 19th century, many states permitted commitment based on a wide range of behaviors associated with mental illness, not only dangerous behavior. Forms of these statutes remain in effect in most states. During the 1930s through the 1950s, the trend was away from strict procedural commitment and hearings. The power to commit an individual to an institution was entrusted to one or two physicians.

    Shortly after passage of the Community Mental Health Center Act of 1963, civil rights lawyers began to challenge the treatment of mentally ill persons. Judicial activism began with concern about the treatment of the mentally ill and maintenance of their rights. Commitment to mental hospitals was no longer only a medical decision, but one entrusted to a neutral decision maker, such as a judge. Many laws were changed to encompass not only mental illness, but also dangerousness.

By 1992, large numbers of hospitalized individuals were released into the community, and concerns were raised that community facilities and services be adequate to care for these persons. Many states have developed programs using crisis mobile teams. Respite stabilization units and short-term inpatient facilities are now available in some areas so that a person does not have to be hospitalized for long periods of time. In addition, managed care is decreasing the length of hospital stay.

- **UNLESS A COURT HAS FOUND AN INDIVIDUAL INCOMPETENT TO MANAGE PERSONAL MATTERS AND A GUARDIAN HAS BEEN APPOINTED, THE PERSON DOES NOT LOSE THE RIGHT** to make personal or business decisions when admitted, voluntarily or involuntarily, to a psychiatric facility. It was in the 1960s that most states separated the issue of competency from commitment in the commitment statutes.

In an inpatient or outpatient setting, a nurse should know whether the patient has been declared incompetent. If the patient has a copy of the court order, it should be obtained and documentation established as to who has the authority to consent to treatment or authorize release of records.

- **THE LEAST RESTRICTIVE ALTERNATIVE** is a concept in the delivery of mental health care. When professional caregivers plan mental health care, they focus on a treatment program that can be implemented in the least restrictive environment. If a person can be treated in a halfway house or at home, it is a preferable to involuntary commitment on a locked ward in a psychiatric hospital. This doctrine is based on the principle that the state may have a legitimate reason for wanting to treat an individual, but treatment must be provided in a manner that is least restrictive but that provides sufficient care for the patient's needs.

- **ONE OF THREE TYPES OF ADMISSION TO INPATIENT PSYCHIATRIC HOSPITALS** is generally followed:

Voluntary admission of a patient who is mentally ill and in need of inpatient care first involves the patient's willingness to seek admission. In addition, the patient must consent to all treatment. After a patient requests release that patient must be released in a reasonable period of time (specified by state law), or a petition for judicial commitment should be initiated. In some states parents may authorize the voluntary admission of their children (under 18 years of age); in some states the courts have to do the authorization.

Emergency involuntary admission occurs when an individual is thought to pose an immediate threat of serious harm to self or others as a result of mental illness and is unwilling to seek treatment; commitment for a short time is permitted without a court order.

Indefinite involuntary (judicial commitment) involves both immediate danger to self or others, as well as more passive types of danger that can result from a person's inability to avoid or protect self from harm because of mental illness.

- **A DILEMMA HAS ARISEN ABOUT WHAT TO DO WITH INDIVIDUALS WHO, WHEN DISCHARGED** from an inpatient facility, are continuously noncompliant. Because hospitalization tends to be for shorter periods, a movement has begun toward mandatory outpatient treatment, also called preventive or involuntary outpatient treatment.

- **CERTAIN LEGAL RIGHTS ARE MAINTAINED WHEN AN INDIVIDUAL IS ADMITTED TO A PSYCHIATRIC HOSPITAL**, although the patient may be deprived of the freedom to leave the hospital. The patient's rights are sometimes defined by state law. Consequently, mental health professionals should be familiar with what rights patients have in the jurisdiction where they practice. Unless a patient has been declared incompetent, the individual maintains the rights of any citizen; for example, he or she has the right to vote, manage financial matters, and execute legal documents. A patient is also permitted to communicate with an attorney in person, by letter, and by telephone. In addition, the patient may receive mail, without interference or censorship; may have visitors; and may not be denied the basic necessities of life in the name of treatment.

A patient right that emerged in the late 1960s was the right to treatment once hospitalized. Treatment should not degenerate to punishment (Rouse v. Cameron,1967). Treatment must provide realistic opportunities for cure and have three charcteristics (Wyatt v. Stickney,1971).

- It must be provided in a humane psychologic and physical environment.
- Qualified staff in sufficient numbers should provide treatment.
- Treatment plans should be individualized.

The state cannot constitutionally confine without treatment a nondangerous individual who is capable of surviving safely in the community alone or with the help of a willing and responsible family member or friend (O'Connor v. Donaldson, 1975).

- **ADULTS WHO ARE OF SOUND MIND, THAT IS, MENTALLY COMPETENT, HAVE THE RIGHT TO DETERMINE WHAT WILL BE DONE TO THEIR BODIES.** Moreover, a person must not only give consent for a procedure to be carried out, but that consent must be based on sufficient information provided to him or her by the health care team. When a patient enters a hospital for a mental illness, the right to consent to treatment is not abdicated. A voluntarily admitted patient should also have the right to refuse any kind of treatment.

Patients who are involuntarily committed and who are competent have the same right of informed consent. When the patient has been found incompetent by a court of law, an appropriate consent should be obtained from a formally appointed substitute.

The guidelines for how to manage an incompetent involuntarily committed patient follow several courses. A court-appointed guardian will make a decision using one or a combination of both of the following guidelines: What treatment is in the best interests of the patient? What would the patient want if he or she were competent (substitute judgment decision)?

- **A PATIENT'S RIGHT TO REFUSE PSYCHOTROPIC MEDICATIONS AS WELL AS TREATMENT** has been addressed in several lawsuits during the past few years. Because of the drugs' potentially incurable side effects, such as tardive dyskinesia, patients were motivated to file suit to protect their right to refuse medication.

When managing the care of a patient who refuses medications, state systems or individual facilities should take certain steps. Procedures should be established about how to intervene. Guidelines for managing the involuntarily committed patient who refuses medication should incorporate state law, case decisions, rules and regulations, and consent decrees of the particular jurisdiction where the facility is located. There is, however, no substitute for a therapeutic relationship between a patient and a mental health professional to resolve issues about medication. An ongoing dialogue over several days can assist in assessing the patient's reasons for refusing medications.

- **TO BE CAREFUL AND THOROUGH IN OBTAINING VALID CONSENT FOR PARTICULAR INTRUSIVE PROCEDURES, SUCH AS ELECTROCONVULSIVE TREATMENT (ECT),** is especially important. The competent patient should be fully informed of all the facts about the treatment, including side effects. The patient can refuse the treatment.

Conducting research on psychiatric patients in an institutional setting is controversial and should be reviewed by an institutional review board, which is convened to protect the rights of human subjects. All professional disciplines and consumers from the community should be represented on the professional review board.

- **SECLUSION AND RESTRAINT** have been the subject of much clinical and legal debate during the last two to three decades. The rates of seclusion and restraint vary greatly, even within the same state. Generally, only a psychiatrist or qualified physician with specialized training can order nonemergency seclusion and restraint. Then, usually, the patient must be monitored every 15 minutes. In an emergency situation, generally, a qualified registered nurse is authorized to give a seclusion and restraint order if no doctor is available. The nurse must evaluate the situation and record the observations. This authority is usually limited to one hour. A physician must see the patient within a specified period of time.

- **ACCURATELY RECORDING TREATMENT AND NOTING WHY THE DECISION WAS MADE TO PROVIDE A SPECIFIC KIND OF CARE** is important in the care of a mentally ill individual. An overall psychosocial assessment should be made of each patient and a treatment plan developed and updated as needed. The treatment process should be accurately recorded. It is better to describe an event (behavioral responses) in detail than to label the behaviors.

  Another important issue to document is a patient's crisis episode and the therapeutic intervention. The nurse's assessment of the crisis and the intervention should be recorded not only to protect the patient, but to protect the nurse, especially if the patient later responds to the crisis situation with self-inflicted injury or follows through on threats that were made.

- **ALL PRESCRIBED MEDICATIONS MUST BE DOCUMENTED**, including the continued use of medication throughout the treatment. The long-term effects of medications are of concern. Nurses caring for patients in the community should be particularly sensitive to individuals who are on drug therapy and complain of difficulties. It is imperative that any complaints of medication side effects be immediately and accurately recorded and reported to the prescribing physician.

- **MALPRACTICE AND NEGLIGENCE ARE OFTEN USED INTERCHANGEABLY** in health care. The court will analyze all the elements of negligence in relationship to the facts of a case before determining whether malpractice exists. For a nurse to be found liable for negligence, the person bringing the lawsuit must show a causal relationship between the professional's acts and the alleged injury. The causal link must be established, which is often difficult to do. An example of a potential malpractice issue relating to mental health practice relates to the suicide of a patient after discharge from a facility or during off-the-ward activities. Generally courts rule that if the staff had carefully observed the patient and suicidal behavior had not been exhibited, verbally or nonverbally, the mental health team would not be held liable; if, however, the individual had exhibited current suicidal tendencies and was discharged or given a pass, conceivably the ruling would not be in the favor of the staff. It is imperative that communication about a patient's condition be reported verbally and written in the record.

- **COURTS REQUIRE NURSES TO FUNCTION AT A MINIMUM STANDARD** that is equivalent to that of a reasonably prudent nurse delivering care in the same circumstances.

- **A NURSE-PATIENT RELATIONSHIP IS ESTABLISHED** when a nurse initiates a professional relationship with a patient, and the nurse is obligated to give care in an appropriate manner. If the nurse observes an action by another professional that the nurse thinks breaches the standards of care and can predict or foresee possible harm to the patient, the nurse has a responsibility to intervene and prevent injury.

- **CONFIDENTIALITY AND PRIVILEGE** are two often misunderstood concepts that are vitally important to a relationship with a patient. Confidentiality relates to the responsibility of the agency and professional to keep all information, records, and correspondence confidential and private and allow third parties access to these records only under specifically defined circumstances. Privilege, on the other hand, specifically refers to the relationship of a particular professional to a patient and the protection of information obtained from the patient as a result of this relationship. Each state defines by law which professionals have privilege and whether that privilege is absolute; the nurse should be familiar with the law where he or she practices.

- **THE RANGE OF PATIENTS SERVED AT THE COMMUNITY LEVEL** has expanded. Fewer patients can be referred to hospitals when problems arise. More potentially dangerous patients must continue to be served in the community and more severely and persistently mentally ill patients must be supported in that setting.

    When it is determined that a patient in the community must be referred for inpatient care, appropriate treatment should be discussed with the patient so that, if possible, he or she can make an informed decision concerning hospitalization. If, based on the mental illness, the individual does not pose a threat of serious harm, it may not be possible or desirable to force the community-based patient to be hospitalized against his or her will. If, however, the individual is unwilling to seek inpatient care as a voluntary admission or is posing an immediate threat of harm to self or others, a decision must be made concerning involuntary commitment to a psychiatric inpatient facility.

    Another issue involving the care of individuals in the community is the potential danger to third parties and the responsibility of the therapist to warn of the potential danger (Duty to Protect). It is important for mental health practitioners to know the laws in the states where they practice—when it is required to report conduct of a patient that might harm a third party and when to commit a patient to prevent harm.

- **BOUNDARY VIOLATIONS** have been written about a great deal in recent years. When someone transgresses a patient's boundaries, e.g., a therapist has sexual relations with a patient, the person, or victim, can be devastated for years. Therefore, basic information on ethical prohi-

bitions should be made available to all trainees (students), including all people in the helping professions. The helping process, one of the bases for health care, has special significance in providing mental health care for patients. Information about abuse of power and breach of trust, including theory on victimology, should be provided. Issues relating to identity, self-esteem, and self-image must be thoroughly discussed. Managing countertransference issues is very important and attraction to a patient should be openly discussed, without fear, with supervisors. The patient's welfare must be kept as the driving force. Dealing with sexual feelings and sexual acting out by the patient should also be discussed in the supervisory sessions.

- **THE AMERICANS WITH DISABILITIES ACT** protects individuals who have mental health problems that limit them in one or more major activities. When an individual is seeking employment, he or she cannot be asked about prior mental health treatment as part of the pre-employment evaluation process. Once an individual with a limitation is hired, the employer is expected to make reasonable accommodations for the employee.

- **THE COURTS MAY ASK HEALTH PROFESSIONALS** to evaluate individuals who have emotional problems and who have been charged with crimes (forensic services). What information mental health professionals should provide and what issues they should address have been deliberated. One issue that must be addressed is the competency of an individual to stand trial. Determining competency can be done in an inpatient or community-based setting. The second issue relates to the insanity defense (criminal responsibility). The courts may ask a mental health professional to do an evaluation. Several states have adopted a Guilty But Mentally Ill Statute (GBMI), which does not abolish the insanity defense but provides an alternative plan, usually a provision of services, for those defendants who are mentally ill but not insane at the time of the crime.

TAKING ANOTHER LOOK

You are now ready to respond to the questions that were raised in Gaining a Perspective at the beginning of this chapter. After you have written or thought about your responses, you may wish to look at the Suggested Responses on page 322.

12 THERAPEUTIC COMMUNICATION

GAINING A PERSPECTIVE

Think about the questions listed below, and after you have read the Key Concepts for this chapter describe in more detail your thoughts on the subjects queried.

1. What factors influence your way of communicating?

2. Why is it that quite often there are misunderstandings between what a person says and what another person hears?

3. How do you feel therapeutic communication differs from social communication (conversation)?

4. In what situation might you, in your professional role as a nurse, use silence as a therapeutic communication technique?

KEY CONCEPTS

• **COMMUNICATION IS A CONTINUOUS ACTIVITY OF GENERATING, EXCHANGING, AND PROCESSING INFORMATION.** Communication is essential for the maintenance and evolution of all life forms and essential to growth and development. Not only does the concept organize our thinking about patterns of maintenance and change, it also broadens our scope to recognize that, in human terms, communication goes beyond the spoken and written word.

• **FACTORS THAT INFLUENCE COMMUNICATION**

Culture. Anthropologists believe that culture determines language and gesture. Cultures vary in the "rules" they apply to expression of emotional behavior; rules governing intimacy vary. Unspoken gestures take on cultural meanings and are emblems. The nurse's and the patient's cultural backgrounds can have a profound effect on therapeutic communication. Customs, beliefs, values, and knowledge guide behavior and communication.

Gender. Patterns of communication tend to vary between the sexes. In the United States, women express more emotion in their verbal and facial expressions than men. The relative influence of gender on communication is debated: Do differences arise out of cultural determinants or innate determinants?

Socioeconomic background. Education, vocabulary, personal experiences, and relative status position become important factors in variations in patterns of communicating and provide an experiential basis for differences in interpreting spoken and nonspoken behavior.

Social distance. Age, status, and, at times, gender dictate the degree of familiarity with and receptivity to communication. In the mental health field, the concept of social distance (closeness) and its relationship to a free flow of communication was recognized and the development of indigenous workers came about.

Power relationships. Ascribed and prescribed power in interpersonal relationships is most evident in the type, direction, frequency, and content communicated. Relative levels of power are ascribed by tone of voice, body posture, and phrasing of words. Strength and weakness are inferred by communication behaviors.

Number of receivers. The size of the group determines how often a person speaks, what is said, and what patterns of initiating, confirming, negating, and speaking freely are used.

Language. Language and the individual's use of words are directly and inextricably linked to therapeutic communication. Language is the tool and the nurse will need to recognize the patient's level of language use and ability. Nurses need to clarify interpretation of words, validate meaning, and search for shared thoughts. The nurse's awareness of nonverbal communication is critical when the nurse and the patient do not share a common language. Attitudes and perceptions affect the nurse's abilities to perceive and interpret communications.

Past experiences. People's backgrounds influence their ability to communicate; for example, some people are supported and encouraged to verbalize their thoughts. One's own experience with self-disclosure, freedom of expression, and feelings of self-esteem affect communication.

Level of expertise. The process of therapeutic communication can be influenced by the level of nursing expertise. Nurses who have a good understanding of self and the theories and principles of interpersonal communication, and who have experience relating to patients, may be more effective communicators.

Internal state. How one feels greatly influences patterns of communication. Part of knowing people is learning what their behavior is in relation to their statements concerning their internal state.

Drugs. Drugs affect communication, including sending, receiving, and processing information.

Other considerations. A poor state of health, including loss of sensory abilities, can alter expectations regarding communicating behavior. Age is another factor. Recognizing differences in the communication processes of young children, adolescents, and older people may facilitate relationships.

- **SPOKEN AND UNSPOKEN BEHAVIORS** are two broad categories of communication.

Spoken behavior can be studied from the following perspectives:

- **Phonology.** The study of how sounds are put together to form words.
- **Syntax.** How words are put together to form clauses, phrases, sentences, etc.
- **Semantics.** The study of the meaning of words.

  DENOTATION refers the general meaning of a word.

  CONNOTATION refers to the meaning of a word suggested by a person, a meaning different from that specifically assigned to the word.

  That words have a potential for more than one meaning (public and private) and that the choice of words is influenced by the context in which a person finds him or herself suggest great room for misunderstanding.

- **Pragmatics.** Deals with the relationship of linguistic expressions and the user.
- **Paralanguage.** Nonverbal aspects of speech, such as tone, rhythm, and tenor of the voice (aspects that probably convey emotion).

Nonspoken behavior used in communication is also studied from several perspectives:

- **Body language.** The gestures, mannerisms, and movements used by a person to communicate with another
- **Writing.** Handwriting analysis (graphology) is an area that needs more research. Diaries, journals, and biographical sketches may be used.
- **Spacial behavior** (proxemics). The psychological use of space, for example, who sits and who stands or who sits where.
- **Autonomic nervous system responses.** Tear-

ing, blushing, crying, pallor, gastrointestinal sounds, and breathing patterns. Measuring tics and other nonspoken mannerisms during discussions may give clinicians clues that a topic has more significance than might be consciously apparent to patient.

- **Clothing and symbols.** The care and appropriateness of dress is part of assessment. Wearing jewelry, for example, a wedding ring, conveys information. Dress may tell about social group conformity.

Spoken and nonspoken behavior are related. We have an internal response to the total communication experience with another person. Much of what a person communicates may be well out of the consciousness of that person. Understanding another in the process of communication is enhanced in recognizing the potential for confusion. Being sensitive to feedback may cause one to adjust communication patterns. It has been realized that an internal system of communication has physiological consequences, and physiological experiences have psychological consequences.

- **GENERAL THEORIES OF COMMUNICATION** are closely related to the theories of learning. The most simplistic theory of communication emphasizes the sender and receiver (Hullian, 1952). The theory assumes that (1) there is a correct message and (2) the sender and receiver are relatively independent of one another, having little influence on the meaning of the message, but great responsibility for sending it and the skills to receive it. The denotation aspects of words, syntax, and semantics are emphasized, and skill is based on selecting words and their appropriateness.

Reciprocity in interaction is emphasized at the next level of theorizing. It is emphasized that each person has a perspective, and it is important for each to step into the meaning framework of the other. This theory leads to the expectation that one person can know the experience of another in a direct way, and it is assumed that words carry this directness of information.

The next level of theory development moves communication from the level of an action and interaction to the level of a transaction, which takes into account the pragmatics of conversing and the complexity of meaning. Behavior is a result of the personal perception of experience. Perceptions serve a decisive functional role in the behavior generated from experience.

The most complex theory is that the meaning of communication is derived from personal psychological constructs. The theory resulting in the symbolic interactionist model of communications involves input (any stimulus that engages the individual in an interpersonal interaction for some specific goal) and covert rehearsal (a cognitive map that is the structure of how meaning is derived for the person). The map contains stored resources for filtering and interpreting messages from without and within. Covert rehearsal also includes the processes that generate behavior: delivering the message, generating new information, and the goal response. Success is a function of the person's criteria.

Whatever is communicated at a point in time cannot be repeated. Communication is ongoing and complex. Meaning is not transferred, it is inferred and negotiated.

- **WHEN COMMUNICATING THERAPEUTICALLY WITH A PATIENT,** the nurse is focused on the patient's feelings, experiences, and ideas. Therapeutic communication is well-planned and patient-focused, with goal-directed interactions. Components of therapeutic communication include:

Therapeutic use of self. Focus is on the patient, not the nurse; patient is made to feel safe; nurse is engrossed in the patient's level of comfort; ability to engender trust requires the nurse to keep promises and be reliable, consistent, and accepting of the patient's behaviors.

Empathy. Nurse's ability to place self in the patient's position without losing objectivity; nurse shares patient's frame of reference; responds to patient in a reflective sensitive mode; uses active listening skills (see Study Guide Table 12-1).

Table 12-1
ACTIVE LISTENING BEHAVIORS

FACILITATE COMMUNICATION	HINDER COMMUNICATION
direct eye-to-eye contact	avoiding client's eyes
comfortable physical distance	too close or too far apart
leaning toward client to listen	sitting way back in chair
open body posture	folding arms tightly
gentle nodding, gesturing	bored appearance
relaxed manner	fidgeting, nervousness
looking concerned	nonresponsiveness
gentle, reassuring touch	aggressive physical contact

Respect. Conveyed through unconditional positive regard; values the patient; allows patient to feel good about self; conveyed through privacy, confidentiality, and dignity. Respect is indicated by:

- Introducing self and asking how the patient wishes to be addressed
- Clarifying roles and duties with the patient
- Establishing a time frame for interactions, including the length and location of the meeting
- Creating a secure, private environment
- Reviewing issues of confidentiality with the patient
- Discussing the patient only with the staff
- Protecting the patient's rights, including written records and shared information
- Advocating the patient's dignity by explaining procedures, policies, and activities

Genuineness. Convey true interest, openness, authenticity, and sincerity.

- **COMMUNICATION MAY BE ENHANCED** by means of:

  Nonverbal skills. Simple actions that indicate the nurse is attending; for example, the use of touch or silence as a time for thinking; silence may also convey acceptance.

  Acknowledging. Recognizing patients for who they are: address patient by preferred name; use appropriate distance and touch; maintain an attentive stance.

  Open-ended questions. Allow patient to respond in a variety of ways; permit description,

sharing of information, and changing topic.

Giving information. Offers patient data needed to experience growth; good screening questions necessary so that nurse knows what information patient needs and why.

Focusing. Assists the patient to pursue an idea or emotion further and eliminates peripheral communication that prevents discussion of specific information.

Probing. Questions and statements encourage patient to express more information; sometimes interpreted as invasive or insensitive ("Tell me more").

Paraphrasing. "Translates" for the patient what the nurse thinks the patient is communicating ("In other words..." or "I hear you saying...").

Clarifying. Ensures understanding of the communication ("I'm not sure I understood what you are saying" or "Could you repeat?").

Exploring and questioning. Not simply seeking information, rather more involved with the patient's personal issues; occurs only after therapeutic relationship is established; in atmosphere of trust the client is able to respond to more personal questions; exploring senstive issues promotes patient's healing and growth.

Confronting. Demonstrates for patients the incongruencies, discrepancies, or inconsistencies in their communication and behavior; not aggressive or an attack; expands self-awareness and behavioral change; includes feedback as to how behavior and actions affect the nurse. Constructive confrontation includes the following elements:

- Active listening with special attention to non-verbal behaviors
- Use of "I" statements
- Acknowledging that changing behavior is difficult
- Focused feedback statements that point up the incongruencies and inconsistencies in the patient's feelings, thoughts, and/or behaviors
- Supportive statements that challenge the patient to action, including being responsible for his/her own behavior and accountable for his/her feelings
- Integration of patient-identified coping responses to foster confidence that change is possible

Reflecting. Helps the patient explore his or her own feelings; responding to patient's feeling tones or affective statements explores the meaning of the communication; states the implied.

Summarizing. Verbally captures the essence of a transaction; allows the patient to hear what is recalled about the interaction and experience being heard; terminates session and sets tone for the next.

- **INEFFECTIVE VERBAL COMMUNICATION TECHNIQUES** include:

  Blaming. Attacks the patient's behaviors or actions ("You caused...")

  Advice giving. Offering opinions is ineffectual ("I think you should..." or "In my view...")

  Falsely reassuring and approving. Used when nurses do not want to confront the real meaning of an interaction ("Don't worry...")

  Judging. Behavior is judged ("good" or "bad")

  Rationalizing. Attempts to explain away patient's feelings ("Everyone feels like that...")

  Changing topics. May meet the needs of the nurse who has anxiety about a topic

  Other nonfacilitative actions

  - Leading patient to a response nurse desires
  - Moralizing
  - Asking multiple questions without waiting for a reply
  - Patronizing, using immature language

TAKING ANOTHER LOOK

You are now ready to respond more confidently to the questions raised in Gaining a Perspective at the beginning of this chapter. After you have written or thought about your responses, you may want to look at the Suggested Responses on page 322.

SECTION III

CLINICAL DISORDERS ON THE STRESS-CRISIS CONTINUUM

The mental disorders described in the following section are classified on a seven-level stress-crisis continuum. The first levels in the continuum include high physical symptomotology with an identified or an unclear stressful event. The event may increase anxiety, which provokes coping behaviors; however, a crisis state is not necessarily triggered. At the upper end of the continuum, the individual has preexisting psychiatric conditions that complicate the stressful situation and require psychiatric intervention and case management for the acute and long-term phases. In advancing from level 1 to level 7, the internal biopsychosocial conflicts of the patient and family increase in maladaptive coping behaviors. This typology is designed to assist in assessing patients, identifying nursing diagnoses, and developing care plans.

Assessing stress in terms of seven levels along a stress-crisis continuum is an adaptation of the work of Peplau (1952), Baldwin (1978), and Burgess and Roberts (1995).

The seven levels are:
Somatic distress
Transitional stress and altered self-regulatory patterns
Traumatic crises
Relational and family crises
Serious mental illness
Psychiatric emergencies
Cataclysmic crises

13 SOMATOFORM DISORDERS

TERMS TO DEFINE

body dysmorphic disorder

conversion disorder

hypochondriasis

pain disorder

somatization disorder

GAINING A PERSPECTIVE

Think about the situations described below, and after you have read the Key Concepts for this chapter answer the questions in more detail.

1. When would you as a nurse be likely to come in contact with a patient with a somatization disorder? Describe one intervention that might help the patient.

2. How would you as a nurse respond in the following situation?

   The parent of a 24-year-old patient diagnosed as having one of the somatoform disorders says to you, "I knew it was all in her head. She is always complaining of physical pain, but now I know the pain is not real."

Key Concepts

- **IN THE FIVE SUBTYPES OF SOMATOFORM DISORDERS SYMPTOMS SUGGEST A PHYSICAL DISORDER** and can cause clinically significant impairment or distress in social, occupational, or other areas of functioning. Unlike in malingering, symptoms are not intentional. Laboratory testing does not confirm any pathophysiological process. Patients do not perceive themselves as having a psychiatric problem.

  Patients who have persistent, troubling somatic symptoms without identifiable etiology may be expressing psychological distress in bodily terms. These disorders are more likely to occur among patients with a recent decline in self-esteem, those undergoing serious life stresses, and those whose characteristic coping patterns and defense mechanisms are failing (see Study Guide Table 13-1).

- **IN SOMATIZATION DISORDER** patients have physical symptoms with no findings to support subjective complaints (called hysteria in Freud's time). The DSM IV (1994) includes the following criteria:

  A history of many physical complaints or a belief that one is sickly, beginning before age 30, persisting for several years, and interfering with social, occupational, and other important areas of functioning.

  Symptoms from four groupings

  - Four pain symptoms. A history of pain from at least four body sites.
  - Two gastrointestinal symptoms, not pain.
  - One sexual symptom other than pain, for example, sexual indifference, erectile dysfunction, excessive menstrual bleeding.
  - One pseudoneurological symptom. Suggests a neurological condition not limited to pain, for example, conversion symptoms such as impaired balance, localized weakness.

Table 13-1
SOMATOFORM DISORDERS

	Somatization Disorder	Conversion Disorder	Somatoform Pain Disorder	Hypochondriasis	Body Dysmorphic Disorder
Key Features	Multiple physical symptoms with no organic basis, causing the individual to seek medical care or medications	Loss or change of physical function caused by psychological conflict. Usually single symptom or sign.	Preoccupation with pain. Symptom in the absence of physical findings, or in excess of what would be expected with findings.	The fear of having, or belief that one has, a serious physical disease	Preoccupation with an imagined body defect
Epidemiology	One-year prevalence; 0.2% women>men	Rare Women> men	Common Women> men	Common in women and men	Common in men and women
Treatment	Consolidation of care under single supportive doctor. Identification of psychosocial stressors. Psychotherapy	Behavioral therapy. Psychotherapy	Consolidation of care under single supportive doctor. Behavioral therapy, pharmacotherapy with tricyclic antidepressants	Consolidation of care under single supportive doctor. Psychotherapy	Seeks out dermatologists or plastic surgeons

Physical symptoms may differ across cultures. Prevalence rates differ according to the interviewers' gender and profession. The disorder is presumed to be psychological in origin. Pathological identification with a parent, immature efforts to deal with dependency needs, and maladaptive resolution of intrapsychic conflict have all been proposed as a mechanism by which symptoms similar to those seen in somatization disorder are produced (see Study Guide Figure 13-1).

- **CONVERSION DISORDER (CONVERSION HYSTERIA)** is characterized by loss or alteration of physical functioning that suggests a physical disorder, but is apparently an expression of psychological conflict or need. The problem is not under voluntary control and cannot be explained by any physical disorder or known pathophysiological mechanism. The DSM IV (1994) criteria include:

One or more symptoms of deficits affecting voluntary motor or sensory function that suggest a neurological or other general medical condition.

Psychological factors are judged to be associated with the symptoms because the symptoms are preceded by conflicts or other stressors.

The symptom is not intentionally produced or feigned.

The symptom cannot be explained by a physical disorder, a substance, or a culturally sanctioned behavior.

The symptom causes clinically significant distress or impairment in social, occupational, or other areas of functioning.

The symptom is not limited to pain or sexual dysfunction.

Conversion disorder is more common in rural populations, among women patients of lower socioeconomic status, and among patients who

Figure 13-1

Critical Pathway for Patient with Somatization Disorder

Expected Length of Treatment: _____

Nursing Diagnoses: Ineffective individual coping

Altered work role performance

Altered family role

Related to: (check at least one)

☐ Repressed anxiety   ☐ Unmet dependency needs

☐ Low self-esteem   ☐ Focus on self and symptoms

☐ Sporadic work performance   ☐ Dysfunctional family

☐ Other

Outcomes: Patient will demonstrate ability to cope with stress by means other than preoccupation with physical symptoms by discharge.

Patient will verbalize an understanding of the relationship between emotional problems and physical symptoms.

Interventions: _____

Day:_____**Date :** _____

Planned	Completed	
_____	_____	1. Monitor ongoing physical assessments, lab data, diagnostic data, etc.
_____	_____	2. Recognize the physical complaints constitute the symptoms of the psychiatric disorder.
_____	_____	3. Identify gains that the physical symptom is providing for the patient: increased dependency, attention, distraction from work and family problems.
_____	_____	4. Prioritize patient's dependency needs.
_____	_____	5. Gradually withdraw attention to physical symptoms.
_____	_____	6. Encourage patient to verbalize fears and anxieties. Reduce attention if rumination about physical complaints begins.
_____	_____	7. Give positive reinforcement to adaptive coping strategies.
_____	_____	8. Assist patient to identify ways to achieve recognition from others without resorting to physical symptoms. Review patient's interpersonal relationships.
_____	_____	9. Teach patient relaxation techniques and assertiveness skills.
_____	_____	10. Teach patient how physical symptoms can arise in response to psychosocial stressors. Review patient stressor.

Figure 13-2
Critical Pathway for Patient with Conversion Disorder

Expected Length of Treatment: _____

Nursing Diagnosis: Sensory-perceptual alteration

Related to: (check at least one)

☐ Repressed anxiety   ☐ Unmet dependency needs

☐ Low self-esteem   ☐ Loss/alteration of physical functioning without organic
                                    cause

Outcomes: Patient will demonstrate recovery of loss function and verbalize an understanding of relationship of emotional problems by discharge.

Patient will be able to verbalize adaptive methods of coping with stress and community support systems.

Interventions: _____

Day:_____**Date :** _____

Planned	Completed	
_____	_____	1. Monitor physical assessments, lab reports, diagnostic studies.
_____	_____	2. Identify gains the physical symptom is providing for the patient: increased dependency, attention, distraction from other problems.
_____	_____	3. Fulfill patient's needs related to ADLs with which physical symptoms are interfering.
_____	_____	4. Do not focus on the disability. Allow patient to be as independent as possible.
_____	_____	5. Encourage patient to participate in therapeutic activities to the best of his/her ability.
_____	_____	6. Gradually minimize patient's use of the disability; withdraw attention if patient continues to focus on physical limitation.
_____	_____	7. Encourage patient to verbalize fears and anxieties; teach patient to recognize that physical symptoms appear in times of extreme stress and are a coping mechanism.
_____	_____	8. Teach patient to identify coping mechanisms that he/she can use when faced with stressful situations.
_____	_____	9. Teach assertiveness techniques.
_____	_____	10. Identify community resources and a support system for the patient.

are less psychologically minded. Two mechanisms explain why a person may have a conversion symptom. In one mechanism, the individual achieves a "primary gain" by keeping the psychological conflict out of conscious awareness. In the second mechanism, the individual achieves "secondary gain" from the symptom by avoiding a particular painful activity (see Study Guide Figure 13-2).

- **PAIN DISORDER** is essentially the same as conversion disorder except the symptom involved is limited to physical pain of at least six months in duration, in the absence of explanatory physical findings. The DSM IV (1994) criteria include:

Pain occurs in one or more anatomical sites and warrants clinical attention.

Pain disrupts social, occupational, or other functional areas.

Psychological factors are judged to have an important role in the onset, severity, exacerbation, or maintenance of the pain (see below).

Pain is not intentionally produced or feigned.

The pain is not accounted for by another disorder.

Pain disorder appears to be relatively common. The etiology of pain is believed to be psychological in origin. That the cause of pain is psychological is indicated by the following:

- a temporal relationship exists between an external stressor and pain
- the pain enables a person to avoid a distressing activity
- the pain enables a person to obtain added support from the environment

It is suggested that patients with pain disorder may be less able to experience and verbalize feelings directly; the implication is that emotions are translated into physical pain (see Study Guide Figure 13-3).

- **HYPOCHONDRIASIS** is the fear of having a serious illness. A "hypochondriac" is a person who complains about minor physical problems, worries unrealistically about serious illness, per-

sistently seeks professional care, and consumes multiple over-the-counter remedies. Minor bodily symptoms are exaggerated. This chronic disorder usually begins in adolescence, but may not begin until the fourth decade in men and the fifth decade in women. The DSM IV (1994) criteria include:

Preoccupation with the fear of having, or belief that one has, a serious disease, based on the person's misinterpretation of bodily symptoms.

The preoccupation persists despite medical evaluation and reassurance.

Duration of the disturbance is at least six months.

Hypochondriasis is believed to have its origins in maladaptive attempts to cope with unmet psychological needs or unconscious psychological conflicts (see Study Guide Figure 13-4).

- **BODY DYSMORPHIC DISORDER** is characterized in two DSM IV (1994) criteria:

Preoccupation with some imagined defect in appearance. If a slight physical anomaly is present, the person's concern is excessive.

The preoccupation causes clinically significant distress or impairment in social, occupational, or other important areas of functioning.

Psychological factors are a critical etiological factor. The disorder usually begins in adolescence, but may not be diagnosed for many years due to the individual's reluctance to reveal symptoms. Uncertainty about the etiology of body dysmorphic disorder is reflected in the diversity of treatments: medication, for example, antidepressants such as serotonin-reuptake blockers; psychotherapy; and cosmetic surgery (see Study Guide Figure 13-5).

Figure 13-3
Critical Pathway for Patient with Pain Disorder

Expected Length of Treatment: _____

Nursing Diagnosis: Pain

Related to: (check at least one)

    ☐ Repeated health visits   ☐ Repressed anxiety

    ☐ Dependency issues   ☐ Denial psychological issues

    ☐ Other

Outcomes: Patient will demonstrate ability to intervene as anxiety increases, to prevent onset or increased severity of pain.

Patient will verbalize an understanding of the relationship between pain and emotional problems. Patient's normal social and occupational functioning increases.

Interventions: _____

Day:_____**Date :** _____

Planned	Completed	
_____	_____	1. Observe and record the precipitants, duration, and intensity of pain.
_____	_____	2. Teach measures to reduce pain-related behavior.
_____	_____	3. Use of milieu or group interventions.
_____	_____	4. Assist patient to connect symptoms of pain to times of increased anxiety and to identify specific situations that cause anxiety to increase.
_____	_____	5. Encourage patient to identify alternative methods of coping with stress.
_____	_____	6. Teach patient ways to intervene as symptoms begin to intensify (i.e., visual/auditory distractions, guided imagery, breathing exercises, massage, application of heat or cold, relaxation techniques).
_____	_____	7. Reinforce adaptive coping and behaviors.
_____	_____	8. Refer to an interdisciplinary treatment center or support group for patients with chronic pain.

Figure 13-4
Critical Pathway for Patient with Hypochondriasis

Expected Length of Treatment: _____

Nursing Diagnoses: Self-care deficit
                            Impaired physical mobility

Related to: (check at least one)

    ☐ Paralysis of body parts   ☐ Inability to speak

    ☐ Inability to see   ☐ Pain, discomfort

    ☐ Inability to hear   ☐ Other

Outcome: Patient will recover mobility of body part and/or sensory deficit.

Interventions: _____

Day:_____**Date :** _____

Planned	**Completed**	
_____	_____	1. Assess patient's level of disability—note areas of strength and impairment.
_____	_____	2. Allow and encourage patient to perform normal ADLs to his/her level of ability.
_____	_____	3. Encourage independence, but intervene when patient is unable to perform.
_____	_____	4. Convey nonjudgemental attitude.
_____	_____	5. Provide assistance with ADLs prn.
_____	_____	6. Offer positive reinforcement for ADLs performed independently (i.e., verbal praise, increased privleges). (Identify_____.)
_____	_____	7. Encourage patient to discuss feelings regarding the disability and the need for dependency it creates.
_____	_____	8. Teach relationship of physical symptoms in response to psychosocial stressors.

Figure 13-5
Critical Pathway for Patient with Body Dysmorphic Disorder

Expected Length of Treatment: _____

Nursing Diagnosis: Body image disturbance

Related to: (check at least one)

     ☐   Repressed anxiety   ☐   Preoccupation with bodily functioning

     ☐   Low self-esteem   ☐   Unmet dependency needs

     ☐   Other

Outcomes: Patient will verbalize perception of own body that is realistic to actual structure/functioning.

Patient will demonstrate acceptance of changes in bodily structure and/or function as evidenced by expression of additional feelings, willingness to perform self-care activities independently, and a focus on personal achievements.

Interventions: _____

Day:_____**Date :**_____

Planned	Completed	
_____	_____	1. Establish trusting relationship with patient.
_____	_____	2. Identify misperceptions/distortions patient has regarding body image. Correct inaccurate perceptions in a matter of fact, nonthreatening manner.
_____	_____	3. Withdraw attention when preoccupation with distorted image persists.
_____	_____	4. Assist patient to recognize personal body boundaries.
_____	_____	5. Provide positive reinforcement for patient's expressions of realistic bodily perceptions.

TAKING ANOTHER LOOK

You are now ready to respond to questions that were raised in Gaining a Perspective at the beginning of this chapter. After you have written or thought about your responses, you may want to look at the Suggested Responses on page 323.

14   ANXIETY DISORDERS

TERMS TO DEFINE

agoraphobia

anxiety

anxiety disorder

fear

malevolent transformation

obsessive-compulsive disorders

panic attack

phobic disorders

post-traumatic stress disorder

situationally bound panic attack

situationally predisposed panic attack

unexpected panic attack

GAINING A PERSPECTIVE

Think about the following two queries, and after you have read the Key Concepts of this chapter describe your answers in more detail.

1. How would you, as a nurse, handle a patient who is beginning to have panic attack?

2. How would you initially respond to a friend who said he was terribly fearful of bears and wondered if it meant he was psychiatrically ill?

Key Concepts

- **ANXIETY DISORDERS ARE AMONG THE MOST COMMON** psychiatric disorders in the general population. Nurses will encounter patients with the symptoms of anxiety disorder.

- **EVERYONE EXPERIENCES ANXIETY; HOWEVER, PEOPLE VARY IN THEIR ABILITY TO TOLERATE** the feelings and cope with anxiety-producing situations. Anxiety is both a psychological and physiological experience. Psychological evidence includes apprehension, panic, inability to concentrate, and uneasiness; physiological manifestations include anorexia, sexual dysfunction, pallor, shortness of breath, and urinary frequency. Anxiety is an unpleasant emotional state. The sources are less easily identified than those of fear where there is usually a recognized external threat.

Theoretical Understanding of Anxiety

- Genetic theory. Anxiety disorders are more common among female relatives of patients; familial influences have been found for panic disorders, agoraphobia, and obsessive-compulsive problems. Genetic effect can be modified by environment.

- Psychodynamic theory. According to Freud, anxiety signaled threats that could potentially overwhelm the ego. Most anxiety, however, reflects unconscious signals of early dangers.

- Interpersonal theory. Human behavior is positively directed toward goals of collaboration and mutual satisfaction and security, unless interfered with by anxiety [H.S. Sullivan, Interpersonal Theory of Psychiatry, NY: Norton, 1953]. Sullivan believes that anxiety is the chief disruptive force in interpersonal relationships and the main factor in the development of serious difficulties in living.

Hildegard Peplau defines anxiety as "energy; a secondary behavior following an experience; a subjective experience; an emotion with a specific object; anxiety is reaction and fear expression in objectivated form; inability to achieve self-realization;threat to some value and danger to self-respect." It is important that nurses know what effect — biopsychosocial, cognitive, or perceptive — anxiety has on observable behavior. Nurses need to remember that anxiety is communicated interpersonally, and thus be aware of own level of anxiety during patient interactions.

- Biochemical theory. Anxiety may be evident in changes in physiological functions: increased heart rate and respiration, higher blood lactate levels, increased urinary urgency, dryness of mouth, cold sweat, and fluctuating blood pressure. The dysfunctional process of increasing a stimulus to the midbrain nucleus, which supplies much of the norepinephrine neurons to the central nervous system, is associated with increased anxiety.

- **ANXIETY DISORDERS ARE DEFINED IN TERMS OF COGNITIVE, SOMATIC, AND BEHAVIORAL SYMPTOMS.** Cognitive features include fears, worries, intrusive thoughts, obsessions, preoccupations, dissociation, and numbing. Somatic symptoms include motor tension, the startle response, autonomic hyperarousal, and other physical sensations and complaints. The behavioral aspects include avoidance of stress stimuli, compulsions, rituals, and compensatory behaviors.

Four clinical types of anxiety disorder are identified:

I. Anxiety as the dominant problem

II. Anxiety experienced if the individual attempts to confront the threatening situation (e.g., phobic disorders)

III. Anxiety experienced if the individual tries to resist thoughts and feelings (e.g., obsessive-compulsive disorder)

IV. Anxiety experienced after an unusual traumatic event (e.g., post-traumatic stress disorder)

I. Anxiety as the Dominant Problem, as in generalized anxiety disorder and panic attacks or panic disorder

- **Generalized Anxiety Disorder (GAD):** Person experiences persistent anxiety for at least six months; signs of motor tension (e.g., shakiness, jumpiness, sighing respirations, tension, fatigue); autonomic hyperactivity (e.g., sweating, heart pounding, cold hands); apprehensive expectation (e.g., feels anxious, worries, anticipates dread); and vigilance and scanning (e.g., feels impatient, on edge, sleep is interrupted).

Patient must experience three of the following six symptoms: muscle tension, restlessness, easy fatigability, difficulty concentrating or "mind going blank" because of anxiety, trouble falling or staying asleep, or irritability.

The anxiety or worry significantly interferes with a person's usual routine and activities or it causes marked distress, which is not due to substance abuse or anxiety disorder or to a general medical condition or other psychiatric disorder. The worry is out of proportion to the likelihood that the feared events will occur.

Epidemiology. Lifetime prevalence rate is about 5%; slightly more common among young to middle-aged women, nonwhites, unmarried people, and those in lower socioeconomic class.

Etiologic factors and family patterns. First-degree biologic relatives have an increased rate of GAD. Involves a conditioned response to a stimulus that becomes associated with danger; the stimulus, it is believed, evolves from the cumulative effect of several stressful events.

Age of onset and course. Onset age is variable but generally between 20 and 30 years. Course is chronic and worsens as stress increases.

Impairments. Individuals are impaired socially and in their occupational and other functional areas.

Nursing assessment and diagnosis. GAD is often diagnosed when another disorder is present. The key factor involves assessing whether the excessive and uncontrollable worrying causes functional impairments and is out of proportion to the actual impact of the feared event.

Interventions. Interventions include:

- Identifying the precipitant.
- Educating the patient. The patient is in need of ego mastery, a sense of control: inform patient of diagnosis and that anxiety attacks are self limiting.
- Cognitive reframing. The nurse and patient together can review and rehearse the thoughts that lead to anxiety attack; the patient can pace the attack; timing symptoms shifts the patient's thinking to a positive action.
- Treating the patient. Combined treatment using biofeedback, relaxation, and cognitive therapy tends to diminish anxiety. Most antidepressants are ineffective.

- **Panic Attacks:** Primary feature is a distinct period of intense fear or discomfort in which four of 13 somatic or cognitive symptoms suddenly develop and peak within 10 minutes. The 13 symptoms are palpitations, trembling, choking feeling, sweating, fear of losing control, dizziness, feelings of unreality, fear of dying, paresthesias, nausea, chest pain, shortness of breath, and chills or hot flashes.

  The attacks are of three different types:

  Unexpected. Occurs without any situation trigger and is required for patient to be diagnosed with panic disorder.

  Situationally bound. Occurs immediately after exposure to or in anticipation of the situational trigger; characteristic of social and specific phobias.

  Situationally predisposed. May occur on exposure to a situational trigger, but does not necessarily occur immediately after the exposure; common for panic disorder and occasionally for specific and social phobias.

- **Panic Disorder and Agoraphobia:** DSM-IV definition — anxiety about being in a situation from which escape might prove difficult or embarrassing or for which help may be absent should one have a panic attack.

  Disorder may lead to severe restrictions on lifestyle and interpersonal functioning. Panic disorder, with or without agoraphobia, includes recurrent, unexpected attacks followed by at least one month of consistent concern about having another attack, or worry about the consequences of an attack, or experiencing a significant behavioral change as a result of the attacks. Individual has a sudden onset of intense apprehension, terror, and fear accompanied by physiological symptoms; attacks generally last minutes. They are not due to direct effects of a substance or a general medical condition, and are not better accounted for by another anxiety disorder. Frequency and severity of attacks vary. Individuals usually present at a hospital thinking that they are having a stroke, heart attack, or other serious problem. Fear is continually present after the first attack; individuals become afraid of situations that they associate with the attack.

  Panic disorder with agoraphobia (agoraphobia: the abnormal fear of being helpless in an embarrassing or unescapable situation [Webster's Collegiate Dictionary]; in current psychological terms, a fear of separation from one's source of security) is usually progressive (becoming afraid of such experiences as crowds, bridges, tunnels) until the avoidance behavior dominates the individual's life. Physiological symptoms include difficulty breathing or an epigastric sensation when confronted with feared activity.

  Epidemiology. Prevalence rate is between 1.5% and 3.5%. Women are more likely to experience agoraphobia and panic disorder; men underreport and disguise symptoms with alcoholism. Unmarried people who are not college-educated have a high rate. Childhood separation anxiety was experienced in 20% to 50% of patients.

  Etiological factors and family patterns. First-degree biological relatives are four to seven times more likely to develop panic disorder than persons not similarly related. Panic attack may be derived from an internal, not external, stimulus, and patients associate the somatic symptoms as a threat and respond with anxiety. In agoraphobia, pairing of associated events (having a panic attack and being in an airplane) leads to behavior modification (avoid travel-

Figure 14-1
Individualized Nursing Care Plan

DSM IV: Panic disorder

NURSING DIAGNOSIS: ANXIETY (PANIC).

RELATED TO: (check at least one)

☐ Traumatic experience	☐ Threat to self-concept
☐ Unconscious conflicts	☐ Unmet needs
☐ Situational/maturational crisis	☐ Fears of dying
☐ Phobic stimulus	☐ Other

TREATMENT GOAL: PATIENT WILL LEARN TO DISSIPATE AND CHANNEL ANXIETY APPROPRIATELY.

TREATMENT GOAL CAN BE MEASURED USING THE FOLLOWING EXPECTED OUTCOMES:

1. By discharge, patient will be able to recognize symptoms of onset of anxiety and intervene before reaching panic level.

2. Patient will be able to maintain anxiety at a level at which problem solving can be accomplished.

3. Patient will demonstrate techniques to be used to halt or displace anxiety prior to reaching a panic level. Interventions:

DATE INITIATED   **DATE DISCONTINUED**

_____   _____   1. Maintain calm, nonthreatening manner.

_____   _____   2. Reassure patient of his/her safety and security.

_____   _____   3. Use simple words and brief messages, spoken calmly and clearly, to explain hospital experience to patient.

_____   _____   4. Assess patient's level of anxiety; try to determine the types of situations that increase anxiety.

_____   _____   5. Keep immediate surroundings decreased in stimuli (dim lighting, few people, simple decor).

_____   _____   6. Administer prescribed medication per physician's orders. Assess for effectiveness/adverse reactions. (Identify_____).

_____   _____   7. When level of anxiety has decreased, explore with patient possible reasons for occurrence.

_____   _____   8. Encourage patient to talk about traumatic experience under nonthreatening conditions ; offer support and reassurance to alleviate any feelings of guilt.

_____   _____   9. Teach patient to recognize s/s that increase anxiety and ways to interrupt its progression (i.e., relaxation techniques, deep breathing exercises, physical exercises, brisk walks, jogging). Document teaching/hospital protocol.

Source: Nursing staff at 1st Hospital of Wyoming under the direction of Theresa M. Croushore.

ing in planes). Freud theorized that anxiety was a signal to the ego that it was in a dangerous situation, and agoraphobia was due to recalling an anxiety attack and fearing that a future attack would occur in a situation from which there was no escape.

Age of onset and course. The condition is often seen between adolescence and mid-30s; rarely begins after 40. Occurs within six months of a major life crisis. It is generally chronic, sometimes with periods of remission. Course of agoraphobia and its relationship to the course of panic attacks are variable. Prognosis is poor.

Impairments and complications. Can have marked impact on functioning, depending on frequency of attacks, agoraphobic conditions, and relationship to carrying out normal activities; associated with major depression, other anxiety disorders, and dramatic personality changes. Self-medication may risk substance abuse and alcoholism.

Treatment. Behavioral and pharmacologic therapies:

BEHAVIORAL THERAPY

EXPOSURE involves an actual stimulus that evokes the behavior until the patient is comfortable.

PAIN CONTROL involves breathing retraining, cognitive restructuring, and exposure to cues that trigger the anxiety response. Goal is desensitization to symptoms of panic attacks.

PSYCHOEDUCATION involves providing the patient with information about the diagnosis, symptoms, prognosis, and treatment. Group therapy may also be helpful.

PHARMACOLOGIC THERAPY

Involves an antidepressant to decrease frequency and severity of attacks.

Nursing assessment and plan of care. Evaluating panic disorders is difficult, as panic attacks may occur in many disorders. Once the disorder is identified, an individualized care plan should be developed (see Study Guide Figure 14-1).

Interventions. Severe panic attacks may benefit from the following:

- Relax patient and break the cognitive pattern (internal dialogue the patient is having, "I feel my heart is racing. I know what is the matter").
- Have patient put his or her mind on another issue; suggest taking deep breaths to break physiologic pattern.
- Talk patient down (don't focus on anxiety).

II. Anxiety Experienced If the Individual Attempts To Confront the Threatening Situation, as in phobic disorders

- **The essential feature of phobic disorders** is persistent, irrational fear of a specific object, activity, or situation that results in a compelling desire to avoid what is dreaded. The individual realizes that the fear is excessive or unreasonable. Phobias include the chief defense mechanisms of regression, projection, and displacement. The person fears an external object rather that an internal, unknown source of distress. Phobias are common among children, but can be crippling in adulthood. A diagnosis of phobic disorder is made when avoidance behavior interferes with the individual's social or role functioning. Subdivisions of phobic disorders include:

Specific phobia

Fear of being harmed by a situation or losing control during situation. Response to the phobic stimulus is an anxiety reaction. The subtypes of phobias are situational (confined spaces), natural environments (heights, storms), blood/injury/infection (simple medical procedures), and specific animal or insect.

Epidemiology. About 9% to 11% is the prevalence rate; there are gender differences according to subtypes; females generally have a higher percentage.

Etiological factors and family patterns. Theories relating to a familial link, learned behaviors, and psychoanalytical relationships exist for specific phobias. A high degree of familial transmission exists for specific phobias by type.

OPERANT CONDITIONING may produce a specific phobia.

FREUD BELIEVED that phobias are symptoms of some unresolved unconscious conflict.

Figure 14-2
Individualized Nursing Care Plan

DSM IV: Phobic avoidance (agoraphobia)

NURSING DIAGNOSIS: FEAR.

RELATED TO: (check at least one)

☐ Specific Phobia   ☐ Performing in public

☐ Being alone in public place   ☐ Being the focus of attention of others

☐ Other

TREATMENT GOAL: PATIENT WILL DECREASE ANXIETY AND LEVEL OF FEAR TO BE ABLE TO SUCCESSFULLY FUNCTION AND SUCCESSFULLY CARRY OUT THE ACTIVITIES OF DAILY LIFE.

TREATMENT GOAL CAN BE MEASURED USING THE FOLLOWING EXPECTED OUTCOMES:

1. Patient will be able to demonstrate three adaptive coping techniques to maintain anxiety at a tolerable level.

2. Patient will be able to verbalize three methods to be able to avoid or successfully deal with phobic objects of situations.

DATE INITIATED	DATE DISCONTINUED	
_____	_____	1. Reassure patient of his/her safety and security.
_____	_____	2. Explore patient's perception of threat to physical integrity or threat to self-concept.
_____	_____	3. Discuss reality of the situation with patient in order to recognize aspects that can and cannot be changed.
_____	_____	4. Include patient in making decisions related to selection of alternative coping strategies to foster sense of control.
_____	_____	5. Implement prescribed B-mod program to work on elimination of the fear (i.e., systematic desensitization). (Identify_____).
_____	_____	6. Encourage patient to explore underlying feelings that may be contributing to irrational fears.
_____	_____	7. Assist patient to understand how facing his/her feelings, rather than suppressing them, can result in more adaptive coping abilities.
_____	_____	8. Administer prescribed medication per physician orders. Assess for effectiveness/adverse reactions. (Identify_____).

Source: Nursing staff at 1st Hospital of Wyoming under the direction of Theresa M. Croushore.

Age of onset. Age of onset varies by type, but all specific phobias tend to begin in childhood. Situational type, however, may not begin until the mid-20s. Phobias may occur as a result of traumatic events; if they persist into adulthood they infrequently remit independently.

Impairment and complications. A phobic person will suffer greater impairments the more frequently he or she is exposed to the feared stimulus. Certain medical conditions may be exacebated by phobic avoidance.

Nursing assessment and care plan. Does phobia significantly impair functioning or cause distress? Is the fear unreasonable? There is a need to differentiate between a specific phobia and other anxiety disorders. The plan of care for specific phobias needs to be individualized (see Study Guide Figure 14- 2).

Social phobia

Avoidance of a situation in which exposure to scrutiny by others may occur or fearfulness of behaving in a manner that will be embarrassing or humiliating (fear of speaking or eating in public or of using public rest rooms). Phobia may produce physical symptoms or even a panic attack.

- **Epidemiology.** Prevalence rate of 3% to 13%; may be more common among women than men.
- **Etiological factors and family patterns.** Theories related to familial, behavioral, and psychoanalytical link.
- **First-degree biologic relatives** more commonly show the disorder; some suggest fears are inherited.
- **Evaluating their own performance in social situations** is difficult for social phobics; they are hypersensitive to criticism or about earlier unpleasant social situation(s).
- **Individual has rigid idea of social behavior,** exaggerated awareness of somatic symptoms, and a tendency to experience others as being critical of him or her.

Age of onset and course. Typically, onset is between the ages of 15 and 20 years. Onset may be sudden (humiliating situation) or develop over a lifetime. Disorder usually lasts a lifetime and the individual may experience changes in severity during adulthood.

Impairments and complications. Difficulties with work, school, and social relationships are consistent. Individuals are likely to be underachievers, have a smaller likelihood of marrying, and be isolated, which may trigger substance abuse and depressive problems.

Treatment. Some antidepressants have been effective, and/or behavioral therapy may be used.

Nursing assessment and care planning. Performance anxiety, shyness, and stage fright in school situation, involving unfamiliar people, are commonly experienced and should not be diagnosed as social phobia unless clinically significant distress or impairment occurs. Individualized nursing care is planned (see Study Guide Figure 14-2).

III. Anxiety Experienced If the Individual Tries to Resist Thoughts and Feelings, as in Obsessive-Compulsive Disorder.

- **The two components of obsessive-compulsive disorder** are obsessions and compulsions. Obsessions are repeated, persistent thoughts or impulses that are seen as intrusive and inappropriate, but unavoidable. The thoughts are highly charged with emotional significance.

Compulsions are the action components, that is, the repetitive, purposeful behaviors, recognized as unreasonable, but nonetheless followed through with to suppress or neutralize the obsessions. This disorder is viewed as a defense against anxiety. Ego defenses used by the individual include repression, isolation, reaction formation, and undoing.

Commonly described obsessions are:

Thoughts of violence, e.g., ideas of stabbing, shooting, maiming, hitting.

Thoughts of contamination, e.g., images of germs, dirt, feces.

Repetitive doubt and concern that something is not right, that a tragic event may occur, or that perfection was not achieved.

Repeating or counting images, words, or objects in the environment.

Figure 14-3
Individualized Nursing Care Plan

DSM IV: Obsessive compulsive disorders

NURSING DIAGNOSIS: INEFFECTIVE INDIVIDUAL COPING

RELATED TO: (check at least one)

☐ Situational crisis   ☐ Inadequate support systems

☐ Maturational crisis   ☐ Fear of failure

☐ Ritualistic behavior   ☐ Unmet dependency needs

☐ Obsessive thoughts   ☐ Other

TREATMENT GOAL: BY DISCHARGE, PATIENT WILL DEMONSTRATE FLEXIBILITIES IN ACTIVITIES OF DAILY LIFE.

TREATMENT GOAL CAN BE MEASURED USING THE FOLLOWING EXPECTED OUTCOMES:

1. Patient expresses three feelings of self confidence.

2. Patient demonstrates use of three adaptive coping skills.

3. Patient is able to interrupt obsessive thoughts and avoid ritualistic behaviors when required to successfully deal with activities of daily living.

DATE INITIATED	DATE DISCONTINUED	
_____	_____	1. Assess patient's level of anxiety and try to determine types of situations that increase anxiety.
_____	_____	2. Assess patient's mood; observe for suicidal behaviors and report same to physician.
_____	_____	3. Initially meet patient's dependency needs as required.
_____	_____	4. Slowly encourage independence and give positive reinforcement for independent behaviors (i.e., verbal praise, increased privileges). (Identify_____).
_____	_____	5. Allow time for rituals.
_____	_____	6. Support patient's efforts to explore the meaning and purpose of the behavior.
_____	_____	7. Provide structured schedule of activities. (Identify _____).
_____	_____	8. Gradually begin to limit amount of time allotted for ritualistic behavior as patient becomes increasingly involved in unit activities.
_____	_____	9. Offer positive reinforcement for nonritualistic behaviors. (i.e., verbal praise, increased privileges). (Identify _____).
_____	_____	10. Teach patient to recognize situations that provoke obsessive thoughts and/or ritualistic behavior. Also teach methods to interrupt these thoughts and behaviors (i.e., thought-stopping techniques, relaxation techniques, exercise, play/diversional activities). Document teaching/hospital protocol.

Source: Nursing staff at 1st Hospital of Wyoming under the direction of Theresa M. Croushore.

Commonly described compulsions are:

Touching, usually repetitive, often combined with counting.

Washing, especially hands.

Doing and undoing, opening and closing doors, walking backward and forward, changing order or organization.

Checking, essentially to make sure that no disaster has occurred and that no one has been injured.

The intent of obsessions and compulsions is to minimize and deflect anxiety and anger, but they produce both. Not only do the rituals fail to provide a sense of security, they burden the individual with further symptoms. The person recognizes that the obsessions are products of his or her own mind, not imposed from without and not simply excessive worry about real-life problems. Individuals who have compulsions recognize that their behavior is excessive and unreasonable. The obsessive-compulsive disorder causes marked distress, is time-consuming, and/or significantly interferes with normal routine, occupational functioning, social activities, and relationships with others.

Epidemiology. Prevalence rate is 2.5%; equally common in males and females

Etiologic factors and family patterns. Etiologic factors include familial/genetic, psychoanalytic, cognitive, behavioral, and neurobiologic factors.

- High rates of obsessive-compulsive disorders among first-degree biologic relatives of an individual with this disorder; link may also be to mood disorders.

- Disorder may evolve from a disturbance in the anal-sadistic phase of development.

- Patients are viewed as having a defect in their cognitive information-processing mechanism, producing a mismatch between beliefs and sensory data.

- Obsessions result from associating mental stimuli with anxiety-producing thoughts. Compulsions are formerly benign behaviors that are now linked to anxiety reduction and are reinforced.

- Dysfunction is found in the brain serotonin neural system.

Age of onset and course. Onset is usually be-tween adolescence and adulthood; may occur in childhood; males between 6 and 15 years of age, females 20 to 29 years. Gradual onset. Course is chronic, and symptoms are exacerbated by stressful life events. Prognosis is not good.

Impairments and complications. The individual is significantly impaired in occupational and social functioning. Patients may have sleep disturbances, abuse alcohol and sedatives, and have marital problems. Suicide risk is high.

Treatment. Therapeutic gains have been made in treating obsessive-compulsive disorders with the medication clomipramine and behavioral therapies; however, patients do not fully recover.

Nursing assessment and care planning. Recurrent or intrusive thoughts or behaviors may occur in the context of many other psychiatric disorders. An individualized care plan is necessary (see Study Guide Figure 14-3).

Interventions. Close observation for increase in intensity and severity of symptoms and emergence of depression and psychosis; reality testing for patients who have exaggerated or grandiose thoughts connected with the performance of rituals; symptom substitution, which is a method to interrupt obsessive patterns (e.g., the patient yells "STOP" in the middle of the obsession); and goal-oriented interviews to avoid endless discussion of symptoms.

IV. Anxiety Experienced After an Unusual Traumatic Event, as in post-traumatic stress disorder (PTSD) and acute stress disorder

- **Post-traumatic stress disorder (PTSD)** provides a conceptual bridge linking a variety of traumatic events such as war, terrorism, natural disasters, and rape to a set of specific symptoms. In PTSD, the individual has experienced a traumatic event that threatens serious injury, or death, or is a threat to one's own physical integrity or someone else's. The person reacts with horror, extreme fright, or helplessness. Then the individual repeatedly reexperiences the event or avoids anything that evokes memories of it, experiences a sense of emotional numbing or unresponsiveness, or has symptoms of hyperarousal. Persons with PTSD commonly have intrusive thoughts and memories of the event, suffer flashbacks, feel emotionally detached and blunted, startle easily, and have trouble sleeping and difficulty concentrating while awake. PTSD can be further specified by its duration: acute, less than three months; chronic, three months or longer. In addition, it may have a delayed onset of six or more months after the stressor.

Epidemiology. Prevalence varies from 1% to 14%; however, for at-risk individuals (combat veterans) rates are from 3% to 58%. Risk factors for PTSD on exposure to traumatic events are family history of psychiatric disorders, being male, extroversion, and history of conduct disorder problems and neuroticism. Risk of developing PTSD after experiencing trauma is increased when the individual has a family history of anxiety, was separated from parents in childhood, is female, and has preexisting anxiety, depression, or a history of antisocial behavior.

Etiologic factors and family patterns. Two theories:

- Psychobiological. Patients with PTSD have heightened autonomic or sensory nervous system arousal when reminded of the trauma.

- Behavioral. The two-factor learning theory involves aversion conditioning to a neutral stimulus that has been paired with a trauma reaction. Further conditioning leads to instrumental learning, whereby behaviors are acquired to avoid anxiety from conditioned stimuli. Additional factors interfere with extinction occurring naturally.

Age of onset and course. No particular age of onset is noted. Months or years can transpire between the trauma and the onset of PTSD. Complete recovery within three months for about 50%. Relapse can occur.

Impairments and complications. Individuals with PTSD often experience painful guilt about surviving when others did not or what they had to do to survive. Avoiding similar situations (even symbols of them) may interfere with interpersonal relationships, and lead to marital discord, divorce, or job loss. A formerly happy productive person becomes hostile, withdrawn, and self-destructive. Higher risk exists for impulse behavior and suicide.

Assessment. Questions are asked about any life trauma; reaction may be normal or patient may have true clinical symptomatology. Diagnosis is based on level of distress, degree of impairment, and duration of symptoms.

Treatment. Effective therapy has been coupling pharmacological measures, such as administering fluoxetine (Prozac) to alleviate physiological symptoms, and nonpharmacological therapies, such as cognitive therapy that involves relaxation, thought stopping, breathing control, communication skills, and cognitive restructuring.

In acute stress disorder, symptoms are similar to those of PTSD, with acute distress from the trauma and functional impairment; however, symptoms last only two to four weeks. Symptoms must occur within four weeks to be classified as acute stress disorder.

TAKING ANOTHER LOOK

You are now ready to respond to the queries that were raised in Gaining a Perspective at the beginning of this chapter. After you have written or thought about your responses, you may want to look at the Suggested Responses on page 323.

15 DISSOCIATIVE DISORDERS

GAINING A PERSPECTIVE

Consider the situation described below, and after you have read the Key Concepts for this chapter respond to the query.

1. What one characteristic sign or symptom of a patient diagnosed as having a dissociative identity disorder (DID) would require that the nurse do a careful assessment so as to protect the patient? Describe that sign or symptom.

Key Concepts

• **THE DISSOCIATIVE DISORDERS ARE A GROUP OF PSYCHIATRIC SYNDROMES CHARACTERIZED BY** a sudden, temporary disruption of some aspect of consciousness, identity, or motor behavior. In dissociation, certain mental contents are separated from the usual flow of consciousness. Individuals often mobilize dissociation to protect themselves from being overwhelmed by intense pain and trauma. They split off clusters of distressing thoughts, feelings, and memories from conscious awareness, thereby altering their state of consciousness. As a result, the individual feels "detached" from his or her surroundings.

The functions of memory, personal identity, and motor behavior are critical for the integrated operation of the personality— a complex set of mental and behavioral activities. The syndromes, which are statistically uncommon, present a dramatic clinical picture, when they occur, of severely disturbed personality functioning. In their pathology, the disorders are presumed to share the defense mechanism of dissociation.

The four types of dissociative disorders (see Study Guide Table 15-1) are:

Dissociative amnesia is a loss of memory for significant personal information, often of a disturbing nature; not simply forgetting; not due to other psychiatric or medical conditions or the use of drugs. The symptoms cause disruption in social, occupational, and other areas of functioning.

Dissociative fugue is characterized by sudden, unexpected "flights" from work or home and then assumption of a new identity. There is an inability to recall one's past, and when the episode resolves, the fugue state is not remembered.

Depersonalization disorder is the occurrence of persistent or recurrent episodes of deper-

Table 15-1

DISSOCIATIVE DISORDERS

	Dissociative Amnesia	Dissociative Fugue	Multiple Personality Disorder	Depersonalization Disorder
Key Features	Memory loss following a stressful or traumatic life experience.	Memory loss, travel to new location, and assumption of new identity.	Coexistence of two or more distinct personalities in the same individual.	Sudden temporary loss of sense of one's reality causing social or occupational dysfunction.
Epidemiology	Rare More common in adolescents and young adults.	Rare	Exact incidence unknown but may be more common than previously believed. More common in adolescents and young adult women.	Incidence unknown
Differential	Memory disturbance in organic disorders such as alcoholic blackouts, postconcussion amnesia, transient global amnesia. Dissociative fugue Multiple personality disorder Malingering	Wandering as a result of dementia Dissociative amnesia Multiple personality disorder Malingering	Dissociative amnesia Dissociative fugue Schizophrenia Malingering	Medication side effects. Neurological diseases, such as epilepsy, brain tumor. May occur as symptom of another mental disorder, such as anxiety and affective disorders, schizophrenia, substance abuse.
Treatment	Amobarbital interview Psychotherapy	Amobarbital interview Psychotherapy	Psychotherapy	Treat underlying condition when present.

Source: MacKay, S. and Purcell S.D., Somatoform & Dissociative Disorders. In Goldman H. Review of General Psychiatry. Appleton & Lange, Norwalk, CT, 1995.

sonalization in which a sudden temporary loss of the sense of one's own reality occurs, accompanied by the feeling of being detached from oneself (feeling "mechanical" or as though one were in a dream).

Dissociative identity disorder (DID), previously known as multiple personality disorder, is a syndrome that involves all the principal el-ements of the other dissociative disorders. DID presumes the existence of two or more distinct personality states or personal identities that recurrently take charge of the patient's behavior. The patient cannot remember important personal information. The disturbance is not due to drugs or a medical condition.

• HISTORY. Cases have been reported since the

17th century. Until the 1970s DID was thought to be nonexistent, rare, or an artifact of hypnosis or other iatrogenic mischief. Presently, the number of individuals diagnosed with interactive DID is increasing.

- GENDER, AGE, CULTURE, AND PREVALENCE. Occurs more in women (5:1 ratio). The mean age of diagnosis 28.5 years with floridly "multiple" clinical presentation during the third and fourth decade. Occurs across all major racial groups and settings.

- ETIOLOGY. Children who are physically and/or sexually abused are at risk, and incest seems to be prevalent. Many abusing adults are first-degree relatives.

- THEORIES OF DID

3-P model (Braun and Sachs, 1985). Predisposing, precipitating, and perpetuating factors are necessary to initiate development.

Two predisposing factors appear to be:
— biopsychological capacity to dissociate.
— repeated exposure to an inconsistently stressful environment (receiving love and abuse from the same parent).

The perpetuating phenomena are interactive behaviors between the abused and the abuser. Separate memories and responses develop, and continued unpredictable trauma reinforces the chaining of memories and associated response patterns. Gradually the different response patterns become functionally separated by amnesic barriers (split personalities).

BASK model (Braun,1988). The event is dissociated into four compartments (behavior, affect, sensation, and knowledge) that function on a continuum and can occur in anyone on all levels. Must have the ability to dissociate, which is the response of a creative mind seeking to escape the saturation of childhood terror and pain. The more severe the abuse, the more fragmented the adult patient's personality and thinking.

Kluft theory (1984). States that the person who develops DID will have four facets:
— capacity to dissociate, which is mobilized for defensive purposes

— life experiences that traumatically overwhelm the nondissociative defenses and adaptive capacities of the child's ego
— shaping-influences and available substrates determine the form of dissociation
— inadequate provision of stimulus barriers, soothing, and restorative experiences by significant others.

- PATIENT PROFILE

HISTORY of several psychiatric or medical conditions.

INCONSISTENCIES in physical behavior, e.g., voice changes, differences in hair style.

PSYCHOPHYSIOLOGIC MANIFESTATIONS such as headache, anxiety, unpredictable responses to medication (e.g., fluctuations in insulin requirements).

EXPERIENCING VOICES "inside" the head talking to one another or to the patient. (Usually, the schizophrenic patient experiences voices originating outside the head.)

DID OR OTHER DISSOCIATIVE DISORDERS or history of abuse in the patient's family; evidence exists for a transgenerational component in DID.

- TREATMENT ISSUES

PAST TRAUMA involving abuse.

PRESENT TRAUMA OF A MULTIPLE PERSONALITY and trying to fit into a society that stresses continuity of time.

FOUR PRIMARY AIMS
— to provide support and safety for the patient.
— to decrease conflict within system and increase cooperation of multiple personalities.
— to uncover and work through traumatic memory and affect, with increased sharing of information and experiences among personalities.
— to develop improved coping skills and reality testing and gradual relinquishment of dissociative defensive processes.

PROGNOSIS is generally good, but actual course of therapy is long and arduous and punctuated with crises.

CONTROVERSY ABOUT HYPNOSIS used to gain access to hidden trauma and memories.

NURSING PROCESS

— Assessment should include questions that provoke information concerning a patient's history of abuse. Question patient about earliest, first-hand memory (not childhood stories told by photographs or other people) of significant events, imaginary friends, lost time or blackouts, voices heard from within the head. If DID is actually suspected, tests are administered.

— Nursing diagnoses that may apply are related to low self-esteem, inability to express feelings, helplessness, potential for self-inflicted injury, difficulty in interpersonal relationships, denial of problems or abuse, disrupted homeostasis, sleep disturbance.

— Treatment interventions for DID are usually on an outpatient basis except when the patient becomes suicidal or if nonsuicidal self-inflicted injury occurs, or if the patient experiences depression or threatens violence. Hypnosis may be used.

— Evaluation of treatment does not end at the point of stabilization, or integration of personalities; rather, nondissociative defense and coping skills should be enhanced.

PHARMACOLOGICAL IMPLICATIONS are that medications are not heavily used unless symptoms are causing sufficient problems.

LEGAL/ETHICAL IMPLICATIONS are many. When one of a multiple alter personalities commits a crime, is it fair to blame or punish the others? What about one of a multiple, but not the others, entering a contract? Ethically, nurses are educated to see humans holistically and should be able to define the person with DID as a living being with needs and purposes.

TAKING ANOTHER LOOK

You are now ready to respond to the query raised in Gaining a Perspective at the beginning of this chapter. After you have written or thought about your response, you may want to look at the Suggested Responses on page 324.

16 LOSS, GRIEF, AND BEREAVEMENT

TERMS TO DEFINE

anticipatory grief

bereavement

chronic mourning

complicated grief and loss reactions

complicated mourning

death

delayed grief

disenfranchised grief

dying

grief

loss

mourning

pathologic grief

GAINING A PERSPECTIVE

Think about the problems presented below, and after you have read the Key Concepts respond to these three questions.

1. How would your culture and that of your family help you cope with grief?

2. How would you, as a nurse, assist a patient who is in a hospice in the terminal stages of an illness? (Focus only on the patient.)

3. What are some ideas about coping that you, as a nurse, might give a caregiver who is caring for a terminally ill friend who has AIDS?

Key Concept

• **THE CONCEPT OF TRANSITION** is prominent in the literature describing family-centered care designed to assist people to cope with changes associated with loss. Adaptive behavior in response to a transition is an opportunity to stimulate developmental growth or dysfunction. Psychological distress is commonly linked to life events that are associated with loss or anticipated loss. Serious illness, divorce, change in residence, retirement, and the death of a loved one are examples of loss experiences that precipitate grief responses and bereavement.

The bereavement process is not linear; rather there are periods of overlap and regression. Each bereaved individual is unique, and the course of bereavement varies (see Study Guide Table 16-1).

Professional nurses, by expanding their knowledge of bereavement care, can enhance their assessment and communication skills and their interventions to create supportive environments for bereaved individuals. Nurses frequently encounter bereaved individuals and families.

• **PERTINENT VOCABULARY**

Loss is a universal experience; it results in deprivation, tangible or symbolic.

Grief is a normal process of psychological, social, and somatic reactions to loss. Symptoms might include guilt, anxiety, sorrow, depression, relief, and sadness. Intensity varies according to person, type of loss, situation surrounding loss, concurrent stressors, social supports, and strength of attachment to the deceased.

Disenfranchised grief is experienced when persons incur a loss that is not or cannot be openly acknowledged, publicly mourned, or socially supported such as prenatal death, abortion, divorce, death of a pet, extra-marital relationship.

Bereavement is the state of loss of a significant other through death.

Table 16-1
SELECTED VIEWS OF GRIEF: 20TH CENTURY

◆ FREUD, S. (1917)
▼ **Psychoanalytic View — Depression Model of Grief**

Psychoanalytic views of mourning were described in case studies of individuals who had experienced major loss events. Descriptions of normal grief responses and pathological expressions or of grief were were offered in an an attempt to differentiate mourning, anxiety and pain resulting from loss. Freud documented expressions of grief in the classic paper *Mourning and Melancholia* (1917/1959) that included anniversary reactions, feelings of guilt and responsibility for the death in an ambivalent relationship, and an explanation of "decathexis" — the process of detaching and modifying emotional bonds so that new relationships can develop.

◆ DEUTSCH, H. (1937)
▼ **Psychoanalytic View — Absent Grief Response**

Absence of grief response in bereaved individuals was recognized as a form of pathological grief. Case studies supported this hypothesis through descriptions of how bereaved individuals expressed their grief in other ways (e.g., neurotic symptoms or narcissistic schizoid character traits).

◆ LINDEMANN, E. (1944)
▼ **Acute Grief Syndrome**

A pattern of psychological and somatic symptoms of acute grief was developed through clinical observations and interviews with bereaved persons. The grief syndrome was characterized by preoccupation with thoughts of the deceased, feelings of hostility and guilt, loss of usual patterns of behavior, and somatic symptoms. Somatic symptoms associated with grief included: sighing, shortness of breath, lack of stength. Term "anticipatory grief" proposed. Three tasks of grief: emancipation from bondage to the deceased; readjustment to the environment without the deceased loved one; and formation of new relationships. Abnormal patterns of grief were described as distorted or delayed grief reactions and were viewed as having potential to influence physical and mental health.

◆ POLLOCK, G.H. (1961)
▼ **Ego-Adaptive View**

The mourning process was described as an ego-adaptive process that attempts to maintain the internal psychic equilibrium. A revised view of mourning was posited to include the theory of adaptation, the concepts of homeostasis, and Darwin's phylogenetic evolution. Responses during the acute stage of grief were conceptualization as shock, acute regression, and immobilization. Hyperactivity, deep despair, sorrow, anxiety, energy impoverishment, and intense psychic pain were also described as grief responses. Integration of the loss experience into reality was thought to be facilitated by adaptive mechanisms in the stage of chronic grief.

◆ CAPLAN, G. (1961)
▼ **Crisis Theory View**

Initially, bereavement was viewed as a life event that had the potential to initiate a "crisis" that could be resolved in a relatively short span of time (4 to 8 weeks). Crisis theory suggested a more inclusive view of the balance between the person's available resources and stressors. A crisis was viewed as a pivotal time when an individual had an increased desire for help, and could be more readily influenced by others.

◆ ENGEL, G.L. (1961, 1964)
▼ **Biochemical/ Physiological View**

A medical model approach advanced that grief was a multidimensional phenomenon with biochemical, physiological, and psychological aspects. Engel suggested a theory of grief that included the following stages: shock and disbelief; developing awareness; restitution; and resolution. Successful mourning was signaled by the bereaved individual's "ability to remember comfortably and realistically both the pleasures and disappointments of the lost relationship" (1962). Engel identified the predictors of difficult mourning: individuals who want to cry but are unable to, identification with the negative traits of the deceased, and an exaggerated desire to fulfill the wishes of the deceased.

◆ PARKES, C.M. (1964, 1972)
▼ **Life Transition View**

Grief is viewed as a process that requires bereaved individuals to change their relationship with the deceased. Parkes' systematic observations of individuals' adjustment after spousal loss contributed to the description of grief as a major life transition. The phases of grief that are included in this life transition are: numbness, yearning and protest, disorganization, and reorganization. Antecedent and concurrent variables were tested for ability to predict mental and physical health outcomes of bereaved individuals. A profile of high-risk factors for bereavement recovery included: low socioeconomic status, concurrent multiple losses, sudden unexpected loss, relationship characterized by ambivalence, and early severe distress.

Table 16-1 (continued)
SELECTED VIEWS OF GRIEF: 20TH TO 21ST CENTURY

◆ BOWLBY, J. (1969, 1980)
▼ **Attachment Theory View**

Attachment theory was developed on extensive clinical observations of adults and children in scientific and medical settings. Attachment was viewed as a basic biological mechanism that protects the survival of the individual and the species. Bowlby's theory (1981) integrates concepts from psychoanalytic theory and ethology. Adult response to loss was described as a four-phase process that included: numbing; the urge to recover the lost object (yearning and searching); disorganization and despair; and reorganization. Bowlby described the state of "chronic mourning" as unusually intense, prolonged emotional responses that include anger and self-reproach, and sorrow is conspicuously absent.

◆ KRUPP, G. (1972)
▼ **Intrapsychic/Ecological View**

In a paper that describes intrapsychic maladaptive reactions to grief, Krupp discussed family systems dynamics and how unresolved mourning can characterize an entire family. Grief reactions of an individual that permeate all members of a family unit require both individual and family level intervention. There is also reference to societal influences on grief resolution, such as the smaller circle of close relationships, and fewer opportunities to express and resolve intense emotions characterizing life in the later part of the 20th century.

◆ BUGEN, L. (1977)
▼ **Human Grief Model**

This conceptual model of grief posits that the intensity and duration of grief is best predicted by the magnitude of closeness within the relationship (central or peripheral) and the degree to which survivors perceive that the death was preventable. Within this view, intense bereavement response would be anticipated in a mourner who feels responsible for the loved one's death.

◆ RAPHAEL, B. (1983)
▼ **Lifespan Development View**

In a review of bereavement literature, Raphael summarized the forms of human grief resulting from lost relationships across the lifespan. Implications for providing comfort, consolation, and facilitating recovery for the bereaved are offered in the comprehensive work entitled *The Anatomy of Bereavement*.

◆ MARTOCCHIO, B. (1985)
▼ **Theory of Grieving**

According to Martocchio's framework, grief is defined as the process of moving through the pain of loss. The process of grief is characterized by complex thoughts and emotions, and is a time for healing, adaptation, and growth for the bereaved.Martocchio, a nurse researcher, described clusters of reactions that are not bound in time, and may overlap. The clusters that form the framework include: shock and disbelief; yearning and protest; anguish, disorganization, and despair; identification in bereavement; and reorganization and restitution. The time line for grief resolution defined by Martocchio is variable. Periods of time that grief resolution may occur are defined as ranging from shorter to much longer than one year. Martocchio asserted that loss reactions may last a lifetime. Anniversaries and holidays may be times that are particularly difficult for survivors as they recall memories of the deceased loved one. The goal of successful grief work, according to this framework, is to be able to remember the loved one without major emotional pain and to reinvest emotional energy in living.

◆ STROEBE, W. & STROEBE, M. S. (1989)
▼ **Deficit Model of Partner Loss**

This framework applies the general psychological stress model to the experience of conjugal loss. Widowhood results in situational demands and loss of coping resources previously available in the conjugal relationship such as instrumental support, validational support, and emotional support. The loss is thought to have a negative inpact on the surviving partner's definition of self and social identity.

◆ SANDERS, C. (1989)
▼ **Integrative Theory of Bereavement**

This perspective includes both biological and psychological factors. An individual's psychological health and successful use of coping strategies in the past will influence the abilities to cope with the loss of the loved one. External factors such as the availability of social support systems, the circumstances surrounding the death, the relationship to the deceased, socioeconomic status, and concurrent stressors influence bereavement patterns. Internal mediators included in this theory are: age, gender, personality, health, and feelings about relationship with deceased loved one. There is wide variation in the ways people grieve and in the time required to get through the phases of the grief process. The phases of the bereavement are: shock, awareness of loss, conservation-withdrawal, healing, and renewal.

◆ **THEORIST**   ▼ **View of Grief**

Mourning represents culturally defined rituals and behaviors that are usually performed after a death.

Death is a process that may last a few hours, days, or months. It has four dimensions:

- SOCIAL DEATH. Symbolic death that occurs because of lifestyle changes brought on by illness
- PSYCHOLOGICAL DEATH. Withdrawal of certain aspects of a dying individual's personality; causes include loss of autonomy, biochemical changes (drug or illness related), decline in functional or cognitive abilities
- BIOLOGICAL DEATH. Consciousness and awareness no longer exist
- PHYSIOLOGICAL DEATH. Cessation of all vital organ functioning

Anticipatory grief is the anticipation of a future loss and includes many of the symptoms and processes of grief following a loss; may be experienced by the dying patient as well as the family and friends of the terminally ill; includes psychosocial and somatic reactions to predicted future loss such as depression, intensified concern for the terminally ill person, rehearsal of the impending death, and attempts to adjust.

Chronic mourning is usually an intense, prolonged emotional response to loss that is accompanied by anger, self-reproach, and absence of sorrow. Depression is the principal symptom and is concurrent with anxiety, agoraphobia, hypochondria, or alcoholism.

Complicated mourning involves a compromise, some distortion, or failure to successfully engage in the complete process of mourning. The bereaved individual attempts to deny, repress, or avoid aspects of the loss, and hold on to and avoid relinquishing the lost loved one.

Complicated grief and loss reactions may occur in persons who have experienced multiple deaths of significant people in a relatively short period of time. Families with the following characteristics are also at risk:

- Low socioeconomic status
- Poor health status

- Sudden death or death following a short illness
- Perceived lack of available social support
- Lack of support from religious belief system
- History of psychiatric illness
- Multiple concurrent losses
- Dysfunctional family relationships
- Geographic distance from extended family
- Guilt within family relationships
- High level of dependency among survivors
- Ambivalent relationships within the family

Pathologic grief criteria are based on unusually severe or prolonged manifestations of grief or conversely, inhibited manifestations of normal grief. Three variants are:

- Delayed grief. Typical manifestations are delayed for more than two weeks after the loss; then it becomes absent grief.
- Inhibited grief. Expected typical responses of grief are diminished.
- Chronic grief. The intensity of separation anxiety does not diminish during the first year.

- **EPIDEMIOLOGY**

Psychiatric complications of bereavement are among the most common disorders of patients in outpatient and consultation psychiatric settings. Pathological grief, major depressions, anxiety disorders, and post-traumatic stress disorder are complications of bereavement that require professional intervention.

Two million deaths occur a year (800,000 lose a spouse), resulting in 8 to 10 bereaved family members per death — a potential for 5 to 6 million new cases of pathologic grief; estimates of bereavement complications during the first year following loss are about 20%.

Bereavement is an important cause of depressive complications.

- **SOCIOCULTURAL ISSUES**

These issues — diverse personal values and beliefs, socioeconomic status and cultural backgrounds, religious or existential beliefs — influence bereaved individuals' grief processes.

Spiritual assessment is gaining information about how an individual's or family's belief system influences the process of grief. Questions may include:

- What gives meaning to your life?
- Is religion or God significant to you?
- What is your source of strength and hope?
- Are there spiritual practices that help you (prayer, meditation)?
- Is there someone (clergy, church members, etc.) that I may contact for you that could assist you with your spiritual practices?

In addition, nurses need to be aware of their own spiritual beliefs to assist the bereaved individual and family.

- Know yourself as a spiritual being.
- Understand that spirituality is not limited to definitions of God or Ultimate Being.
- Encourage and share in reminiscing; experience the present moment — whatever joy, pain, or grief it may hold.
- Recognize the importance of "being present with" patients as they describe the meaning of pain in their lives.
- Know that ambiguities, struggles, and searching are aspects of spirituality that may remain unanswered questions.
- Recognize that each individual is the "expert" of his or her own life journey.

Cultures have different mourning traditions. Members of cultural groups may have certain expectations of the newly bereaved, in terms of participating in festivities, forming new attachments, and mourning traditions (clothing, periods of mourning, memorial rituals).

Expressions of loss and grief vary across cultures.

- Orthodox Jews. Highly structured participatory mourning rituals for one year; supportive of the bereaved. "Shiva" refers to the first seven days of mourning, when community members visit and assist with household duties. Then after 30 days during "Shiloshem" (end of ritual mourning), individuals can return to more active involvement in work and life. Prior to the first death anniversary, a commemorative stone is unveiled. On subsequent death anniversaries and certain holidays the deceased is remembered by survivors. Excessive grief is not viewed favorably.

- Native Americans. This population is comprised of a broad diversity of cultures, encompassing more than 500 recognized entities. Most Native Americans value self-reliance, but there is a tradition of shared decision making among extended family members. Many Native Americans are death-accepting and view life and death in a circular fashion. Children are taught that death is a part of life. Dying is usually accepted stoically. Navajo Americans limit expression of mourning to four days and set expectations for individuals to return to normal roles. They express fear of death and the ghost of the deceased.

- African-Americans. Many in this population believe in immortality; funeral rites are characterized as a celebration of life. Members of the extended family have strong multigenerational ties. Open expression of grief is valued. May perceive better control over their own lives after death (due to years of oppression imposed by the dominant culture). Extended family, friends, family, and church members openly demonstrate expressions of support. Death is perceived as a reunification of those who have died and their passage to a better life.

- Americans of European descent. This population is dominant within the U.S. culture. Expressions of sadness and grief are learned within the family and vary across this group of Americans. Stoicism may be displayed; usually a death-denying group. Less visible because of decline in multigenerational living. Many of European heritage believe in immortality; variations in spiritual beliefs and traditions. Family closeness highly valued.

- Hispanic Americans. Diverse cultures are represented, such as Mexican-Americans, Latinos, Spanish-Americans, and Chicanos. Each may differ in traditional beliefs and practices in care of dying. Death, which is accepted, is a family event. Children are full participants. Religiosity is noninstitutional; rather, it is centered in the home. Symbols and rituals are comforting and important. Open expressions of grief are expected in women, not men.

• Asian-Americans. The subgroups, with diverse values and beliefs, are represented by Chinese, Japanese, Koreans, Filipinos, Cambodians, Hmong, Latinos, and Vietnamese. They share a holistic conception of health and illness in which physical and mental functioning are intimately linked. Many believe in both Eastern and Western medicine. Past generations of ancestors are revered; ritual ceremonies that honor dead ancestors are incorporated into the care of the dying. Families, not individuals, play a key role in decision making about medical care.

Cultural assessment is important in planning for death and dying. It is inappropriate to make assumptions about patients and their families based solely on an awareness of their cultural heritage. The family's cultural background is assessed, and family roles, life style, developmental level, authority patterns and resources, and strengths and weaknesses within the family system/network are all considered.

• **ASSESSMENT OF BEREAVED INDIVIDUALS** often reveals feelings of anxiety, loneliness, spiritual distress, depression, and guilt; displaying a flattened or inhibited affect is common. The time that these feelings occur among family members may not coincide; therefore each family member needs different support at different times. Bereaved individuals may experience a combination of somatic, psychologic, and cognitive responses during normal grief. Rando's scheme of grief and mourning may be used to guide assessment. The mourner will probably move back and forth between the phases delineated by Rando (see Study Guide Table 16-2).

Assessing normal grief responses. Bereaved individuals typically experience symptoms characteristic of a major depressive episode (e.g., sadness, insomnia, poor appetite, weight loss). Important to differentiate sadness from reactive depression; depression should be treated.

Assessing complicated grief. Some symptoms of grief and depression overlap. Feelings of persistent low self-esteem, unworthiness, and reduced capacity for pleasure and enjoyment may signal depression in bereaved persons. Discussion of suicide should not be avoided.

Table 16-2
RANDO'S SIX "R" PROCESSES OF MOURNING

AVOIDANCE PHASE

1. **Recognize** the loss
   • Acknowledge the death
   • Understand the death

CONFRONTATION PHASE

2. **React** to the separation
   • Experience the pain
   • Feel, identify, accept, and give some form of expression to all the psychological reactions to the loss
   • Identify and mourn secondary losses

3. **Recollect and reexperience** the deceased and the relationship
   • Review and remember realistically
   • Revive and reexperience the feelings

4. **Relinquish** the old attachments to the deceased and the old assumptive world

ACCOMMODATION PHASE

5. **Readjust** to move adaptively into the new world without forgetting the old
   • Revise the assumptive world
   • Develop a new relationship with the deceased
   • Adopt new ways of being in the world
   • Form a new identity

6. **Reinvest**

Printed with permission from: Rando, T.A. (1993). Treatment of Complicated Grief. Champaign, IL: Research Press, p. 45.

Diagnosis of major depressive disorder is generally not made unless the symptoms persist for two months after the loss. Symptoms include:

• Guilt about things other than actions taken by the survivor at the time of death.
• Thoughts of death other than the survivor feeling that he or she would be better off dead or should have died with the deceased person.

- Morbid preoccupation with worthlessness.
- Marked psychomotor retardation.
- Prolonged, marked functional impairment.
- Hallucinating experience other than thinking that he or she hears the voice of or transiently sees the image of the deceased person.

Pharmacologic and psychotherapeutic modalities are effective treatments for depression.
- **INTERVENTIONS FOR BEREAVED INDIVIDUALS AND THEIR FAMILIES** will help to improve their quality of life.

Terminally ill individuals may be helped to deal with anticipatory grief reactions. A decrease in physical and mental symptoms may occur if appropriate interventions are available at the right time.
- Individuals can be helped to engage in activities (e.g., recording, journal writing) that will keep their memory alive for friends and family.
- Patients are encouraged to convey preferences about, for example, types of care and procedures, estate planning, funeral.
- Active listening and being with a patient facilitate an environment in which the individual defines the context and meaning of his or her own life; hope is fostered and thereby, the coping process.

Having hope helps the patient to face the shortness of life constructively. Several factors may foster hope.
- Interpersonal connectedness
- Attainable goals
- A spiritual base
- Personal attributes
- Lightheartedness
- Uplifting memories
- Affirmation of worth

Caring relationships may be fostered by the nurse in providing physical and emotional support networks for the patient, family, and friends; information about hope and dying; and encouragement in creating an environment of closeness and belonging.

In anticipatory grief reactions of family members each family member has a subjective experience of loss. In addition, the family as a whole experiences dynamic shifts in expected roles and responsibilities due to the patient's illness. Caring for the patient at home may strain physical, psychosocial, and financial resources. Disequilibrium within the family is common. Parts of family life that are not illness related should be emphasized.

Informing patient and family about support services is an essential intervention. Federal Family Medical Leave Act (1993) offers working family members unpaid leave benefits for 12 months. Family-based interventions should be provided to support family members providing terminal care at home. Examples of appropriate information would be that concerning all aspects of the patient's illness, how to deal with school-age children, the meaning of illness for all family members, and problem-focused services. Anticipatory guidance should be provided.

Children's needs are also addressed. Children are sensitive to changes in family dynamics; they may develop depressive symptomatology and anxiety. Appropriate referrals may be needed to support the family. Guidance must be age-specific. Parents need to discuss changes in the family, including those that are expected, and be aware of differences in children's and adult's grief reactions. Children may seem insensitive, but it may be in keeping with their growth and development. Children's fantasies about death decrease if appropriate information is provided to the children.

Teaching coping strategies is an intervention directed toward families, especially caregivers to help them cope and manage feelings of loss and grief. Such strategies include taking some time away from caregiving responsibilities; having a "one day at a time" attitude; using a social support network; employing stress management techniques (imaging and progressive relaxation); living fully "in the moment"; defining attainable goals; and engaging in spiritual practices.

For normal grief, no single therapeutic approach is effective. The mourning process is

Table 16-3

ORIGINS AND TREATMENT STRATEGIES FOR COMPLICATIONS OF BEREAVEMENT

ORIGINS	RECOVERY	TREATMENT
Physiological Stress/arousal (corticotropin-releasing hormone, locus coeruleus, norepeniphrine)	Homeostasis	Possibly alprazolam Stress management
Norepeniphrine dusregulation	Homeostasis Substitution (remarriage) Self-care	Antidepressant drugs Cognitive and interpersonal psychotherapy Mutual supports
Behavioral Learned helplessness	Effective coping	Antidepressant drugs Cognitive and interpersonal psychotherapy Psychoeducation Mutual supports
Insecure attachments	Substitution Growth Grief work	Brief, dynamic psychotherapy
Poor health practices	Healthy lifestyle	Health education Psychoeducation
Social Social isolation/loss of care	New interests New friends	Social services Mutual supports
Decline in socioeconomic status	Work Recognition	Social services Mutual supports
Psychosocial transitions	Effective coping New identity New assumptions about the world Future orientation	Psychoeducation Brief, dynamic psychotherapy Mutual supports

Reprinted by permission from: Jacobs S. (1993). Pathologic Grief Maladaptation to Loss, Washington, D.C.: American Psychiatric Press, p. 218.

complete with the completion of the specific tasks.

- Accepting the reality
- Working through the pain of grief
- Adjusting to the world without the loved one
- Reinvesting emotional energy in a new relationship

Nurses can review with family members simple health promotion activities to maintain personal, emotional, and physical well-being, e.g., dealing with uncertainty and anxiety, exercising, contacting friends.

For complicated grief, three methods of therapy are used (see Study Guide Tables 16-3 and 16-4).

- Client-centered therapy facilitates expressions of feeling; relies on building a trusting

Table 16-4

GOALS OF TREATING PSYCHIATRIC COMPLICATIONS OF BEREAVEMENT

MODALITY	GOALS
PSYCHOTROPIC DRUGS	— Treat major depressions and anxiety disorders — Alleviate symptoms that are subjectively overwhelming or that interfere with functioning — Facilitate the natural healing of grief
PSYCHOTHERAPY	— Counter demoralization — Provide psychoeducation — Solve problems — Clarify interpersonal problems — Elucidate maladaptive relationship patterns — Clarify pessimistic cognitive schemas — Desensitize the phobic avoidance
MUTUAL SUPPORT GROUPS	— Provide membership and friendship — Exchange information about grief, coping, and community resources — Offer a milieu for practicing social skills — Empower through publicity and advocacy — Promote self-esteem

Reprinted with permission from: Jacobs, S. (1993). Pathologic Grief Maladaptation to Loss, Washington. DC: American Psychiatric Press, p. 238.

relationship and uses nondirective techniques that enable the therapist to act as a "mirror" to the patient's feelings.

• Gestalt therapy guides the patient to "relive" the loss as fully as possible in the present; use of the "empty chair technique" in which the patient is asked to have a dialogue with the deceased.

• Cognitive and behavioral therapies, such as rational-emotive therapy (RET) and transactional analysis (TA), are directed toward teaching patients to think rationally. Behavior modification interventions are directed toward specific behaviors and acquiring new skills to become more self-sufficient.

Hospice bereavement services have several goals: to support the physical, emotional, social, and spiritual needs of the patient until the end of life. Activities preserve human dignity, maintain comfort, and provide the dying individual with autonomy and the power to make decisions. Family and friends are helped to cope with the reality of terminal illness.

Surviving family members often require interventions that will help them to avert marital dysfunction, family dysfunction, and poor school performance by children.

In group bereavement counseling survivors receive mutual support. Groups are offered through community and hospital-based hospices, mental health agencies, and religious and community organizations. Their goal is to provide a social organization to meet the needs of the bereaved and a forum for valuable information and mutual support. Groups provide the following key elements:

- person-to-person exchange based on identification and reciprocity
- access to a body of information
- an opportunity to share coping techniques and increase sense of personal worth
- a forum for advocacy, change, feedback on performance, and a "reality check" with peers

Pharmacologic interventions may include psychotropic drugs to treat complications of bereavement (e.g., major depressions and anxiety disorders) or to alleviate overwhelming symptoms that interfere with the ability to function or the natural healing of grief.

Legal and ethical implications of dying are many.

- The constitutional right of individuals to engage in decision making regarding medical intervention at the end of life is now protected through federal legislation (Patient Self-Determination Act addresses all Medicare- and Medicaid-funded facilities).
- A living will offers competent individuals a mechanism to document what medical interventions they do and do not want should they become medically incompetent and require medical technology to keep them alive.
- Durable power of attorney provides for an individual to control the process and content of decision making in case of mental incapacity or death.
- Wills give freedom to distribute the individual's property according to the will's terms.
- Will-substitutes transfer property prior to death; state regulations guide the transfer.

TAKING ANOTHER LOOK

You are now ready to respond to the questions that were raised in Gaining a Perspective at the beginning of this chapter. After you have written or thought about your responses, you may want to look at the Suggested Responses on page 324.

17 CHILDHOOD DISORDERS

TERMS TO DEFINE

attention deficit hyperactivity disorder (ADHD)

autism

conduct disorder (CD)

encopresis

enuresis

mental retardation

mood disorders

oppositional defiant disorder (ODD)

pervasive development disorder (PDD)

phobia

rumination disorder

separation anxiety disorder

specific developmental disorders

GAINING A PERSPECTIVE

Think about the problems and issues presented below, and after you have read the Key Concepts about childhood disorders write a more complete response.

1. How would you, as a nurse, be likely to feel when children who have conduct disorders (CDs) exhibit such behaviors as defiance, poor impulse control, and physical aggression? Think of strategies that would help a nurse deal with these feelings.

2. What nursing interventions seem universally appropriate when dealing with children who have emotional disorders?

Key Concepts

• **THE FIRST CHILDREN TO RECEIVE PSYCHIATRIC ATTENTION IN THE U.S.** were troubled adolescents. Child psychiatry was greatly influenced by the psychoanalytic school of thought. Freud emphasized the crucial nature of childhood experiences in adult mental health. Anna Freud and Melanie Klein used play therapy to communicate with children and to foster their understanding. Jean Piaget studied the development of the child's perceptual and sensorimotor systems. The behaviorists Pavlov, Watson, and Skinner contributed the idea of stimulus-response, which has been used to modify behavior in troubled children. Binet and Catell pioneered the field of measuring intelligence in children. Child guidance clinics were established in the 1920s and 1930s.

• **THE CONCEPTS OF MENTAL HEALTH AND MENTAL DISEASE IN CHILDREN** are different from those applicable to adults, depending, for example, on a child's particular stage of development and the nature of current family transactional operations.

• **THE COMPLEX MULTIDIMENSIONAL ETIOLOGY** of mental illness in children includes: **Genetic background** and family history. **Surface conflicts between children and parents** that arise from adjustment tasks, such as the four listed below.
  • Relationships with siblings, school situation, social and sexual development.
  • Deeper conflicts within the child; so-called neuroses.
  • Difficulties of physical handicaps and disorders.
  • Severe mental disorders, such as psychosis.

- **IN ATTENTION DEFICIT HYPERACTIVITY DISORDER (ADHD)** children are described as restless, inattentive, distractable, impulsive, and fidgety. The three subtypes of ADHD are: attention deficit only; hyperactivity only; and both attention deficit and hyperactivity, which is the most common form.

  Epidemiology. The condition is more common among boys; estimated 14% to 20% preschool/kindergarten boys, 5% to 7% preschool/kindergarten girls, and 3% to 10% elementary students have ADHD.

  Etiologic factors and family patterns. Prevalence rates are higher in the immediate families of children with ADHD. Possible causative factors that have been named include neurotransmitter abnormalities, delayed or abnormal maturation of frontal lobes, pregnancy complications, maternal smoking or alcohol, prolonged labor, malnutrition in infancy, lead poisoning, and phenylketonuria.

  Age of onset and course. ADHD begins no later than age 7. Symptoms must persist for at least six months; they are not present all the time, but often.

  Impairment and complications. Symptoms and behaviors may include restlessness, distractibility, difficulty staying seated, difficulty waiting in lines, impulsive speech, difficulty following instructions, short attention span, doesn't seem to listen, forgetfulness, difficulty organizing, losing things and constantly making mistakes, and impaired school performance. Side effects are depression, low self-esteem, and difficulty forming friendships.

  Nursing assessment and diagnosis
  - Input from teacher and parents, standardized tests to evaluate IQ and identify specific developmental disorders.
  - Possible nursing diagnoses
    - Ineffective individual coping
    - Risk for violence (self or others)
    - Impaired social interactions
    - Self-esteem disturbance
    - Ineffective family coping

  Nursing interventions
  - Keep the patient safe. Hold child responsible for rules that are agreed on.
  - Medication management. Ritalin may be drug of choice; important to assess for side effects (depression).
  - Group therapy. Relationships in group will mimic family peer relationships; may learn social skills.
  - Individual therapy. Focus is on anger control and problem solving.

- **PERVASIVE DEVELOPMENTAL DISORDER (PPD)** is characterized by very early distortions (based on the child's chronological and mental ages) in the development of three areas: social interaction; behavioral patterns; and communication, including attention, perception, and reality testing. Children with autism often appear physically normal and come from loving families, but they behave in a very peculiar and disturbing way. This PPD section focuses on autism.

  Epidemiology. Autism occurs in four out of 10,000 children; boys are more likely (3 or 4 to 1) to be autistic. Other PPDs occur in 10 to 20 per 10,000 children.

  Etiologic factors and family patterns. Autism has biological causes (fragile X syndrome). Some cases of PPD stem from maternal infection (rubella) or trauma to the fetus's developing central nervous system. There is a genetic link where family history includes PPD, dyslexia, lung disorders, and mental retardation. Families with one autistic child are at a somewhat higher risk of having another child with the disorder. Three fourths of children born with the disorder are also mentally retarded; one fourth develop seizures in later childhood.

  Age of onset and course. Autism is seen in infancy or early childhood; some children appear normal till age 2 or 3 years. Child has an aversion or indifference to being hugged or held; no social play, clings to inanimate objects. Usually has delayed or abnormal language and speech; shows hand-flapping and head-banging tics.

Nursing assessment and intervention. Children with PPD generally exhibit more bizarre or uneven behavior than children who are mentally retarded. It is hard to differentiate between autism and schizophrenia in very young and/or nonverbal children; rule out sensory deficits, metabolic disorders, or degenerative disease.

Nursing problems are complex and require many levels of intervention. Emphasis is on supporting ego development; a child is encouraged to perform appropriate behavior, decrease clinging, and reduce anxiety. Reducing sensory stimulation and establishing a daily routine may help. Most effective treatment for autism is a specialized education program that the child can begin by the age of 2 years (early intervention); a focus is helping the child avoid institutionalization.

- **MENTAL RETARDATION** is defined as significantly subaverage intellectual functioning originating during the developmental period, accompanied by impairment in at least two of the following areas: communication, self-care, home living, social skills, community use, self-direction, health and safety, functional academics, leisure, and work. The IQ is 70 or less. Some children may test within the retarded range because they are severely neglected, have specific developmental disorders, and/or are emotionally disturbed.

There are four degrees of retardation:

MILD. IQ 50-55 to 70; 85% of retarded population

MODERATE. IQ 35-40 to 50-55; 10% of retarded population

SEVERE. IQ 20-25 to 35-40; 3% to 4% of retarded population

PROFOUND. IQ below 20-25; 1% to 2% of retarded population

Epidemiology. 1% to 3% of population in US; in 1983 six million retarded people.

Etiologic factors and family patterns
- Mild retardation. Parents may be at intellectual low end. Psychosocial forces such as poverty are factors.
- Moderate to profound retardation. General-

ly linked to genetic abnormalities (Down syndrome) or metabolic trauma and toxic causes.

Age of onset and course. Usually before age 18 years; mildly retarded individuals have difficulty in school. Limitations are specific to individual's degree of retardation. Many retarded individuals function well in society.

- **SPECIFIC DEVELOPMENTAL DISORDERS (SDDs)** among children are characterized by a developmental delay that leads to functional impairment. SDDs are generally centered around reading, arithmetic, language, or articulation. A child usually has more than one disorder.

Etiologic factors. Genetic factors are suggested; it is presumed that there is a delay or abnormal maturation of areas within the cerebral cortex. Etiology is complex and not clear.

Age of onset and course. No information is available regarding onset, but generally first seen when child reaches school age and shows developmental delay. Children do not outgrow disorder and may experience difficulties in adulthood.

Impairment and complications. Secondary symptoms of SDD are behavioral problems and low self-esteem.

Nursing assessments. Diagnostic tools include IQ test; academic achievement tests; and language, speech, and motor functioning tests. Tests are necessary to rule out visual and hearing impairments.

Recommended treatment. Care is delivered by a specialized multidisciplinary team. Nurses provide support for the patient in coping with the disability.

- **CONDUCT DISORDER (CD).** Children with conduct disorders have a repetitive, persistent pattern of disruptive, willfully disobedient behavior. Some of the children will become substance abusers or develop antisocial personality disorder.

Epidemiology. 3% to 7% of children have conduct disorders; most common complaint in referrals to child psychiatric clinics and hospitals.

Etiologic factors and family patterns. No known single cause and no particular combination of factors are present in every case. Some combination of the following factors generally results in the development of a conduct disorder. Three or more of the etiologic factors are required for the diagnosis.

- The child's temperament shows poor adaptability, high activity level, and intense reactivity.
- Parental attention focused on problem behavior rather than good behavior; discipline ineffective and inconsistent, too lax or too punitive
- Poor peer group identification; part of a delinquent group of children
- Genetic predisposition
- Modeling of parent's negative behavior
- Poverty
- Parental marital problem
- Placement outside the home at an early age
- Low IQ

Age of onset and course. Conduct disorder is usually diagnosed in school-aged children. Their behavior usually violates rules and includes stealing, lying, drug use, running away, low achievement in school, truancy, fire-setting, vandalism, cruelty to animals, bullying, forcing sexual activities on others, and physical aggression.

Impairment and complication. Children seem to lack appropriate feelings of remorse, guilt, empathy, and responsibility for their behavior. Poor social skill with peers and adults is common.

Nursing assessment. Assessment is difficult, as children may have a false bravado and tough exterior, attempt to "con" people, and be unwilling to let their guard down.

Treatment. Multifaceted group and play therapy (e.g., creative art, drama, and music); consistency is important; setting of limits. Feelings evoked among staff members by these children include anger, fear, and frustration. Staff need to identify their feelings and express them in supervision to prevent acting them out with the patient. Therapeutically, it is essential that patients believe that staff can limit their inappropriate behaviors.

- **SEPARATION ANXIETY DISORDER** involves a reaction beyond expected developmental levels, often panic, that occurs when a child is separated from parents, another attachment figure, or home or other familiar surroundings.

    Epidemiology. 2% to 15% of children have anxiety disorders, with separation anxiety being the most common; slightly more prevalent among girls.

    Etiologic factors and family patterns. Strong familial link with anxiety disorders. Families of these children tend to have other disorders, including panic disorders, agoraphobia, depression, and alcoholism.

    Age of onset and course. Usually develops prior to age 18, with early onset before 6 years. Must be of at least four weeks' duration. Prognosis is better when disorder appears in a younger child.

    Impairment and complications. Child may be reluctant to go to school, fear being alone or sleeping alone, or have separation nightmares. Depression and other anxiety disorders may also be present.

    Treatment. Goal is to lower anxiety. Basic trust must be established; using a minimum number of caretakers is important. Play therapy and stories may be helpful.

- **OPPOSITIONAL DEFICIT DISORDER (ODD)** is a condition in which children exhibit characteristics that are milder forms of conduct disorder. A child exhibits behavior that is in opposition to authority figures.

    Epidemiology. 6% to 10% of youth have ODD; males with the disorder outnumber females 2or 3 to 1.

    Etiologic factors and family patterns. Possible link to an inherited difficult temperament and children imitating parental behavior that is similar to that seen in the disorder. Parents do not reward good behavior or set clear, consistent limits.

    Age of onset. Negative behavior and tantrums after the age of 3 years; if it only occurs in school, other diagnoses are pursued.

    Impairment and complications. Children with

oppositional deficit disorder chronically display stubbornness, negativism, provocativeness, hostility, and defiance. Difficult to manage at home and school; will not comply even if it is in their best interests.

Nursing assessment. Difficult to assess when child is calm, relaxed, with no demands placed on him or her, and if the child is not with familiar people.

Treatment. Requires caregiver's patience and continued acceptance of child, regardless of negative behavior; structuring a corrective life experience through behavior modification; reinforcing good behavior and offering appropriate alternatives to negative behaviors.

- **PHOBIA** is a fear that is specific and persistently out of proportion to the danger. A phobia leads to difficulty in functioning in school or social situations.

  Epidemiology. Girls report more phobias.

  Age of onset and course. Determination of a phobia depends largely on how the child responds to the fear, not the object feared. Some fears are quite normal and age-appropriate.

  Nursing interventions. Goal is to decrease fear and anxiety. All who are involved in treatment should have a consistent approach to the child.

- **ENURESIS** is repeated, involuntary urination after a child reaches 5 years of age.

  Epidemiology. Among 5-year-olds, 14% of boys and girls urinate involuntarily once a month; at age 14 years, 1% of boys and 0.5% of girls remain enuretic. The spontaneous remission rate is high.

  Etiologic factors and family patterns. It is linked to family genetics, psychological disorders, and physiological problems.

  Age of onset and course. Children 5 years or older experience incontinence two times a week for three consecutive months or a sudden marked impairment.

  Impairment and complications. Enuresis may result in significant family conflict, the child feeling ashamed, peer teasing, and low self-esteem.

Assessment. It is a psychological or physiological problem.

Treatment. Requires that the caregiver be patient and support the child. Child should be allowed some control over the situation (e.g., changing soiled sheets). A system of rewards may be tried.

- **ENCOPRESIS** is an involuntary pattern of passing feces after the child has reached the age of 4 years. Feces may be passed in clothing or other inappropriate places, for example, on the floor or in a closet.

  Epidemiology. Bowel control is usually accomplished; 1.5% of children experience encopresis after age 5. Boys outnumber girls 6:1; 25% of these children are also enuretics.

  Etiologic factors and family patterns. Most cases are physiological — a genetic abnormality, or severe constipation; 15% of encopretic children have fathers who had the problem. May be secondary to sexual abuse or other disorders or temporarily due to a severe stressor.

  Age of onset and course. Onset after 4 years of age; rarely occurs during sleep.

  Impairment and complications. Encopretic children suffer from peer rejection and school and family problems.

  Nursing assessment and treatment. A complete medical, psychological, and toilet-training history must be taken. Nurse can help the child explore feelings regarding soiling behavior. Parents avoiding punitive response can improve the child's recovery and self-esteem.

- **MOOD DISORDERS** can be serious, long-lasting, and recurrent. Generally involve varying degrees of depression, elation, or irritability. Children tend to be irritable and lose weight; the disorders encompass depression and bipolar disorders.

  Epidemiology. Incidence is on the rise, with a declining age of onset for bipolar disorders; 2% of children experience major depression; prior to puberty more common in girls.

  Etiologic factors and family patterns. Strong familial genetic links exist, especially with bipolar disorders.

Age of onset and course. Can occur at any age. Difficult to diagnose in young children who cannot communicate thoughts and feelings.

Impairment and complications. Behaviors of depressed children vary by appropriate developmental level. Poor school performance, decreased desire to interact with other children, boredom, stomachaches, and headaches may arise from mood disorders. Major depression could be indicative of a bipolar disorder.

Assessment and treatment. In interactions with child, age-appropriate language is used and the possibility of suicide is evaluated. Supportive individual and/or family therapy and medications may be beneficial.

- **RUMINATION DISORDER OF INFANCY** is repeated voluntary regurgitation and rechewing of food with weight loss or failure to gain weight. Child does this to release tension or as a source of pleasure.

  Epidemiology. More prevalent among males by 5:1

  Etiologic factors and family patterns. One third of infants have mothers who experienced obstetrical complications; one fourth of infants have developmental delays. Disorder is linked to neglect, harsh handling, and maternal depression.

  Age of onset and course. Occurs between ages 3 months and 1 year, usually in infants with moderate to severe mental retardation.

  Impairment and complications. When not ruminating, child may be withdrawn and apathetic or irritable and fussy or may appear normal.

  Assessment and treatment. Hospitalization is usually required. Supportive therapy for parents and parenting education may be needed.

TAKING ANOTHER LOOK

You are now ready to respond in greater depth to the issues and problems that were raised in Gaining a Perspective at the beginning of this chapter. After you have written or thought more about your responses, you may wish to look at the Suggested Responses on page 325.

18 ISSUES IN ADOLESCENT MENTAL HEALTH

GAINING A PERSPECTIVE

Think about the situations presented below, and after you have read the Key Concepts of this chapter address the questions in greater detail.

1. Describe your feelings about your own adolescence.

2. How would you, as a nurse, handle a teenager who tells you that she wants to kill herself?

3. Discuss how you, as a nurse, would go about arranging the interviews described in the situation below.

> You are a nurse in a psychiatric clinic and have been assigned to interview a newly admitted adolescent patient. His parents are present. It is the policy of this clinic for the same nurse to interview both the patient and parents, each in an individual interview.

Key Concepts

• **MISCONCEPTIONS AND MYTHS** have been perpetuated about the adolescent experience. Nurses who work with adolescents need to be aware of recent studies and resist the pull of theoretical "sacred cows" and ethnocentric assumptions.

• **IN DECISION MAKING, THEORIES GUIDE** a nurse's interpretation and evaluation of what is appropriate patient behavior, environment, and development. A theory may be thought of as a compass for decision making. Although some scholars focused on biological influences and others on moral development, personality theorists have dominated adolescent psychology. Historically, several theories of personality development have been relevant to the study and treatment of adolescents.

Psychoanalytic theory (Sigmund Freud)
Interpersonal theory (Harry Stack Sullivan)
Psychosocial developmental theory (Erik Erikson)
Cognitive development theory (Jean Piaget)

The theories stress that developmental events taking place in the present are systematically linked to past events and that development is a consistent process.

More recent approaches to adolescent psychology and psychiatry are accompanied by significant developments in psychobiology and behavioral biology. Studies suggest that biology will have a greater role in approaches to personality development and adolescent mental health than it has had in the past.

• **ADOLESCENCE IS A PERIOD DISTINCT FROM** childhood and adulthood. It is marked by ever-changing influences and conditions, including physiological changes, that make it difficult for intergenerational understanding.

During adolescence, certain tasks must be completed: becoming physically and sexually mature, acquiring skills to carry out adult roles, and gaining increased autonomy from parents. At the same time, adolescents need to establish and realign their social interconnections with peers.

- **EARLY, MIDDLE, AND LATE ADOLESCENCE** are common divisions of the period.

  Early adolescence (prepubescence) and puberty (ages 10-14)
  - Most girls have a growth spurt at 9-1/2 years of age; changes in girls during early adolescence, before puberty, include increased estrogen levels, breast development, pelvic widening, and growth of pubic and axillary hair. Menarche denotes the onset of puberty.
  - In most boys the growth spurt is two years later than the girls and physical changes begin about one year after the testes begin to secrete testosterone. Boys' shoulders broaden, genitals enlarge slightly, voice deepens, and pubic, axillary, facial, and chest hair (in that order) grows. Seminal emissions (spermarche) denote onset of puberty.
  - Male and female reactions to puberty differ.
  - Adolescence is a confusing time in that the effects of maturational timing are different for different individuals; if an adolescent's pubertal maturation comes at a time different from that of his or her peers, the consequences could potentially be negative.
  - Peer group becomes increasingly significant as a socializing context; family influence is reduced, but not eliminated. The primary influence on educational aspirations and occupational plans appears to remain with parents. As importance of parental approval wanes with increasing importance of peer approval, high achievers may be faced with a dilemma.

  Middle adolescence (ages 14-15 to 15-17) is a time for increasing independence.
  - Some individuals mark the end of adolescence if they complete schooling or become emancipated.
  - Time to come to terms with maturing body and sexual identity. Gender role identification intensifies.
  - Peers have special significance as the effort to separate from parents takes place.

  Late adolescence is an indefinite period from age 18 years to the mid-20s, depending on individual factors such as educational goals. Task in this period is to define who they are and what their future direction will be.

- **ADOLESCENT HEALTH ISSUES** differ over time. Today's issues and experiences can not be compared with those of the past. In the 1970s, consensus was that young people were victims of social forces beyond their control. In the 1980s, young people were found to be the source of problems that they created for themselves. Adolescents often feel like outsiders in modern Western societies. Their well-being seems to have declined, and problem behavior seems to have increased (rising rate of academic failures, delinquency, suicide, and sexual license). Some professionals suggest that parental influence has decreased primarily because parents have chosen to withdraw from the lives of their youngsters; this lays the groundwork for feelings of abandonment and alienation. Health status of the adolescent has declined. Morbidity and mortality among adolescents are attributed primarily to social, environmental, and behavioral determinants rather that biomedical facts. Mortality rates of adolescent females are half those of adolescent males; life expectancy is lowest among African-American males. Violence continues to pose the greatest health risk for young people. The major declines in health status are also linked to:

  Substance abuse. Studies show that:
  - marijuana use among eighth graders has more than doubled since 1991.
  - drug use has increased among all teenagers.
  - alcohol consumption was reported by 92% of high school seniors.
  - 18% of high school seniors report cigarette smoking.
  - drug and alcohol abuse present a variety of

clinical pictures. The drug experience affects and is affected by the adolescent's developmental phase.

Negative consequences: memory impairment; developmental lag in cognitive, moral, and psychosocial domains; a pattern of apathy.

Negative reactions of family and others can lead to: development of negative identity, social alienation, and estrangement at a time when social support is needed.

Accidents

- More than one half of all deaths of people 10 to 19 years of age are due to accidents; most involve motor vehicles (speeding, tailgating, using drugs and alcohol). Driving under the influence of alcohol is involved in over half of the fatalities; high rates of intoxication are also found among samples of adolescents who die as pedestrians or while using recreational vehicles.
- Nonfatal injuries resulting from vehicular accidents account for the largest number of hospital days among adolescents between ages 12 and 17.

Sexual activity

- By age 19 years, more than 77% of males and more than 62% of females have engaged in sexual intercourse.
- 25% of sexually active adolescents become infected with sexually transmitted diseases (STDs) during high school. STD rates are higher among black teenagers. Risk factors include multiple partners and failure to use condoms.
- One million adolescents in the U.S. become pregnant every year (many within six months of becoming sexually active), and 50% of these teens give birth.

Fads have the potential to cause illness and injury.

- Body marking includes body piercing, scarring, and tattooing and may cause infection.
- Moshing (slam dancing) includes body surfing, hurling oneself into a crowd, and stage diving, all of which can cause injury.

- **ADOLESCENT MENTAL HEALTH DISORDERS,** the literature indicates, run the entire range of psychopathology experienced by adults. Overreporting or diagnostic confusion may occur because of the difficulty of distinguishing between normal adolescent turmoil due to family dysfunction and incipient mental problems. Overall, rates do not differ by sex; however, females are more often given the diagnosis of depression and males the diagnosis of conduct disorder. The types of disorders seen in adolescents are described below.

Adjustment disorder is a pathological reaction to an identified or external stressor, which may range from physical illness to parental divorce. The disorder persists for up to six months and impairs adolescent social functioning. Symptoms may include defiance, aggression, outbursts of rage, or drug and alcohol use; the symptoms vary depending on developmental phase, previous patterns of coping, and the familial or environmental circumstances of the adolescent. Adjustment disorder, of which there are subtypes, is linked with one of several specifics: academic inhibition, anxiety, physical complaints, conduct disturbances, depression, or social withdrawal.

Eating disorders typically refer to the syndromes of anorexia and bulimia nervosa. The two syndromes may coexist. Some dispute exists as to whether the disorders are increasing in number or whether they are being acknowledged, recognized, and diagnosed more extensively. From 1965 to 1985, the incidence of anorexia nervosa doubled. Anorexia occurs in about 0.5% of females aged 12 to 18 years. The prevalence of bulimia is increasing (5% to 18% of young women in high school are afflicted). Bulimia also occurs in males. Sociocultural values (i.e., the high value placed on thinness) have been implicated in the genesis of this disorder.

- ANOREXIA NERVOSA

  ADOLESCENT PERCEIVES herself as overweight, which in reality may not be true.

  RAPID, EXTREME WEIGHT LOSS is achieved by restricting caloric intake, purging (vomiting), fasting, using laxatives or diuretics, and through excessive physical activity.

Highest reported morbidity and mortality rates (10% to 15%) of all psychiatric illnesses.

Physical problems involve all body systems and include cardiac arrhythmias, renal failure, anemias, and endocrine imbalances (amenorrhea).

Hallmarks are secretiveness, massive denial that problem exists, and resistance to therapy or any treatment that will cause weight gain.

- Bulimia nervosa typically develops in late adolescence (ages 17 to 25).

  Weight control of concern; young women have tried many diets and failed.

  Binging on large amounts of foods, usually high caloric and starchy, then inducing vomiting, using diuretic or laxative, or fasting.

  Dental enamel erosion, electrolyte imbalances, and esophagitis usually develop.

- Obesity occurs in 15% of adolescents; usually caused by overeating.

- Depression and low self-esteem often develop; may become vulnerable to cognitive and emotional disturbances or maladaptive behaviors.

Depression may be a temporary, situational reaction, or a chronic condition.

- Incidence difficult to calculate because of different definitions and measurements; may be that 5% to 7% of high school students have experienced severe depression, and 21 to 27% moderate depression.

- Defined as a debilitating affective state characterized by dysphoric mood or loss of interest or pleasure in usual activities.

- Symptoms include hopelessness; irritability, or "feeling blue or sad"; poor academic performance; restlessness; and aggressive or sexual acting-out behavior; may appear bored or engage in high-risk behaviors, such as drug and alcohol use.

- Depression may lead to suicide.

Suicide

- Accounts for 6% of deaths among 10- to 14-year-olds and 12% in the 15 to 19 age group.

- Usually more than one attempt.

- Clinical risk factors include major psychiatric disorder (e.g., bipolar disorder, schizophrenia) and a family history of suicide or psychiatric illness.

- Common stressors among vulnerable youth are family conflicts, rejection by peers, or a romantic situation.

- About 30% of adolescents who commit suicide are substance abusers.

- Traits considered common risk factors are poor mood regulation, intense rage, impulsive behavior, and limited tolerance for frustration.

- Hotlines and other crisis services reduce suicide attempts among white women.

Oppositional disorder is a controversial diagnostic category that includes persistent disobedient, negativistic, and provocative opposition to authority figures; rule violation; argumentativeness; provocative behavior; and stubbornness. Oppositional behavior can be due to a situational crisis and is seen in depressed teens. Diagnosed more often in males; long-term prognosis is poor.

Conduct disorder is the most common psychiatric diagnostic category in referrals to child mental health services.

- The condition occurs more commonly in male adolescents, especially those who come from lower socioeconomic backgrounds and environments in which harsh punishment and domestic violence are frequent.

- Two subtypes: one aggressive, in which the adolescent is asocial and isolated; the second involves the organized pathology of gangs.

- Characterized by academic problems, overt and covert hostility, disobedience, physical and verbal aggressiveness, quarrelsomeness, vengefulness, and destructiveness.

- Powerful association with later substance abuse.

- Etiological factors seem to include parental skills deficit, parental alcoholism, sociological factors, social immaturity, and aggressiveness; personality traits may have a biological component.

- Therapy is likely to be ineffective; 50% later exhibit antisocial personality disorder.

Schizophrenia most often appears for the first time between the ages of 15 and 25 years.

- Presents itself slowly; often difficult to diagnose.
- Enormously problematic for the family. Families may have to relinquish hopes they had for their child. They often feel isolated, embarrassed, and blame themselves. May become extremely overprotective of the child.
- Recent research shows schizophrenia is not a degenerative disease. Early treatment of schizophrenia with antipsychotic drugs not only cuts short the psychotic episode, but may improve long-term outcome.

Deviance and delinquent behavior

- Delinquent behavior ranges from truancy to serious criminal offenses and is highly correlated with drug and alcohol abuse.
- Explanations of adolescent deviance generally focus on social and community factors that influence opportunities, as well as biological susceptibilities, personality and character traits, parental inadequacies, vulnerability to peer influence, and negative consequences of premature adolescent emancipation from parental control.
- Treatment indicates that imprisonment fails to deter crime, and diversional programs and preventive techniques (job programs and counseling) appear ineffective.

Violence in all forms is a greater killer of children in the U.S. than disease.

- Victimization includes physical assault and sexual abuse. Studies indicate 25% of 10- to 16-year-olds have experienced an assault or sexual abuse.
- Homicide is the leading cause of death among black males, particularly those living in impoverished urban areas. It accounts for 33% of deaths among all 15- to 19-year-olds.
- Children exposed to violence have thoughts that frequently provoke enduring anger or self-blame and post-traumatic stress disorder which may seriously affect cognitive, emotional, and interpersonal development.

Running away from home is done by up to two million young people in the U.S. each year, and another 500,000 have no home. Studies indicate 60% are thrown out of their homes. Almost 50% reported physical or emotional abuse at home, and 10% reported sexual abuse.

Cults, social psychologists believe, flourish in times of violence, social disorganization, and great uncertainty. For their adherents, they offer security and absolute truth. The adolescents belonging to cults come from families that show high tolerance for deviant behavior and whose members have unresolved, unspoken conflicts from which they prefer to distance themselves. Generally, adolescents who join cults are thrill seekers who have low self-esteem and poor social skills.

- **TREATMENT IS PROVIDED FOR ADOLESCENTS** in a variety of settings: residential schools for long-term therapy, hospitals for acute psychiatric emergencies, day hospitals and clinics, and community health centers. Nurses are often the first professionals an adolescent encounters in the hospital or outpatient setting. Working with adolescents can be intensely rewarding and frustrating. Nurses must be aware of their own feelings and reactions to difficult behavior and not overreact or project their own insecurities. Nurses should practice effective stress management to deal with their own day-to-day reactions.

Most adolescents come to treatment manifesting obvious distrust and hostility. They are likely to try to embarrass and provoke their parents and attempt to antagonize and humiliate the nurse. The nurse should anticipate this and be as good-humored and low-keyed as possible. Respect and understanding are essential elements in communicating with adolescent patients. Adolescents respond to firmness, honesty, genuine affection, and consistent behavior on the part of authority figures.

Because adolescents value their independence and having a sense of control, it is crucial that nurses, as often as possible, communicate directly with the adolescent, not through intermediaries. Nurses must thoroughly explain confidentiality and clearly delineate what issues it entails and excludes.

Adolescents with a history of violent, impulsive behavior pose a special challenge to nursing staff. Warning signs of potentially explosive episodes are a loud strident voice, tense posture, fist clenching, or an inability to sit still. In the initial contact with a potentially violent adolescent, the nurse and patient should not be alone together. From the beginning, the nurse must calmly state that violent acting-out will not be tolerated. Offering a soft drink or snack can sometimes help to reduce the adolescent's agitation.

Involuntary treatment, regardless of its structure or setting, poses many obstacles. Part of the difficulty is that involuntary treatment heightens the disparity in power between an adolescent patient and staff member and exacerbates already existing conflicts over authority. To develop a meaningful and mutually respectful relationship, nurses must concentrate on helping the adolescent; emphasizing verbally and through action that their obligation is primarily to the adolescent and his or her welfare.

• **IN CARING FOR ADOLESCENT PATIENTS,** nurses must be aware of the developmental needs of adolescents and the key issues that are unique to that age group, such as puberty. A comfortable environment in which to talk should be created.

Assessment, or gathering information, is important, particularly information about sexuality, sexual behavior, and any need for knowledge about sexual issues. Both adolescents and parents should be interviewed; it is useful to express an awareness that points of view will differ and the professional is willing to listen to all views.

Diagnosis is analyzing the data collected. Diagnoses are labels that identify problems or risk factors. Diagnoses may be useful, but they say nothing about a patient's assets or strengths.

Planning involves prioritizing problems, with safety being of paramount importance to enable intervention. Planning should look at an adolescent's strengths and assets, as well as liabilities. It is goal directed and based on desired outcome objectives that can be measured. Discharge planning and strategies for inpatient or outpatient care are included. Planning must be a collaborative process, with adolescents maintaining a sense of control. Presenting a forced choice may instill a sense of autonomy and self-direction. A multidisciplinary team reduces fragmentation and offers a more holistic approach to patient care.

Interventions assist people to achieve their goals or function more effectively. The purpose of intervention may be remedial, preventive, or developmental (education to increase functioning or coping ability). Interventions for adolescents include counseling, psychotherapy, and psychopharmacology. Generally, therapy focuses on flexibility of approach, present function, directiveness, and directness. Family therapy and group therapy may also be helpful if used properly.

Evaluation is determining whether outcomes that were initially agreed upon by adolescent, nurse, and treatment team were met. The implementation processes of the treatment program should also be evaluated.

• **RESEARCH CONCERNING ADOLESCENTS HAS BEEN FLAWED** in many respects, most specifically in terms of sampling; girls and minorities have been underrepresented.

Nurses who work with hospitalized adolescents are conducting research that significantly contributes to the care of adolescents.

TAKING ANOTHER LOOK

You are now ready to respond to situations that were described in Gaining a Perspective at the beginning of the chapter. After you have written or thought about your responses, you may wish to look at the Suggested Responses on page 325.

19 AGING AND MENTAL HEALTH

TERMS TO DEFINE

autonomy

delirium

dementia

depression

ego integrity versus despair

electroconvulsive therapy (ECT)

grief

incompetency

informed consent

loss

mental status exam

monoamine oxidase inhibitors (MAO-I)

neuroleptics

pharmacodynamics

pharmacokinetics

physical restraint

polypharmacy

presbyopia

reality orientation

reminisce therapy

respite care

senility

sundowning

tricyclic antidepressants

GAINING A PERSPECTIVE

Think about the following five questions, and after you have read the Key Concepts for this chapter consider more comprehensive responses.

1. How would you, as a nurse, respond initially to an elderly person who is concerned about forgetting?

2. How do you think it would feel to retire?

3. What type of questions would a nurse probably ask an unmarried, emotionally and mentally well older woman in order to determine her functional status?

4. Why is depression often unnoticed in the elderly, and what implications does the oversight have for you, as a nurse?

5. What would you, as a nurse, do if a co-worker says that an elderly patient who is confused needs to be placed in restraints?

Key Concepts

• **AMERICANS ARE LIVING LONGER.** Statistics reveal that 12.5% of Americans are elderly. The stereotyped image that American society has of its older adults represents them as frail and heavily dependent on others. This portrait, however, is far from accurate. No age group is immune from emotional problems. Nurses may encounter the elderly in a wide variety of settings, such as acute care hospitals, personal care homes, adult day care, psychiatric hospitals, outpatient clinics, geriatric evaluation clinics, community mental health centers, primary care, physicians' offices, and even in the streets.

• **THE FINAL STAGE OF ERIKSON'S EIGHT STAGES OF MAN IS THE ACHIEVEMENT OF EGO INTEGRITY VERSUS DESPAIR.** During this stage, older adults review their life for meaning, purpose, and a sense of worth. If they feel reasonably pleased with the way they have lived, the developmental task has been successfully accomplished; if instead they face many regrets and resentments, then despair leading to depression may ensue.

- **NORMAL AGING DOES NOT INVOLVE DRASTIC PERSONALITY CHANGES**, rather established personality styles are strengthened. Confusion is not a part of normal aging. What is normal are occasional forgetfulness, especially of the recent past, and needing more time to process information. Older adults may take longer to respond to questions and requests and to process multiple stimuli. They also may experience shorter sleeping periods and may complain of insomnia. Hearing is the most common, most disabling sensory problem. Visual changes include presbyopia, but cataracts and glaucoma are more serious problems. Normal changes need to be assessed early so that interventions, such as eyeglasses, hearing aids, and appropriate communication methods, can be implemented if needed.

- **THE LOSSES AND STRESSES THAT ELDERLY PEOPLE MUST DEAL WITH** include death of family members and friends, decreased income, or caring for an ailing spouse. A loss of independence may be particularly disturbing to an older adult. Crime and violence are especially frightening. Another source of stress is relocation, such as from home to apartment or nursing home. The elderly may feel a loss of control when decisions regarding relocation are made without considering their choice or preference.

TABLE 19–1.
THE GERIATRIC ASSESSMENT

Chief complaint/reason for interview
Demographical information
Medical and psychiatric histories
Current overall medical health
Physical examination and laboratory tests
Medication inventory and compliance
Drug and alcohol use
Mental status examination
Stressors and coping style
Nature of support system
Functional status
Cultural and spiritual assessments
Tests/screening tools as needed
Patient concerns and goals

Retirement is usually viewed as a loss, with changes in role, time structure, and financial status. Retirement is likely to be stressful when related to such negative events as illness or firing. Retirement planning is a worthwhile intervention best taken during middle- to late-middle age.

- **THE PSYCHOLOGICAL ASSESSMENT** of the older patient is much like that of younger individuals (see Study Guide Table 19-1).

Symptoms of physical disturbances mimic symptoms of emotional problems. In later life, physical illness, especially multiple illnesses, does increase the risk of emotional problems. Assessment of mental status should include the following elements:
  General appearance
  Reaction to the interview
  Level of consciousness
  Orientation
  Consistency and appropriateness of behaviors
  Mood and affect
  Thought content
  Judgment and insight
  Recall and memory
  Intellectual function
  Comprehension
  Concentration and attention
Warning signs of mental illness in the elderly include:
  Significant personality changes
  Confused thinking
  Strange or grandiose ideas
  Prolonged and severe depression
  Apathy
  Extreme mood changes
  Severe anxiety
  Extreme fear
  Suspiciousness
  Blame of others
  Withdrawal
  Isolation
  Denial

Suicidal ideation

Suicide talk

Exaggerated anger

Psychosis

Drug and alcohol abuse

Inability to cope with daily living

Assessment of patients' support systems, including kin, friends, neighbors, organizations, and professional helpers, is important. Does the patient have someone with whom to share problems? Social supports may act as a "buffer," mediating the influence of stressful life events. Functional status must also be explored. To plan care, a patient's ability to care for self and mobility are critically important assessments.

Customs and beliefs affect attitudes toward health, illness, aging, death, health care providers, gender role differences, and family roles. A patient's cultural background and value system influence how, or if, symptoms are reported. In some cultures, depressive-type symptoms ("nerves" and headaches in Latino and Mediterranean cultures) may not be revealed without gentle probing. Some older adults may be wary of the health care system because of experiences with discrimination.

After the patient is asked about personal concerns, preventive measures and anticipatory guidance are implemented. The patient's goals and ideas must be assessed and seriously considered. Helping the patient to set realistic goals is an important nursing function.

Psychiatric nurses have many screening tools to aid assessments and provide more objective data (see Study Guide Table 19-2).

Building rapport and a trusting therapeutic relationship helps the patient feel comfortable enough to discuss concerns openly and honestly and thereby assists in obtaining accurate test results. Some considerations for interviewing and testing are:

Late morning may be a time of optimum cognitive function, but functioning may be tested at various times.

A quiet environment should be selected to minimize anxiety and sensory overload, which interfere with memory and learning.

Explain the purpose and length of the interview and screening tests.

Prescribed sensory aids should be worn by the patient to reduce impact of sensory deficits.

Speak clearly; avoid medical terminology and slang.

Allow adequate response time and clarify as needed.

Demonstrate patience, comfort with silence, and a nonjudgmental attitude.

The patient's physical comfort is important; give stretch breaks if the testing tool permits.

- **DEPRESSION IS THE MOST PREVALENT EMOTIONAL DISORDER** plaguing older Americans and is believed by some to have the most disturbing symptoms. Depression is the most treatable mental disorder in later life, but is often undetected. The consequences are suffering, mental anguish, and suicide. Health care professionals all too often conclude that depression is a normal consequence of old age, much as physical illness, economic difficulties, and social problems. Symptoms may be labeled part of the aging process.

Clinical manifestations of depression include loss of appetite, disturbed sleep, decreased energy and enjoyment, and a range of physical symptoms; they may be more evident than a depressed mode. Symptoms may be determined by interviewing family and caregivers and using sound screening tools (Study Guide Table 19-2).

Risk for depression in the elderly is the same as for younger adults; most at risk are women, unmarried (especially widowed) individuals, and persons who experience stressful life events or who have no supportive social network. There is also a connection between physical illness and depression. In reviewing one's life during old age, negative thoughts, or regrets, may lead to depressive emotions.

Depression must be distinguished from bereavement. Loss may lead to depression; bereavement and depression are not identical. Bereaved adults generally see themselves positively: there is not a morbid preoccupation with worthlessness as in depression. There is no suicidal ideation. Generally treatment during bereavement is supportive.

TABLE 19-2. LIST OF TESTS/SCREENING TOOLS

Test/Scale	Author(s)	Year	Measures
ADLs/Functioning:			
CADET	Rameizl	1983	Self-care
Geriatric Functional Rating Scale	Grauer and Birnbom	1975	Functioning, to determine need for institutional care
Index of Independence in Activities of Daily Living	Katz, Ford, Inoskowitz, Jackson, and Jaffe	1963	Asks about behaviors most people encounter daily
Instrumental Activities of Daily Living Scale	Lawton and Brody	1969	Self-maintaining and instrumental activities of daily living
OARS Instrument	Duke Univ. Ctr. for the Study of Aging and Human Develop.	1978	Functional ability
Townsend's Activities of Daily Living Scale	Townsend	1979	Functional status
Depression:			
Beck Depression Inventory (BDI)	Beck	1961	Depression
The Geriatric Depression Scale	Yesavage Brink, Rose, Lum, Huang, Adey, and Leiter	1983	Depression
Zung Self-Rating Depression Inventory (SDS)	Zung	1965	Depression
Dementia:			
Blessed Dementia Rating Scale	Blessed, Tomlinson and Roth	1968	Dementia
A Dementia Rating Scale	Lawson, Rodenberg and Dykes	1977	Dementia
FROMAJE	Libow	1981	Dementia, depression
Mental Status/Cognition:			
Assessment of Confusion	Vermeersch	1986	Presence/severity of acute confusion
Confusion Rating Scale	Williams, Ward, and Campbell	1988	Subtle manifestations and rapid changes of acute confusion
The Face-Hand Test (FHT)	Fink, Green, and Bender	1952	Adjunct in assessment of organic mental disorders, to distinguish patients with brain damage from those who are psychotic without an organic cause
Mental Status Questionnaire (MSQ)	Kahn	1960	Severity of brain syndrome, a gross measure of mental status and cognitive function changes
The Mental Status Questionnaire for Evaluation of Brain Dysfunction in the Aged	Kahn	1971	Mental status
Mini-Mental Status Examination	Folstein and McHugh	1975	Cognitive function
Nurses' Observation Scale for Inpatient Evaluation (NOSIE)	Honigfeld and Hendricks	1981	Patient behaviors, incl. factors of social competence and interest, cooperation, and psychotic depression
Sandoz Clinical Assessment-Geriatric (SCAG)	Shader, Harmatz, and Salzman	1974	Mental status, mood, motivation, social ability, fatigue, and anxiety
Short Portable Mental Status Questionnaire (SPMSQ)	Also, Duke University	1978	Mental status: intact to severe impairment
Others:			
Delighted-Terrible Faces Scale	Andrew and Withey	1976	Current and overall life satisfaction
Elders Life Stress Inventory (ELSI)	Aldwin	1990	Stress of events of past year
General Health Questionnaire (GHQ)	Goldberg and Williams	1988	Psychiatric morbidity
Neugarten's Life Satisfaction Scale Index A	Neugarten, Havighurst, and Tobin	1961	Current and overall life satisfaction
PACE II	U.S. Dept. of Health, Educ. and Welfare	1978	Physical health of nursing home patients
Social Network Scale	Hirsch	1980	Network size and type
	Stokes	1983	

TABLE 19–3.
NURSING CARE PLAN: DEPRESSION

Providing an Accepting, Comforting Atmosphere	Problem Solving
Establish rapport	Include family therapy when indicated
Display empathy	
Encourage expression of feelings	Teach relaxation techniques to decrease anxiety
Allow time for responses, show patience	Assist with utilization of constructive problem solving process
	Assist with structuring of daily activity
	Assist with realistic goal formation
	Deemphasize importance of unrealistic goals

Maintaining Safety	Increasing Self-Esteem
Assess suicidality carefully and repeatedly	Assist to reduce negative thoughts via examination of perceptions/conclusions
Hospitalize when necessary	Limit negative self-criticism
Provide close supervision as needed	Stimulate participation in activities/hobbies
Assess and maintain physiological status	Encourage exercise, adjusted to health level
Assure that self-care needs are met	Encourage independence
Encourage appropriate expression of anger	Provide positive feedback
	Encourage socialization
	Assist with life review

TABLE 19–4.
ANTIDEPRESSANTS: SIDE EFFECTS PROFILE

Tricyclics	
Anticholinergic effects:	**Other effects:**
Dry mouth	Lightheadedness
Blurred vision	Dizziness
Tachycardia	Sedation
Urinary hesitancy/retention	Photosensitivity
Constipation	Headache
Nausea	EPRs
Vomiting	Hypotension
	Cardiac rhythm disturbances

MAO-Is
Restlessness, jitteriness, hyperactivity
Insomnia
Fatigue
Weakness
Dizziness
GI disturbances, i.e., anorexia, nausea, diarrhea, abdominal cramping
Headache
Dry mouth
Blurred vision
Orthostatic hypotension
Cardiac rate and rhythm changes
Risk of hypertensive crisis

Suicide risk is highest for elderly white men. Precipitants for suicide in the elderly are ill health, loneliness, and bereavement; studies also indicate fear of being placed in a nursing home, pain, interpersonal difficulties, incapacity, finances, and remorse as other reasons. Preventing suicide is more likely when reasons can be identified and dealt with.

Etiology involves many theories. An imbalance in the brain of the neurotransmitters norepinephrine and serotonin may cause depression. Special attention is being paid to sites where neurotransmitters attach to the postsynaptic neuron; these receptors may be "down regulated" in depressed people.

Clinical management for depression in later life has the following goals (NIH, 1992): to de-crease symptoms, decrease risk of relapse, increase quality of life, increase medical health, and decrease health care costs and mortality.

- "Talking" therapies — counseling and supportive care — should be offered. Having empathy will encourage the elderly individual to express feelings. Life review and reminiscing are two helpful approaches; each gives the elderly person a chance to reorganize and resolve issues. A general nursing plan for older individuals with depression is presented in Study Guide Table 19-3.
- Medications — antidepressants — act to increase the concentration of chemical mes-

TABLE 19–5.
CONTRAINDICATIONS TO USE OF ANTIDEPRESSANT MEDICATIONS IN OLDER PATIENTS WITH PHYSICAL ILLNESS

Relative contraindications

Symptoms of urinary obstruction
  benign prostatic hypertrophy
  urinary retention due to outlet obstruction

Delirium

Marked sedation or agitation

Use of multiple drugs with anticholinergic side effects
  antipsychotics, antiparkinsonian agents
  antihistamines
  atropine-containing drugs

Use of other drugs with the potential for serious interactions with tricyclics
  guanethidine, methyldopa, clonidine
  antiarrhythmics, such as quinidine or pronestyl

Orthostatic hypotension

Severe hypertension

Moderate to severe congestive heart failure

Unstable angina

Conduction disturbances—any combination of two of the following:
    first-degree heart block
    left anterior hemiblock
    left or right bundle-branch block

Poorly controlled seizures

History of allergy to a tricyclic antidepressant

Absolute contraindications

Recent myocardial infarction (within six weeks)

Acute ischemia on electrocardiogram

Acute angle closure glaucoma (rare)

Second- or third-degree heart block

New bundle-branch block following initiation of tricyclic treatment

Increased ventricular arrhythmias following initiation of tricyclic treatment

Reprinted from Koenig HG, Breitner JCS: Use of antidepressants in medically ill older patients. *Psychosomatics* 1990; 31: p. 24.

sengers (neurotransmitters) in the synaptic clefts. Because of the pharmacokinetics of the elderly, judicious use of any medication is imperative; potential adverse side effects may occur (see Study Guide Tables 19-4 and 19-5).

Several newer drugs, such as trazadone, bupropion, and fluoxetine, produce fewer anticholinergic and cardiovascular side effects. Considerations in addition to side effects include the patient's medical status, previous response, symptom pattern, and lifestyle, functional ability, and knowledge base. Conservative dosing, that is, starting low and increasing gradually, is key to success. Elderly patients may take six to twelve weeks to respond to drug. Treatment should continue for six months after the first episode, and for twelve months following the second or third episodes. Because compliance with drug regimen may be a problem, a thorough assessment and effective teaching about medication, including a return demonstration, are key components of therapy.

- Electroconvulsive therapy (ECT) may be the treatment of choice for older depressed patients when delusions, catatonia, or life-threatening behaviors are also present. ECT may be safer than antidepressants. There seems to be an increased risk for post-ECT confusion in older age; it may be reduced by performing ECT unilaterally. Six to ten treatments are usually required.

TABLE 19–6.
ALTERNATIVE NAMES USED TO LABEL DELIRIUM

Acute brain failure	Clouded states	Subacute befuddlement
Acute brain syndrome	Exogenous psychosis	
Acute cerebral insufficiency	ICU psychosis	Sundown syndrome
Acute confusional state	Metabolic encephalopathy	Toxic confusional state
Acute organic psychosis	Pseudosenility	Toxic delirious reaction
Acute organic reaction	Postcardiotomy delirium	Toxic encephalopathy
Acute organic syndrome	Rapid-onset confusion	Toxic psychosis
Acute psycho-organic syndrome	Reversible brain syndrome Reversible dementia	Transient impairment
Cerebral insufficiency	Reversible toxic psychosis	Transient impairment syndrome

Reprinted with permission from Rosen SL: Managing delirious older adults in the hospital; Med Surg Nurs, 1994; 3: 181–189.

- **DELIRIUM** is a syndrome that goes by many names (see Study Guide Table 19-6). The names imply that delirium is a temporary illness and the individual will return to normal functioning. Delirium is often unidentified in the elderly.

Clinical manifestations include changes in cognition, such as difficulties with memory, concentration, focusing, registration, and directed thinking, that tend to fluctuate throughout the day in an unpredictable manner. Orientation may be disturbed. Psychomotor behavior may be either hyperactivity, hypoactivity, or a combination (see Study Guide Table 19-7).

The variability in signs and symptoms may account in part for underdetection. Diagnostic criteria are listed in Study Guide Table 19-8. Pathogenesis involves four basic theories:

- A generalized cerebral insufficiency related to a decrease in the mechanisms for cerebral oxidation.
- Changes in the neurochemical mechanism, with a decrease of acetylcholine synthesis.
- A reaction to acute stress, with an accompanying mediation of increased plasma levels of cortisol.
- Acute brain lesions, especially in the right hemisphere.

Risk factors include substance abuse, polypharmacy, surgery, structural brain pathology, chron-

TABLE 19-7.
CHARACTERISTICS OF HYPERACTIVE VERSUS HYPOACTIVE VARIANTS OF DELIRIUM

Hyperactive	Hypoactive
Increased psychomotor activity	Decreased psychomotor activity
Mixed fast and slow frequencies on EEG excitability, hyperarousal of autonomic system	Diffuse slowing on EEG
	Decreased alertness, arousal, excitability
Agitated, belligerent, restless	
Pressured speech, loud	Lethargic, drowsy, quiet, calm
Psychotic tendencies	Responds slowly to questions

Reprinted with permission from Rosen SL: Managing delirious older adults in the hospital; *Med Surg Nurs*, 1994; 3: 181–189.

TABLE 19-8.
DIAGNOSTIC CRITERIA FOR DELIRIUM DUE TO MEDICAL CONDITION

- Disturbance of consciousness (i.e., reduced clarity of awareness of the environment) with reduced ability to focus, sustain, or shift attention.
- A change in cognition (such as memory deficit, disorientation, language disturbance) or the development of a perceptual disturbance that is not better accounted for by a preexisting, established, or evolving dementia.
- The disturbance develops over a short period of time (usually hours to days) and tends to fluctuate during the course of the day.
- There is evidence from the history, physical examination, or laboratory findings that the disturbance is caused by the direct physiological consequences of a general medical condition.

Diagnostic and Statistical Manual of Mental Disorders ed. 4. Washington, DC, American Psychiatric Association, 1994, p. 129.

ic illness, impaired vision, sleep deprivation, advanced age, social isolation, unfamiliar environment, and weakened psychological defenses.

Etiology
- Physiological components include primary cerebral disease stemming from vascular insufficiency; CNS infection, trauma, or tumors; entracranial diseases, such as cardiovascular (congestive heart failure, arrhythmias); pulmonary abnormalities (pneumonia); systemic infections; metabolic disturbances; drug intoxications; endocrine problems; malnutrition and anemia; and disruption in temperature regulation.
- Psychological factors include anxiety, depression, fatigue, pain, and grief.
- Environmental factors might be unfamiliar surroundings, sensory overload or deprivation, and sleep deprivation.

Underdetection may be the result of several factors: an attitude that some degree of disorientation is normal; high incidence of hypoactive and mixed variant behaviors; the variety of names used for the syndrome; not performing comprehensive examinations; and ageism, which gives a low priority to the mental health needs of elderly individuals.

Delirium is a medical emergency. Recovery is inversely related to age and duration of syndromes. Undiagnosed patients are at risk for falls, fractures, and head injury. Delirium can progress to chronic brain impairment followed by death. Patients require a comprehensive initial assessment and ongoing assessments. Prompt diagnosis is more likely when nurses ask the questions. **Clinical management** is to first determine the underlying cause of the confusion and then aggressively treat it.

- Physiological Support. Significant attention must be given to maintaining hydration, nutrition, and electrolyte balance. As a means of assisting the patient to adjust to hospital foods, which can affect nutrition negatively, the patient is permitted as much choice as possible. To meet elimination needs provide a call bell; place urinal/bedpan within easy reach. Nursing activities should be planned so that minimal disruption occurs in the usual sleep and activity patterns. (In delirium, the sleep/wake cycle is often impaired.) Sleep-enhancing measures are implemented.

- Environment. The best environment is one that is familiar, provides many orienting clues, has a balance of sensory stimulation, and is safe. Room changes should be kept to a minimum. Family and friends should be encouraged to visit. Visitors should be educated about the patient's condition. For example, they should understand that they may frequently have to answer the same question. They should interact (including touching) as much as possible and encourage the patient to talk about familiar topics. Overnight visits should be considered. Use clocks and calendars to orient the patient to time. DO NOT support the patient's disorientation. Staff should reinforce reality-based behaviors. Control the amount of stimulation. The patient should wear assistive devices (e.g., dentures, glasses, hearing aids). Darkness contributes to confusion; having a small light on at night may be helpful. Avoid producing shadows that may be misperceived. Delirious patient should have a private room. Mechanized equipment should be clearly explained (e.g., the beeps of a monitor). Arrange for rest periods. Use television or radio when human contact is not available.

- Communication. Both content and process require attention. Address the patient by name; introduce self. Wear a name tag as an orienting clue. Have the patient's attention before beginning a conversation. Look at the patient while speaking clearly and distinctly. Do not rush; be relaxed. Assess the patient's understanding. Do not use childish tones or language. The patient will likely be anxious; reassure and support patient through verbalization, gestures, and, when appropriate, touching. Use relaxation techniques. Promote comfort and provide pain relief. Allow the patient as much independence as possible. Give the patient an opportunity to recount events that led to current problem.

- Protection. The patient with the hyperactive variant of delirium may be at increased risk for injury. Too often patients are physically and/or chemically restrained, which leads to increased confusion and greater injuries. A plethora of problems arise from the use of physical restraints, e.g., skin damage, pneumonia, elimination difficulties and other problems of immobility, as well as loss of self-image, psychological dependency, increased panic and fear, increased anger, belligerence, and agitated behavior.

  When the patient seems uncontrollable and in need of restraints for the protection of self and others, first rule out less restrictive measures. If restraints are used, they should be removed as soon as indicated, necessitating frequent reassessment by nursing staff. After restraints are removed, the patient should be questioned (debriefed) about the experience. When restraints are being used, the patient should be in a low bed, and the room should be uncluttered and harmful objects removed. Close observation can often eliminate the need for restraints, as can setting up safe areas for patients.

- Medication. Medication or other treatment modalities can be predisposing factors and/or cause delirium in older adults. Care is needed to determine what medication, how much, and how often. For psychotic components of delirium, medication should be used in an amount that will eliminate the psychotic features without sedating the patient. The butyrophenones, especially Haldol, are suggested. Watch for side effects. In general, barbiturates, sedatives, and hypnotics should be avoided.

TABLE 19–9.
DIAGNOSTIC CRITERIA FOR VASCULAR DEMENTIA

- The development of multiple cognitive deficits manifested by both
- Memory impairment (impaired ability to learn new information or to recall previously learned information)
- One (or more) of the following cognitive disturbances:
  (a) Aphasia (language disturbance)
  (b) Apraxia (impaired ability to carry out motor activities despite intact motor function)
  (c) Agnosia (failure to recognize or identify objects despite intact sensory function)
  (d) Disturbance in executive functioning (i.e., planning, organizing, sequencing, abstracting)
- Significant impairment in social or occupational functioning and a decline from a previous level of functioning.
- Focal neurological signs and symptoms (e.g., exaggeration of deep tendon reflexes, extensor plantar response, pseudobulbar palsy, gait abnormalities, weakness of an extremity) or laboratory evidence indicative of cerebrovascular disease.

Diagnostic and Statistical Manual of Mental Disorders ed. 4. Washington, DC, American Psychiatric Association, 1994, p. 146.

- **VASCULAR DEMENTIA**, also called multiinfarct dementia, is a common type of dementia. Repeated tiny strokes eventually destroy enough brain tissue that memory and other intellectual functions are impaired. Hypertension is associated with this type of dementia. Unlike Alzheimer's disease, whose course is progressive, this dementia is stepwise, producing patchy deficits. Neurological symptoms are usually evident (See Study Guide Table 19-9). Diagnosis is aided by computer tomography (CT) and magnetic resonance imaging (MRI).

- **DEMENTIA OF THE ALZHEIMER'S TYPE** (frequently referred to simply as Alzheimer's disease) is, according to NIH (1991), the most common form of dementia (20% of persons older than 85 years have it); it is the fifth leading cause of disability and the fourth leading cause of death for adult Americans. It causes intellectual impairment.

  Clinical manifestations. Definitive diagnosis of Alzheimer's disease is not possible during life. Criteria for diagnosis are listed in Study Guide Table 19-10, and the characteristics that distinguish delirium from dementia are listed

TABLE 19–10.
DIAGNOSTIC CRITERIA FOR DEMENTIA OF THE ALZHEIMER'S TYPE

- The development of multiple cognitive deficits manifested by both
- Memory impairment (impaired ability to learn new information or to recall previously learned information)
- One (or more) of the following cognitive disturbances:
  (a) Aphasia (language disturbance)
  (b) Apraxia (impaired ability to carry out motor activities despite intact motor function)
  (c) Agnosia (failure to recognize or identify objects despite intact sensory function)
  (d) Disturbance in executive functioning (i.e., planning, organizing, sequencing, abstracting)
- The cognitive deficits cause significant impairment in social or occupational functioning and represent a significant decline from a previous level of functioning.
- The symptoms have a gradual onset and continuing cognitive decline.
- The symptoms are not due to
  - Other central nervous system conditions
  - Systemic conditions that are known to cause dementia (e.g., hypothyroidism, vitamin B_{12} or folic acid deficiency, niacin deficiency, hypercalcemia, neurosyphilis, HIV infection)
  - Substance-induced conditions

Diagnostic and Statistical Manual of Mental Disorders (ed. 4.) Washington, DC, American Psychiatric Association, 1994, pp. 142–143.

in Study Guide Table 19-11.
The symptoms, which at first are mild, are progressive. The two forms of psychosis in demented patients are nonelaborate persecutory delusions and simple auditory hallucinations. Agitation will develop. Average duration of the disease is eight to ten years.

Etiology. In Alzheimer's disease abnormal fibers accumulate in the proteins of the nerve cells in the cerebral cortex of the brain (neurofibrillary tangle). Another contributor to the disease process is the degeneration of groups of nerve endings in the cortex (forming plaques) which disrupts the passage of electrochemical signals between the cells. Other factors that may also be involved are genetic predisposition, decreased levels of neurotransmitters, decreased oxygen as a result of sleep apnea, environmental toxins, dietary habits, and immune system deficits.

TABLE 19–11.
DISTINGUISHING CHARACTERISTICS OF DELIRIUM VERSUS DEMENTIA

Characteristic	Delirium	Dementia
Age of onset	Any	Usually >65, highest >85
Onset	Sudden, usually over a period of hours to days	Gradual
	Frequently during the night	
Duration	Brief, days to months	Long term, months to years
Course	Tends to fluctuate, often worse at night	Relatively stable decline
Consciousness	Clouded	Usually normal
Alertness	Tends to fluctuate	Usually normal
Cognition	Periods of lucidness	Consistent loss
Memory	Recent impaired	Recent and remote impaired
Attention	Ability to maintain or shift always impaired	Usually normal
Affect	Intermittent fear, anxiety, or puzzlement	Flat or indifferent
Judgment/Insight	Good during periods of lucidness	Poor
Sleep-wake cycle	Disrupted sometimes with a complete reversal	Sleep fragmented

Clinical management. Nurses' interventions are similar to those used in working with patients with delirium (see Study Guide Table 19-12).

- Educating the patient's loved ones is particularly important if they are the primary caregivers, but a nursing responsibility whatever their role. Safety is the first priority in education. Potentially hazardous materials need to be removed. Inappropriate clothing is stored out of reach. Clothing should be easy to put on, adjust, and remove. Schedule regular bathroom visits; night ones also. Give the patient simple tasks to do. Caregivers may need direction in finding financial assistance, legal aid, support groups, and educational materials.

- Medication may be used to decrease symptoms; however, there is presently no cure. Psychosis and other symptoms, such as excitement and hostility, may be decreased by neuroleptic use. When drugs are used, nurses must assess for any signs of extrapyramidal reactions. Tardive dyskinesia is thought to be a problem for patients who have dementia.

- **FAMILY MEMBERS MAY RESPOND IN DIFFERENT WAYS** to an ill loved one, depending on their level of coping. Caregiving functions

TABLE 19–12.
NURSING CARE PLAN: DEMENTIA

Demonstrating effective communication

Speak slowly and calmly
Use simple words and sentence structure
Ask only one question at a time
Repeat questions/statements exactly when repetition is needed

Maintaining safety

Be firm but gentle with an agitated patient
Determine the agenda/feelings behind inappropriate behaviors and wandering
Always, use least restrictive means
Provide diversional activity as needed
Be careful not to put unnecessary restraints on independence

Educating patients and family

Describe the usual progression of disease
Inform the patient of his condition/progress when patient is lucid
Teach the family orienting and reminiscing techniques: use role-play
Provide written instructions
Suggest further reading materials
Refer to community resources as needed

may be performed by a spouse, child, grandchild, or another person. Typically, the family is in denial and needs gentle but firm confrontation and education. When anger is present, listening to the family vent may be helpful. When a family feels guilt, it may be due to dilemmas about nursing home placement. Guilt related to abuse or neglect requires special intervention to protect the older adult.

The family may do too little for the elderly patient, leaving that individual vulnerable to injury or disease, or the family may do too much, contributing to the elder's feelings of uselessness. Those family members who are overinvolved may require family sessions with the elder to learn the elder's feelings about not being allowed to do for himself or herself.

Long-term care of older adults is largely maintained within the family system. With many four-generational families existing, the old are taking care of the very old. In the future, this may occur with greater frequency. The family caregiver must be educated about the aging process to help her or him differentiate normal from abnormal. Having this information will enable family members to detect small changes and problems early.

TAKING ANOTHER LOOK

You are now ready to respond to the questions that were raised in Gaining a Perspective at the beginning of this chapter. After you have written or thought about your answers, you may want to look at the Suggested Responses on page 326.

20 MOOD DISORDERS

GAINING A PERSPECTIVE

Think about the three situations described below, and after you have read the Key Concepts in this chapter, respond in greater detail.

1. How are you likely to feel when you are depressed and how do you normally deal with these feelings?

2. How would you, as a nurse, react to a patient on a psychiatric inpatient unit when the following situation occurred?

   The patient is making one telephone call after another, to florists, department stores, etc. The patient is ordering presents for his friends and family. He has a credit card and is giving that number appropriately.

3. How would you, as a nurse, feel about talking with a patient who is to sign a consent in preparation for electroconvulsive therapy?

Key Concepts

- **MOOD,** a prolonged emotion that colors the whole of psychological life, involves either elation or depression. An altered mood does not indicate a mood disorder; such a diagnosis comes from analysis of signs and symptoms that occur over a specific period of time and present a certain level of disability.

- **MOOD DISORDERS** (depressive disorders, bipolar disorders, and disorders based on a medical condition or substance abuse) are disturbances of mood with accompanying symptoms of a depressive or manic syndrome. The disorders are not completely understood by the psychiatric community. Etiology is uncertain.

  Mood disorders are frequently misdiagnosed or underdiagnosed in primary care settings, which may be because of the condition's social stigma, the patient's unwillingness to report or recognize symptoms, or the clinician's unfamiliarity with signs and symptoms. Often, diagnosing the elderly with depression is difficult, as many symptoms are similar to dementia and other common geriatric medical conditions.

  The cost of caring for individuals with mood disorders is about the same as caring for patients with cardiovascular disease, about $44 billion in the U.S. in 1990. About 70% of psychiatric hospitalizations are for individuals with mood disorders. About 15% of those hospitalized with major depressive disorders eventually commit suicide, significantly higher than the general population.

- **THE PERCENTAGE OF THE POPULATION** that will require treatment for a mood disorder is high, 5% to 20% Risk factors include:

Family and personal histories
A concurrent medical disorder
Prior suicide attempts
Being female
Inadequate support systems
Life stress
Substance abuse
A postpartum condition

- **THE CLASSIFICATION OF MOOD DISORDERS** in DSM-IV follows:

  Depressive Disorders (unipolar depression)
  Major Depressive Disorder
  Dysthymic Disorder
  Depressive Disorder Not Otherwise Specified

  Bipolar Disorders
  Bipolar Disorder I
  Cyclothymic Disorder
  Bipolar Disorder Not Otherwise Specified

  Etiologically Based Disorders
  Mood Disorder Due to a Medical Condition
  Substance-Induced Mood Disorder

- **SEVERAL THEORIES OF CAUSATION** have been put forth, including genetic, chemical, psychological, and social.

  Genetic. Studies on the high rates of depression among first-degree biologic relatives have led to the conclusion that most cases of recurrent depression have a biological basis. This does not mean that psychological factors have no role. Although studies suggest a genetic link, the specific mechanism that triggers the disorder is not explained. The rate of first-degree relatives with bipolar disorders is twice that of first-degree relatives with depression. Chromosome linkage studies have found pedigrees with linkage of bipolar disorders to markers on the X chromosome, chromosome 6, and possibly chromosome 11.

  Neurotransmission dysregulation. This theory involves a regulatory disturbance in the biogenic amine neurotransmitter systems, particularly those involving norepinephrine,

serotonin, and dopamine. The biogenic amine hypothesis is widely accepted as the predominant explanation for bipolar illness (see Study Guide Table 20-1).

Another neurotransmission theory with a connection to psychosocial theories is "kindling," a process where neurotransmission is altered by the effects of stress. External stressors trigger internal physiological stress responses, which activate an episode of depression or mania. An electrophysiological sensitivity is created to future stress; therefore, less stress is required to evoke another episode. The implication of the kindling theory is that early treatment can protect the brain from sensitivity changes. Kindling may also alter the process of selective gene expression regulation, which activates certain genes that may initiate episodic symptoms in genetically predisposed individuals.

Neuroendocrine disturbances. The disturbances occur primarily in the hypothalamic-pituitary-adrenal (HPA) axis, thereby impacting physiological responses to stress. The

TABLE 20–1.
HYPOTHESES CONCERNING THE PATHOPHYSIOLOGY OF DEPRESSION

Serotonin hypothesis: Depression is associated with an absolute or functional deficiency of brain serotonin.

Catecholamine hypothesis: Depression results from an actual or functional deficiency of catecholamines.

Dopamine hypothesis: Depression is associated with changes in dopamine metabolism.

Alpha–adrenergic receptor theory: Depression results from an increased alpha–adrenergic receptor sensitivity.

Permissive hypothesis: Diminished serotonin secretion permits a mood disorder and:
  Superimposed norepinephrine deficiency results in depression
  Superimposed norepinephrine excess results in mania

Dysregulation hypothesis: Depression is caused by a failure of the interregulation of neurotransmitter systems.

Gamma–aminobutyric acid (GABA) hypothesis: Depression is associated with changes in GABA metabolism.

Source: Wells, B G: Issues in the diagnosis of major depression. *Formulary 1995;* 30:3–9.

hypothalamus, through its endocrine function, regulates behaviors related to "fight vs. flight" response, feeding, and mating. These behaviors are often altered during a mood disturbance. Another theory is asynchronization of the circadian rhythm oscillator. Disturbance in rhythms (sleep/wake cycles) is associated with depressive symptoms and seasonal affective disorder (SAD). In addition, hormone levels, such as melatonin levels, have a major impact on mood disorders.

Anatomical abnormalities. Nuclear magnetic resonance imaging has revealed lesions in the front or temporal lobes of the brain that may be connected to mania or depression. CT scans have shown enlarged ventricles; PET scans have shown decreased metabolic activity in the brains of bipolar individuals.

Psychologic theories

- **Cognitive.** Individuals who have a cognitive style that focuses on what is wrong or negative tend to experience depressive symptoms at a higher rate than others.

- **Developmental.** Negative resolution of a developmental stage—an early experience within the family environment, such as physical/sexual abuse, parental loss, or alcoholism—may be associated with depression.

- **Psychodynamic.** The beginnings of this theory originated with Freud, who discussed how normal grief shades into the abnormal. Edward Bibring later defined depression as an ego state in which the individual's emotional expression of helplessness and powerlessness occurs and there is loss of self-esteem in reaction to three dynamic issues: (1) the wish to be worthy, loved, and appreciated; (2) the wish to be good, loving, and nonaggressive; and (3) the wish to be strong, superior, and secure. When these aspirations are threatened, self-esteem is lowered and depression develops.

Sociological theory. This theory suggests that depression is usually a response to loss. The problem is in the relationship of the individual and society.

- **DEPRESSIVE DISORDERS** are generally characterized by an inability to concentrate, hopelessness, sadness, dejection, disappointment, and demoralization, not necessarily warranted by reality. The syndrome involves a mood disturbance as well as other psychological, somatic, and cognitive issues that impair functioning. The mood state of depression may occur in a normal person, in a patient with a psychiatric syndrome, or in a medical patient. Whether the mood of depression in normal people differs from the mood of depression in people who have clinical depression has not been decided.

Major depressive disorder

A patient must, during a period of one to two weeks, exhibit at least five of the symptoms listed below that would represent a change from previous functioning. At least one must be the first or second symptom — depressed mood or diminished interest in activities.

- Depressed mood (in children and adolescents may be irritability rather than depression)
- Diminished interest or pleasure in most or all usual activities
- Significant weight loss or gain, or decrease or increase in appetite
- Insomnia or hypersomnia
- Psychomotor agitation or retardation as observed by others
- Fatigue or loss of energy
- Feelings of worthlessness, or excessive or inappropriate guilt
- Diminished ability to think or concentrate, indecisiveness
- Recurrent thoughts of death, suicidal ideation, suicide attempt, or a specific plan for suicide

EPIDEMIOLOGY. The prevalence of major depressive disorder is 5% to 9% of women and 2% to 3% of men; lower among prepubescent boys and girls; and about 13% of elderly in nursing homes. It is the most common psychiatric illness among the elderly

ETIOLOGY AND FAMILY PATTERNS. A strong familial component exists. Additional influential factors are gender and age, ethnic background, marital status, or education. Alcohol dependence in the adult first-degree biologic relatives and attention deficit hyperactivity disorder in their offspring are linked to individuals who have suffered major depression.

AGE OF ONSET AND COURSE. Average age of onset is mid-20s to early 30s. Onset is gradual and does not necessarily follow a stressful event. If untreated, the episode usually lasts from 6 to 24 months; 50% of those who suffer have a recurrence.

IMPAIRMENT AND COMPLICATIONS. The individual likely experiences reduced social, occupational, and interpersonal functioning. Laboratory findings associated with major depression include:

- Sleep electroencephalogram (EEG) abnormalities
- Abnormal dexamethasone suppression test
- Abnormal brain imaging
- Abnormalities in evoked potential studies
- Abnormalities in waking EEG

Complete remission can return, individual to normal functioning; however, those who only partially recover have higher incidences of another episode, poor recovery prognosis, long treatment, and a greater need for both medication and psychotherapy. Some individuals may go several years without an episode; some experience more episodes as they grow older.

NURSING ASSESSMENT AND DIAGNOSIS. Early diagnosis and treatment of major depressive disorder significantly improve prognosis and quality of life. The following steps are taken to assess the patient:

- Clinical interview. The interview helps to determine which, if any, of the nine specific symptoms of depression is present. A direct interview with the individual, self-report ratings, and/or a history from spouse, friend or family are included in the clinical interview. The individual interview is also used to assess the possibility of concurrent substance abuse or medication use triggering depressive symptomatology.
- Physical examination and medical history. Findings are reviewed to assess whether a medical disorder is causing or is associated with the depressive symptoms.

- Evaluation for a concurrent nonmood psychiatric condition. Study Guide Table 20-2 may be used to evaluate whether major depressive disorder or other mood disorders are present.

TREATMENT. Must always be individualized and depends on symptoms (see Study Guide Figures 20-1, 20-2, and 20-3).

- Antidepressant drugs are the primary treatment for major depression (See Chapter 42 for discussion of drugs). The response to drugs is generally positive. Nurses must understand the actions, effects, dosage schedules, interactions, contraindications, and self-care implications of the drug used.
- Electroconvulsive therapy (ECT) is usually performed for patients experiencing severe depression that has not responded to drug treatment (discussed later in chapter).
- Psychotherapy has proven to be as effective as drug therapy for milder forms of depression.
- Educating patients and their families about the disorder's clinical course and treatment enables them to dispel the myth that depression is caused by a weakness or flaw in an individual.

Dysthymic disorder

Dysthymic disorder involves a chronic prevalent depressed mood that lasts for at least two years. It is less severe but of longer duration than major depression. The mood is sadness in adults and irritability in children. Two of the following symptoms must be present:

- Insomnia/hypersomnia
- Appetite changes
- Low energy
- Low self-esteem
- Poor concentration/decision making
- Feelings of hopelessness

EPIDEMIOLOGY. Dysthymia is found in 2.1% to 4.7% of the population; it is twice as high among women (6% of women between the ages of 25 and 64 suffer from dysthymia). Fifteen percent of individuals with this disorder also experience a concurrent mood disorder.

Table 20-2

MAJOR DEPRESSIVE DISORDER SUBGROUPS

Subgroup	Essential Features	Diagnostic Implications	Treatment Implications	Prognostic Implications
Psychotic	Halucinations Delusions	More likely to become bipolar than nonpsychotic types. May be misdiagnosed as schizophrenia.	Antidepressant medication plus a neuroleptic is more effective than are antidepressants alone. ECT is very effective.	Usually a recurrent illness. Subsequent episodes are usually psychotic. Psychotic subtypes run in families. Mood-incongruent features have a poorer prognosis.
Melancholic	Anhedonia Unreactive mood Severe vegetative symptoms	May be mis-diagnosed as dementia. More likely in older patients.	Antidepressant medication is essential. ECT is 90% effective.	If recurrent, consider maintenance medicaiton.
Atypical	Reactive mood Overeating/ weight gain Oversleeping rejection sensistivity Heavy limb sensation Fewer episodes	Common in younger patients. May be misdiagnosed as personality disorder.	TCAs may be effective. MAOIs are preferred. SSRIs are preferred.	Unclear.
Seasonal	Onset, fall Offset, spring Recurrent	More frequent in nonequatorial latitudes. Pattern occurs in major depressive and bipolar disorders.	Medications have efficacy. Psychotherapy has efficacy. Phototherapy is an option.	Recurs.
Postprtum psychosis/ depression	Acute onset (<30 days) in postpartum period. Severe, labile mood symptoms. 1/1,000 is psychotic form.	Often heralds a bipolar disorder.	Hospitalize. Treat medically.	50% chance of recurring in next postpartum period.

Note: ECT—electroconvulsive therapy; TCA–tricyclic antidepressant; MAOIs–monoamine oxidase inhibitors; SSRIs–selective serotonin reuptake inhibitors.
Source: Depression in Primary Care: Vol. 1 US Dept. HHS. 1993.

Figure 20-1
Individualized Pathways Nursing Care Plan

Diagnostic Category: Major Depression

Nursing Diagnosis: DYSFUNCTIONAL GRIEVING

Related to: (check at least one)

    ☐ Denial of loss   ☐ Feelings of guilt

    ☐ Difficulty in expressing love   ☐ Multiple unsolved losses

    ☐ Repressed anger   ☐ Other

Treatment Goal: PATIENT WILL PROGRESS TOWARDS RESOLUTION OF GRIEF AND BE ABLE TO RECOGNIZE THE NORMAL STAGES OF THIS PROCESS AS WELL AS HIS OR HER RELATED POSITION.

Treatment Goal Can Be Measured Using the Following Expected Outcomes:
Patient will no longer manifest exaggerated emotion and behaviors related to dysfunctional grieving and is able to carry out ADLs independently.
Patient is able to:
a. Verbalize normal stages of the grief process.
b. Identify behaviors associated with each stage.
c. Identify own position within the grief process.
d. Appropriately verbalize feelings of grief.

Interventions: _____

Day:_____**Date :** _____

Initiated	Discontinued	
_____	_____	1. Determine the stage of grief which patient is in.
_____	_____	2. Develop a trusting relationship with patient—be empathetic and caring.
_____	_____	3. Convey an accepting attitude.
_____	_____	4. Allow expression of anger.
_____	_____	5. Provide physical outlets for healthy release of pent-up anger (punching bag, exercise, play activities, etc.).
_____	_____	6. Teach patient the normal stages of grief and the behaviors associated with each stage. Document teaching/hospital protocol.
_____	_____	7. Encourage patient to review relationship with lost concept.
_____	_____	8. Communicate to patient that crying is acceptable.
_____	_____	9. Teach adaptive coping skills. Document teaching/hospital protocol.
_____	_____	10. Offer positive feedback for use of adaptive coping skills and independent decision making (verbal praise, increased privileges). (Identify_____.)
_____	_____	11. Encourage patient to reach out for spiritual support during this time.

Figure 20-2
Individualized Pathways Nursing Care Plan

Diagnostic Category: Major Depression

Nursing Diagnosis: SELF-CARE DEFICIT

Related to: (check at least one)

☐ Disabling anxiety   ☐ Obsessive thoughts

☐ Withdrawal   ☐ Other

☐ Excessive ritualistic behavior

Treatment Goal: PATIENT WILL CONSISTENTLY DEMONSTRATE SUCCESS IN THE ACTIVITIES OF DAILY LIVING.

Treastment Goal Can Be Measured Using the Following Expected Outcomes:
Patient maintains optimal level of personal care/hygiene without assistance. (This is to include daily grooming, appropriate dressing, and adequate nutrition.)

Interventions: _____

Day:_____**Date :**_____

Initiated   **Discontinued**

_____   _____   1. Allow and encourage patient to perform normal ADLs at his or her level of ability.

_____   _____   2. Encourage independence, but intervene when patient is unable to perform.

_____   _____   3. Offer recognition and positive reinforcement of independent accomplishments. (i.e., verbal praise, increased privileges. (Identify_____.)

_____   _____   4. Show patient how to perform activities with which he or she is having difficulty.

_____   _____   5. Keep strict records of food/fluid intake.

_____   _____   6. Offer nutritious snacks and fluids between meals.

_____   _____   7. If patient is incontinent, establish routine toileting. (Schedule_____.)

Figure 20-3
Individualized Pathways Nursing Care Plan

Diagnostic Category: Major Depression

Nursing Diagnoses: DISTURBANCE IN SELF-CONCEPT (LOW SELF-ESTEEM)

Related to: (check at least one)

☐ Dysfunctional family system   ☐ Repetitive negative feedback

☐ Unmet dependency needs   ☐ Other

☐ Lack of positive feedback

Treatment Goal: BY DISCHARGE, PATIENT WILL VERBALIZE POSITIVE PERCEPTION OF SELF.

Treatment Goal Can Be Measured Using the Following Expected Outcomes:
Patient will demonstrate ability to manage personal self-care, make independent decisions, and use problem-solving skills.

Interventions: _____

Day:_____**Date :** _____

Initiated	Discontinued	
_____	_____	1. Convey unconditional positive regard for patient.
_____	_____	2. Spend time with patient on a one-to-one basis and in group activities.
_____	_____	3. Assist patient to establish realistic goals—plan activities in which success is likely. (Identify_____.)
_____	_____	4. Encourage and support patient in confronting the fear of failure by attending all therapy activities. (Identify_____.)
_____	_____	5. Assist patient in identifying additional aspects of self and in developing plans for changing the characteristics he or she views as negative.
_____	_____	6. Do not allow patient to ruminate about past failures—withdraw attention if he or she persists.
_____	_____	7. Minimize negative feedback to patient—enforce limit setting in a matter-of-fact manner.
_____	_____	8. Encourage independence in the performance of personal responsibilities, as well as in decision making related to own self-care.
_____	_____	9. Offer positive reinforcement for accomplishments (i.e., verbal praise, increased privileges). (Identify_____.)
_____	_____	10. Assist patient to increase level of self-awareness through examination of feelings, attitudes, and behaviors.

ETIOLOGY AND FAMILY PATTERNS. No universally accepted data exist regarding etiology, but dysthymia is known to be more common among first-degree biologic relatives.

AGE OF ONSET AND COURSE. Dysthymia has a clear onset, usually in childhood or adolescence, with a chronic course. Many who suffer from the disorder develop a concurrent episode of major depression, a condition known as "double depression."

IMPAIRMENT AND COMPLICATIONS. Often, dysthymic individuals can function in society, but are significantly impaired socially and occupationally. They generally experience feelings of inadequacy and insecurity, and suffer from interpersonal problems; they are at increased risk for substance abuse and suicide. A dysthymic individual may suffer from an accompanying nonmood psychiatric disorder or other nonpsychiatric disorders.

TREATMENT. Psychotherapy may be employed in the beginning. In more severe cases, medication can be used as well. Nursing care is individualized depending on symptoms (See Study Guide Figure 20-4).

Depressive disorder not otherwise specified (DNOS)

In DNOS, depressive symptoms are not as severe and of as long duration as in the other depressive disorders. DNOS frequently appears after some distinct stressor (e.g., job loss or divorce) occurs in an individual with poor coping skills and inadequate support systems.

- **IN BIPOLAR DISORDER**, the predominant mood is usually elation, expansiveness, or irritability; associated symptoms of the manic syndrome include pressured speech, hyperactivity, inflated self-esteem, flight of ideas, decreased need for sleep, and excessive involvement in activities that potentially may have painful consequences. The elated mood is often described as cheerful, euphoric, or high, and excessive for the individual. If the expansive quality of the mood is thwarted, the mood may change to irritability. Hyperactive behavior involves excessive planning and participation in multiple activities. The domineering, intrusive, and demanding nature of the interaction is not recog-

nized by the individual. Activities may have a bizarre quality, such as dressing in very colorful clothing or strange garments, wearing excessive make-up, or giving advice to passing strangers. The presence of some form of mania, the opposite of depression, is the key classification tool for bipolar disorders. Bipolar disorders are of three types: bipolar I and II and cyclothymic disorder.

Bipolar I disorder is characterized by one or more manic (or mixed) episodes, which are usually accompanied by major depressive episodes. The true manic episode involves an abnormally and persistently euphoric or irritable mood that lasts for at least one week. The mood disturbance is accompanied by at least three additional symptoms:

Inflated self-esteem
Distractibility
Increased psychomotor agitation
Racing thoughts
Decreased need for sleep
Pressured speech
Involvement in activities harmful to self or others

Depression and hypomania (less severe manic episodes) may be regularly experienced by a bipolar I individual, but are not essential to the diagnosis. Acute mania may include hallucinations or delusions.

Bipolar II disorders are characterized by one or more major depressive episodes accompanied by at least one hypomanic episode lasting at least four days. The symptoms of hypomania are less severely debilitating than those of a manic episode and do not include hallucinations or delusions. If the mood is irritability, not euphoria, then four of the manic symptoms listed above in the bipolar I description must be present.

Bipolar I and II Disorders

EPIDEMIOLOGY, ETIOLOGY, AND FAMILY PATTERNS. Males and females are equally afflicted; family history of the disorder is common.

AGE OF ONSET AND COURSE. Onset is during an individual's early 20s. Untreated manic episodes last six months; depressive episodes

CHAPTER 9

Figure 20-4
Individualized Pathways Nursing Care Plan

Diagnostic Category: Dysthymia

Nursing Diagnosis: IMPAIRED SOCIAL INTERACTION

Related to: (check at least one)

☐ Low self-esteem   ☐ Negative role modeling

☐ Unmet dependency needs   ☐ Discomfort in social situations

Treatment Goal: BY DISCHARGE, PATIENT WILL BE ABLE TO INTERACT WITH STAFF AND PEERS ON THE UNIT WITH NO INDICATION OF DISCOMFORT.

Long Term Outcomes:
1. Patient will seek out staff for social as well as therapeutic interaction.
2. Patient will willingly and appropriately participate in group activities.
3. Patient will verbalize reasons for inability to form close interpersonal relationships with others in the past.
4. Patient will maintain an appropriate interpersonal relationship with another patient.

Interventions: _____

Day:_____**Date :** _____

Initiated   **Discontinued**

_____   _____   1. Develop trusting relationship with patient, being honest and conveying accepting attitude.

_____   _____   2. Offer to remain with patient during initial interactions with others on the unit.

_____   _____   3. Provide constructive criticism and positive reinforcement for effects (i.e., verbal praise, increased privileges). (Identify_____.)

_____   _____   4. Confront patient and withdraw attention when interactions with others are manipulative or exploitative.

_____   _____   5. Act as a role model for patient through appropriate interactions with others.

_____   _____   6. Provide group situations for patient. (Identify_____.)

last eight to ten months. Full recovery usually occurs between episodes. Some individuals experience rapid cycling—four or more mood episodes a year.

IMPAIRMENT AND COMPLICATIONS. Bipolar I individuals experience considerable social and occupational impairment. Unpredictability and chronicity of the disorder can lead to joblessness, divorce, legal issues, and suicide. On the other hand, bipolar II individuals do not experience the same degree of impairment and some see a marked increase in accomplishments, efficiency, and creativity.

NURSING ASSESSMENT AND DIAGNOSIS. Assessment is similar to that done of individuals with depressive disorder, with emphasis being to determine whether mania or hypomania exists. Nursing care is individualized to meet the needs of the patient (see Study Guide Figures 20-5 and 20-6.)

TREATMENT. Lithium is the drug of choice for acute manic and hypomanic conditions. In hypomania, lithium is used alone or with a sedative. In severe mania, a neuroleptic may be added for a brief period to control the psychotic symptoms. Sometimes anticonvulsives and/or ECT is used. For individuals with severe bipolar disorder, lithium may be combined with a tricyclic antidepressant or a monamine oxidase inhibitor (MAO-I).

In pharmacologic management, nurses teach the importance of maintaining medication and the risks of potential side effects and how to handle them. Lithium commonly causes fine hand tremors, nausea, thirst, polyuria, fatigue, and mild muscle weakness.

Cyclothymic disorder

Cyclothymic disorder consists of chronic and cyclical hypomania and mild depressive episodes that last at least two years; one year in adolescents and children. An individual is not symptom-free for more than two months.

EPIDEMIOLOGY. 0.4% to 1% lifetime prevalence.

AGE OF ONSET AND COURSE. Generally begins in adolescence or early adulthood. Onset is insidious and course is chronic. 15% to 50% develop a bipolar disorder. Some individuals function well during periods of hypomania. Some

people view cyclothymic individuals as unreliable, inconsistent, and temperamental. Often patients have marital problems, perform poorly at work, and are promiscuous.

NURSING ASSESSMENT AND DIAGNOSIS. The approach to assessment is similar to that employed for patients with other mood disorders; the emphasis is on determining the severity of manic/depressive episodes, the age of onset, and duration of disorder.

- **IN ELECTROCONVULSIVE THERAPY (ECT)** an electric current is passed directly through the brain to produce a seizure, which may be demonstrated on an EEG. ECT for psychiatric patients has had both favorable and disfavorable periods of popularity. At one time, ECT was performed with the patient alert and awake. Now, the patient is paralyzed to prevent peripheral manifestations of the seizure and anesthesia (sleep) is induced to prevent the frightening sensation of having a seizure.

ECT is first-line treatment for patients who need rapid resolution of life-threatening symptoms or who respond poorly to other treatment. Although ECT is predominately used to treat adults with severe depression (high risk for suicide), it is also used to treat mania, some compulsive disorders, catatonic conditions, and certain schizophrenic syndromes. ECT is used for inpatients and outpatients. As a rule, bilateral ECT is more effective than unilateral.

The procedure is contraindicated in a variety of medical situations. Patients with a history of increased intracranial pressure, recent myocardial infarction, recent intracerebral hemorrhage, bleeding or unstable vascular aneurysm, retinal detachment, or untreated glaucoma need special evaluation.

Why ECT works is unclear. ECT causes changes in EEGs, hypothalamic hormone secretions, calcium metabolism, biogenic amine levels, and receptor sensitivity; it produces amnesia.

Patients usually receive three treatments a week for a minimum of six treatments and an average of nine treatments, with 25 treatments usually being considered the maximum. The treatment must be explained to the patient and

Figure 20-5
Individualized Pathways Nursing Care Plan

Diagnostic Category: Bipolar Disorders

Nursing Diagnosis: INEFFECTIVE INDIVIDUAL COPING

Related to: (check at least one)

☐ Inadequate support systems   ☐ Dysfunctional family systems

☐ Unmet dependency   ☐ Low self-esteem, depressed mood

☐ Depressed mood needs   ☐ Dysfunctional family systems

☐ Unresolved grief   ☐ Other_____

Treatment Goal: PATIENT WILL DEVELOP AND UTILIZE EFFECTIVE AND SOCIALLY ACCEPTABLE COPING SKILLS.

Long-Term Outcomes:
1. Patient is able to successfully resolve problems to such a degree he or she is able to fulfill the activities of daily living.
2. Patient is able to identify reasonable and appropriate skills or methods to be used to cope with stressors.

Interventions: _____

Day:_____**Date :** _____

Initiated	Discontinued	
_____	_____	1. Develop trusting relationship with patient.
_____	_____	2. Encourage patient to discuss angry feelings.
_____	_____	3. Assist patient to identify the true object of the hostility.
_____	_____	4. Provide physical outlets for healthy release of hostile feelings (i.e., punching bag, exercise, play activities, etc.).
_____	_____	5. If depressed, assess suicide potential and report findingd to physician. Document assessment/hospital protocol.
_____	_____	6. Allow patient to perform as independently as possible and provide positive feedback (i.e., verbal praise, increased privileges). (Identify_____.)
_____	_____	7. Assist patient to identify precipitant/stressor to maladaptive coping. If a major life change has occurred, encourage expressions of fears/feelings associated with the change.
_____	_____	8. Teach patient more adaptive coping skills. Document teaching/hospital protocol.
_____	_____	9. Offer positive reinforcement for use of adapting coping skills and evidence of successful adjustment (i.e., verbal praise, increased privileges). (Identify_____.)

Figure 20-6

Individualized Pathways Nursing Care Plan

Diagnostic Category: Bipolar Disorders

Nursing Diagnosis: RISK FOR VIOLENCE, SELF-DIRECTED OR DIRECTED AT OTHERS

Related to: (check at least one)

☐ Low self-esteem   ☐ Repressed anger   ☐ Suicidal threats

☐ Unresolved grief   ☐ Depressed mood   ☐ Hostility

☐ Overt aggressive acts   ☐ Unmet dependency needs

Treatment Goal: PATIENT WILL NOT HARM SELF OR OTHERS DURING HOSPITAL STAY.

Treatment Goal Can Be Measured Using the Following Expected Outcomes:
1. Patient will deny suicidal ideations.
2. Patient will deny homicidal ideations.
3. Patient will control anxiety at a level where he or she feels no need for aggression.
4. Patient will inform staff of inability to control aggressive feelings.
5. Other_____.

Interventions: _____

Day:_____**Date :** _____

Initiated	**Discontinued**	
_____	_____	1. Observe patient's behavior/special treatment procedure as ordered by physician. (Identify_____.)
_____	_____	2. Assess patient for suicide potential/risk and report findings to physician. Document assessments/hospital protocol.
_____	_____	3. Obtain a verbal/written contract from patient agreeing not to harm self and to seek out staff in the event suicidal thoughts occur.
_____	_____	4. Encourage patient to recognize and accept angry or aggressive feelings.
_____	_____	5. Provide safe physical outlets for expression of anger (i.e., punching bag, play, exercise).
_____	_____	6. Remove all dangerous objects from patient's environment.
_____	_____	7. Administer prescribed medication per physician's orders. Assess for effectiveness/adverse reactions. (Identify_____.)
_____	_____	8. Provide seclusion when necessary to decrease stimuli and agitation level.
_____	_____	9. If all other interventions fail, utilize mechanical restraints to protect patient and/or others from injury. Follow special treatment procedure/hospital policy. (i.e., appropriate documentation and prescribed protocol for care of patient in restraints). (Identify_____.)
_____	_____	10. Other_____.

family: the patient will be asleep, receive the treatment, and wake up within an hour with no memory of what happened. The patient is told that a transient memory loss will occur. Medical examination and informed consent are necessary. The steps in preparation and recovery include:

Thirty minutes prior to the treatment, assess vital signs including blood pressure to make sure that they are normal. The patient wears loose fitting clothing, is toileted, and dentures, eyeglasses, and/or contact lenses are removed. If morning treatment is planned, the patient should not have food after midnight of same day.

An intravenous (IV) line is started and 0.8 mg of atropine sulfate is administered subcutaneously 30 minutes prior to the treatment to decrease secretions.

Electrode sites on the patient's scalp are cleansed and electrodes put in place. The patient is oxygenated with an Ambu bag.

The anesthetist administers a quick-acting barbiturate intravenously to induce light sleep. When the patient is asleep, a bite block is inserted to protect the teeth. An IV muscle relaxant (Anectine 10-30mg IV at 0.5-5mg/min) is also administered.

When paralysis is confirmed, the electric stimulus is applied. Patient and vital signs are carefully monitored before and after anesthesia, during the seizure, then periodically, and after recovery. Many ECT machines have a built-in EEG monitor so that the seizure can be directly monitored. The patient usually sleeps for 20 to 30 minutes and is confused for about another 30 minutes.

During recovery, respirations and blood pressure are checked and the nurse stays with the patient to check verbalizations. The patient will need assistance to return to the unit or home.

Modifications include:

• Electronarcosis lasts three to five minutes, stimulates only the brain, and produces loss of consciousness and quivering of the muscles.

• Indoklon administered intravenously or by inhalation induces convulsions.

Nursing care for patients receiving ECT:

• Informed consent is obtained. Patients are entitled to know treatment options and the risks and benefits of ECT. Verbal and written instructions should be provided, as memory loss occurs. Family and/or significant others should also be informed about treatments. The patient should have an opportunity to reexamine and reconsider decisions periodically as ECT treatments continue.

• Education of patients/families is important. Families who understand are better able to support the patient during ECT. The many misconceptions about ECT need to be addressed, e.g., that it can change personality and that it is painful.

• Assessment of the patient's memory and confusion includes, first, a baseline evaluation of memory and cognitive functions. Then, memory is routinely monitored as ECT treatments continue. After each treatment, memory and confusion are monitored for the first 12 to 24 hours and up to 48 hours to determine supervisory needs.

TAKING ANOTHER LOOK

You are now ready to respond more comprehensively to the questions that were raised in Gaining a Perspective at the beginning of this chapter. After you have written or thought about your responses, you may wish to look at the Suggested Responses on page 327.

21 SEXUAL ISSUES, DISORDERS, AND DEVIATIONS

GAINING A PERSPECTIVE

Think about the two situations described below, and after you have read the Key Concepts for this chapter reconsider your thoughts in greater detail.

1. How would you, as a nurse, initially react in the following situation?

   A woman comes to the walk-in mental health clinic. She says she is very depressed and unable to cope with the idea that her 18-year-old son is gay. She says she learned about his sexual preference about two months ago.

2. What information must a nurse have to begin to deal with a woman who says she is having sexual problems with her husband?

Key Concepts

• **SEXUALITY IS A CHALLENGE TO HUMAN INVESTIGATION AND UNDERSTANDING.** The biologist views sexual behavior to be of fundamental significance because it perpetuates the species and thus the continuity of life itself. The psychologist sees, in the sexual impulse of human behavior, motivation that moves people into action and provides the driving force for many day-to-day activities. Sociologists recognize the integrating, cohesive functioning of sex as contributing to the stability of the family unit, and thus the entire structure of the social group. The ethicist finds that problems arise when people attempt to reconcile their basic sexual tendencies with the ideal demands of their sexual group. Although every individual is a sexual being, the expression of sexuality may be altered by personal choice, psychosocial factors, health status, or environment. Nurses encounter patients from various social and cultural groups, of every age, and with various conditions that may threaten the sexual, physical, and mental well-being of those patients.

• **DIAGNOSING SEXUAL DISORDERS TO PROVIDE INTERVENTIONS** has a fairly short history. With the pioneering work of Masters and Johnson in the 1960s, sexual problems became worthy of assessment and treatment. The strong religious influence on sexual behavior dates back to biblical times. Sigmund Freud in the late 19th and early 20th centuries wrote that sexual drives begin in infancy but could be arrested at any stage of development by psychological conflict and trauma. What was repressed at an early age settled into the unconscious; symptoms continued to affect adult behavior or the repressed sexual desire was sublimated into productive aspects of personality function.

- **SEX THERAPY** is a health care specialty that has evolved due to Masters and Johnson (1966). They considered sexual dysfunction, without a medical cause, to be learned behavior fostered by ignorance, performance anxiety, and poor communication. Based on these assumptions, Masters and Johnson developed a system to treat sexual problems through directive psychotherapy, improved communication skills, education, and desensitization.

- **SEXUAL RESPONSE PATTERNS** for males and females consist of four phases: excitement, plateau, orgasm, and resolution. Each phase has specific sex organ and general responses. The length of each phase varies greatly, the longest being excitement and resolution. Orgasmic response in males often differs from that in females.

- **SEXUAL AROUSAL** in humans is expressed in ways that may or may not include orgasmic discharge and does not preclude abstinence and conscious suppression of sexually charged stimuli.

- **HETEROSEXUAL MODES OF EXPRESSION**
  Petting: involves simple kissing to mutual genital stimulation without intercourse.
  Intercourse: insertion of the penis into the vagina.
  Oral genital contact: includes fellatio and cunnilingus.
  Anal sex: insertion of the penis into the anus.
  Autoeroticism: manipulating the genitals with the hand or a mechanical device.
  Abstinence: either total or varying degrees of withdrawal from sexual activity without intercourse.

- **HOMOSEXUAL MODES OF EXPRESSION** for males include massage, mutual masturbation, fellatio, body rubbing, and anal intercourse. Multiple sex, sadomasochism, sexual devices, and pornographic material and stimulants may be used. For lesbians, the emphasis is often tenderness and love and includes cunnilingus and masturbation; dildos may be used.

- **SEXUAL PREFERENCE** refers to sexual attraction. A homosexual is a person whose sexual preference, or orientation, is members of his or her own gender. According to the Kinsey Report (1948), 37% of American men have had at least one homosexual experience and 4% have been exclusively homosexual from adolescence onward; exclusive lesbianism is about 2% to 3%. In 1989 Warren Gadpaille estimated that 6% to 10% of males and 2% to 4% of females may be exclusively homosexual; others say 1% to 2% of the adult population.

The etiology of homosexuality has long been debated: physical and psychological environment or biology. Today research is focused on the part genes play, in contrast to the Freudian focus on resolving Oedipal conflict.

Until 1973, homosexuality was listed in the DSM as a sexually deviant behavior, but in the 1980 DSM it was not included as a mental disorder. Researchers are studying twins and the brain to determine relative roles of genetics and environment. If homosexuality is determined to have a biological basis and be a normal variant of constitution, then it may lose the long-standing moral stigma placed on it by many.

Many families have difficulty accepting that a son or daughter is homosexual. Parents may blame themselves or believe that it is a temporary stage of their child's development. A 1989 U.S. Department of Health and Human Services study indicated that 26% of youths who tell their parents about their homosexuality are ostracized by them. Many youths end up on the streets involved with drugs or prostitution and at risk for AIDS and suicide.

Gay and lesbian people seek counseling for diverse reasons, as other groups do. The role of the psychiatric nurse is to provide the best possible care in an accepting environment where gay and lesbian people are treated with dignity and respect. Homosexual individuals have the same emotional problems as others who seek help. Their sexual orientation is seldom why they seek counseling, as many have come to terms with their homosexuality.

Some gay people may seek counseling for stress they experience in making decisions about their sexual preference. They may lead dual lives. They may be married and have conflicts about revealing their sexual preference, one reason being they may lose custody of their children. The stress is part of the necessary transition of integrating oneself within a family, a social network, and at work.

In an outpatient mental health setting, the psychiatric nurse conducts an initial assessment. The history includes identifying information, the present complaint, psychiatric and social histories, medical history, family background, mental status, formulation of problem, and diagnosis. This process determines the nurse's interventions in diagnosis and treatment planning. The problems that homosexuals have in coping with the demands of life and interpersonal relationships are for the most part similar to those of heterosexuals with the exception of "coming out." Coming out is a process that usually extends over many years. It usually begins in childhood with feelings of being different from others of the same sex. The stages generally are acknowledging one's homosexuality, accepting homosexuality after disclosure to others, and being able to develop intimate sexual relationships with members of one's own sex. During the initial interview and in subsequent meetings with patients who appear uncomfortable with their sexual orientation, it is important to be aware of the underlying feelings of social victimization, suicidal thoughts, and substance abuse. Building and sustaining a sense of self-esteem is a major task in the face of social hostility.

Nurses also need to assess themselves for homophobic feelings, and, if they exist, deal with them in supervision. The nurse must be acutely aware of the tendency to assume all patients are heterosexual. Psychiatric nurses can lead in advocating respect and acceptance of all people regardless of their background, which includes sexual orientation.

- **SEXUAL DYSFUNCTION** is a disruption of sexual behavior or extreme variation of sexual behavior. As a disruption, sexual dysfunction is defined by disturbances in one or more phases of the sexual response cycle, by excessive pain, or by phobic avoidance of sex. As an extreme variation of sexual behavior, sexual dysfunction is defined by the object that is required for sexual arousal and release or by the disregard one has for the rights of, damage to, pain, fear, and sensitivities of another person.

  Biophysiological etiology

  Ill health is one of the greatest detriments to sexual expression. In illness, energy is used to recuperate. In addition, illness often lowers an individual's sense of personal worth and attractiveness.

  - Medical conditions can lead to sexual dysfunction.

    Diabetes causes gradual impotence in about 50% of males and orgasmic dysfunction in 35% of females. It is irreversible.

    Alcoholism results in impotence in 40% of males, decreased libido in 30% to 40%, and retarded ejaculation in 5% to 10%. In females, 30% to 40% have difficulties with sexual arousal and 15% have loss or reduction of orgasmic frequency.

    Renal failure with the use of hemodialysis affects males in that 90% have depressed libido and 80% have erectile difficulties. Among females, 80% have depressed libidos, 70% have difficulty in sexual arousal, and 50% have reduced orgasmic response.

    Cardiovascular disease, if pain or weakness accompanies the disease, may inhibit sexual expression. Following a heart attack, many patients, due to fear or ignorance, restrict their sexual activity.

  - Drugs can create sexual side effects; change of drug or dosage reverses the condition.

    Antihypertensives frequently affect sexual performance.

    Psychotropic drugs
    - MAO inhibitors cause impotence.
    - Tranquilizers create fatigue.
    - Heroin and methadone cause decreased libido in 80% to 90% of users.
    - Barbiturate abuse results in impotence and response difficulties among females.

  - Intrapsychic etiology.

    Fear of
    - Failure (performance anxiety).
    - Displeasing one's partner or being displeased oneself.

- Abandonment or rejection.
- Loss of control.

Traumatic sexual experience.

Cultural or religious taboos.

Severe stress or depression.

Low self-esteem.

Poor body image.

- Interpersonal etiology

Quality of partner's sexual interaction.

Lack of knowledge about sexual anatomy.

Poor communication about sexual preferences.

Nursing diagnosis and intervention

Objective and subjective data are essential. The more closely the objective evidence coincides with a definitive etiology, the more apt the intervention is to be specific. When sexual dysfunction is medical in etiology, nursing care focuses on educating and counseling the patient regarding the dysfunctional process, its treatment, and the patient's response. Nursing intervention is often directed toward both the patient and the partner.

- For medical problems, nursing interventions might include:

Assess and establish existence of intact sexual response patterns and no extreme variation of sexual behavior.

Establish clear definition of primary medical problem (e.g., heart attack).

Establish how sexual behavior influences the medical problem.

Clarify perceptions (the patient's and significant other's) regarding the medical problem's relationship to sexual functioning.

Provide counseling and instruction about focused exercises to enhance functioning.

Evaluate effectiveness of interventions.

- For minor dysfunctions, nursing care includes:

Explaining causal connection between attitudinal set and behavior and its relationship to sexual concern.

Gaining cooperation and agreement to work for change.

Clarifying that change is compatible, comfortable, and acceptable to the patient and partner.

Evaluating outcome. If it is unsatisfactory, reassess the patient and, if necessary, refer for further evaluation or more specific psychiatric treatment of psychological or relationship problem.

Symptoms of sexual dysfunction may be used as defenses by the individual, to avoid commitment and intimacy. When symptoms are removed, an imbalance in the relationship and underlying psychological difficulties may come to the forefront.

- **SEXUAL DYSFUNCTION DISORDERS** are of four major types.

Sexual desire disorders involve lack of sexual desire and aversion to sex.

- Hypoactive sexual desire is the most common complaint of couples.
  - Variety of stressors identified as the cause, e.g., job conflict, marital disharmony, or suppressed homosexual wishes.
  - Medical causes, e.g., alteration in neural hormones.
  - For chronic problem in the physically healthy, functioning individual, psychotherapy and sex therapy may be useful.
  - For short-term problems related to stress and depression, focus on reducing stressors and patterns of avoidance; explore the cause—may be loss of spouse.

Sexual arousal disorders may be caused by psychological or medical problem or substance abuse.

- In female sexual arousal disorder a woman has difficulty with lubrication and swelling response. A persistent lack of sexual excitement and pleasure is reported.
- In male erectile disorder there is a consistent failure to attain erection or maintain it until sexual activity is completed; a lack of sexual excitement and pleasure is reported.

Orgasm disorder

- In female orgasmic disorder orgasm is either delayed or absent following a normal excitement phase.
- In male orgasmic disorder orgasm is either delayed, absent, or premature.
- Nursing intervention should reflect an understanding of the impact of the medical

problem and treatment regimen and focus on rehabilitative measures. Patient education and counseling in conjunction with the medical regimen constitute primary nursing interventions.

- The etiologic condition may be the result of psychological causes. Expectations play a large role in interfering with the sexual response pattern. In providing care, the nurse should present etiologic factors that when considered by the patient may alter some women's sexual response patterns.

Sexual pain disorders

- Dyspareunia, painful involuntary spasm of the outer third of the vagina, interferes with sexual intercourse. Pain is most often not based on organic causes, but nursing intervention must ensure that the patient is thoroughly evaluated for underlying organic causes.

  Nurses may intervene using the cognitive technique of thought stopping and reeducation with patient and partner. Sex therapy provokes anxiety and requires motivation.

- Traumatic events, for example rape, incest, or a brutalizing abusive experience, may cause the patient to later experience sexual pain disorder. Counseling about the unresolved trauma would be a primary intervention. Pain may be a defense against pleasure, and unless acceptance of pleasure is established, removing the pain may provoke intense anxiety and cause withdrawal from counseling.

  Nursing interventions should be appropriate for the cause of the disorder — medical or psychogenic. Interventions may include education, general counseling about personal relationship issues, or focused exercises to alter the cognitive sets or physical behavior. The partner is included.

  Nursing diagnosis may be sexual dysfunction or altered sexual patterns or rape trauma syndrome or others.

- **SEXUAL AVERSION DISORDER** is a persistent or recurring extreme aversion to and avoidance of all or almost all genital sexual contact with a sexual partner. The patient must be evaluated for underlying panic disorder. When panic

response is reduced (medication may be used) and psychotherapy and sex therapy are combined, results may be favorable. Simple phobias respond to psychotherapy or behavior therapy and education. When panic or phobia avoidance is evident, referral is appropriate.

- **SEXUAL DEVIATION** is a variation in behavior in which little or no regard is shown for the welfare of another person. Behavior is compulsive and repetitive, and interventions require a specialist. These individuals are in many settings, e.g., home, prison, and the health care system. Nurses may provide services to the victims of people with this sexual dysfunction or refer victims for services. The victim may need to be hospitalized.

- **PARAPHILIAS** are characterized by arousal in response to sexual objects or situations that are not part of normal arousal activity patterns and that in varying degrees may interfere with the capacity for reciprocal affectional activity. Diagnosis is made only if the person acts on urges or is markedly distressed by them.

  Persons with paraphilia commonly suffer from several varieties such as exhibitionism, fetishism, frotteurism, pedophilia, sexual masochism, sexual sadism, transvestic fetishism, and voyeurism. Criteria for severity are:

  Mild. The person is markedly distressed by the recurrent paraphilic urge but has never acted on them.

  Moderate. The person occasionally acts on the paraphilic urge.

  Severe. The person repeatedly acts on the paraphilic urge.

  It is predominately a male disorder. Common features are an inability to cope with closeness and attachment to other adults and loneliness as part of social separation. Usually individuals cope by withdrawing into a secret, comfortable world of fantasy. Paraphilia involves obsessive-compulsive behavior patterns; clinically it is similar to addiction. Paraphiliacs are unresponsive to nondeviant affectional sexual stimuli; they are dependent on highly specific imaginary or socially inappropriate external stimulation to achieve sexual arousal.

  Addictive components. Paraphiliacs experience an almost "trance-like" sense of relaxation, relief, and homeostasis when involved in the illicit sexual activity and exhibit social distress when not sexually "acting-out." They evidence adolescent-like narcissism. Because of their chronically low self-esteem, self-deprecatory preoccupations, and poor assertiveness skills, paraphiliacs feel victimized. They feel an overwhelming sense of inadequacy and lack of control. These sexual addicts are being pushed by their "sickness" and spend hours each day searching for the right situation to "act out." The "acting out" experience becomes an expression of rage or an attempt at control.

Pedophilia. This sexual deviation involves a sexual act with a nonthreatening child. Because pedophiles' social development has been impeded, they typically verbalize a sense of uneasiness with other adults. Psychosocial trauma has caused a fixation or an impediment to their cognitive maturation; therefore, pedophiles often feel, think, and act like a child.

Incest offenders. Offenders may or may not be paraphiliacs, although many are or are clinically similar. Many incest offenders are pedophiles who have married and continue their pedophilia with greater safety by sexually approaching their own child or a stepchild. The husband-wife relationship in the incestuous family evolves into one of an immature, undifferentiated couple, creating confusion, habitual conflict, and destructive dependent relationships. Homes reflect any combination of chaos, enmeshment, disengagement, and rigidity. The husband or wife is likely to be alcoholic; if nonalcoholic, the offender may display more psychopathology. Some are authoritarian and physically abuse other family members. Usually male incest perpetrators are intimidated by other men; they are uneasy in work and social interactions.

Voyeurism. The voyeur becomes sexually aroused observing unsuspecting people, usually strangers, who are either naked, disrobing, or engaging in sexual activity; no sexual activity is sought. Orgasm is produced by masturbation either during the voyeurism or lat-

er in response to the memory of it.

Transvestic fetishism. An individual has recurrent, intense sexual urges and sexually arousing fantasies involving cross-dressing, lasting at least six months, and usually masturbates while cross-dressed.

Exhibitionism. The exhibitionist, typically a heterosexual man, becomes sexually aroused by exposing genitals to an unsuspecting stranger, usually a woman or girl.

Frotteurism. A frotteur is one who becomes sexually stimulated by rubbing against (and fondling) a nonconsenting person, usually done in a crowded place. Generally the frotteur fantasizes a caring relationship with his victim. The victim does not usually protest, as she cannot imagine such a provocative act in a public place.

Fetishism. The person becomes sexually aroused by an inanimate object, such as shoes or women's clothing. The person may masturbate while holding, rubbing, or smelling the object or ask his partner to wear the fetish object during sexual intercourse. Erectile failure may occur in the absence of the fetish object.

Sexual masochism. Sexual pleasure is derived from being humiliated, beaten, bound, or otherwise made to suffer. Masochistic acts may be fantasized; sometimes they are done with a partner. Hypopilia, a particularly dangerous form, involves sexual arousal by oxygen deprivation and the person escapes asphyxiation before consciousness is lost. Reducing oxygen to the brain achieves an altered state of consciousness, which enhances erotic sensation and fantasy. It may result in an autoerotic death. Other kinds of death that result from masturbation ritual and autoeroticism are often not suspected. The nurse, particularly in the emergency room, may be consulted by police regarding the possibility that the death was autoerotic. The nurse may also be part of an intervention team that provides care to the families of these individuals. The emotional response of the family is particularly traumatic when the body is discovered by family members. The family needs encouragement to share feelings; counseling referrals should be made because the family is at high risk for unresolved grief.

Sexual sadism. Sexual arousal, in sexual sadism, is caused by the suffering of another. It is associated with antisocial personality disorder. The victim is in danger of serious harm or death.

- **GENDER AND SEXUALITY** are extremely complex subjects.

  Gender is distinguished by eight variables:
  - Chromosomal gender: XX in the female; XY in the male
  - Gonadal gender: ovaries in the female; testes in the male
  - Prenatal hormonal gender: estrogen and progesterone in the female; testosterone in the male
  - Internal accessory organs: uterus and vagina in the female; prostate and seminal vesicles in the male
  - External genitalia: clitoris and vaginal opening in the female; penis and scrotum in the male
  - Pubertal hormonal gender: estrogen and progesterone in the female; testosterone in the male
  - Assigned gender: the announcement at birth, "It's a girl" or "It's a boy," based on the external genitals; the gender that parents and society believe the child to be; the gender in which the child is reared
  - Gender identity: the person's private internal sense of maleness or femaleness, which is expressed in personality and behavior, and the integration of this sense with the rest of the personality and the gender roles prescribed by society

    In most cases the variables of an individual's gender are in agreement.

  Sexuality is learned and it is influenced by biology.
  - Biologic influences

  The complex human sexual system, under control of hormones (signaled by chromosomal patterns), begins with gonadal differentiation: male testes and female ovaries. Once the sex of the embryo is established by gonadal development, the ducts of the other sex remain undeveloped in an individual and degenerate. Genetic defects include:

  - Hermaphroditism, which results if a male is deprived of androgens. The hermaphrodite is born with both testicular and ovarian tissue. Pseudohermaphrodites have gonads that match their sex chromosomes but their genitals match the other sex.

  - Klinefelter's syndrome, which is a condition in males in which the male has an extra X chromosome; at maturity testosterone production is reduced, testes are abnormal, and sperm production does not occur. The condition may improve.

  - Turner's syndrome, which is the absence of an X chromosome resulting in nonfunctioning ovaries and the absence of menstruation. Infertility, short stature, and a variety of abnormalities that may involve facial appearance and internal organs occur. Drugs, particularly hormones taken by the mother, could affect the fetus.

Theories about gender and sexuality

- Social learning theory model. Gender development is learned from personal role models and the cultural influences that the child experiences during growth. A child learns sex-typed behavior through combined reward, punishment, and observation of other people.

- Cognitive-development theory. Children form a firm gender identity around 5 or 6 years of age, when they understand that gender is constant. Children learn by observation and imitation to obtain self-identity.

- Biosocial interaction theory. Phases in sexual development influence gender development. They include prenatal programming, psychology, and society's norms and their interactions with biologic factors.

- **IN GENDER IDENTITY DISORDER** individuals are uncomfortable with their actual sex and its gender roles and have a fervent desire to be a member of the opposite sex. For a child to be diagnosed with gender identity disorder the following five criteria must be met:
  - A wish to be of the other sex

- A preference for clothing of the other sex
- Fantasies of being the other sex, or a preference for roles of the other sex
- Wish to engage in the sex play of the other sex
- Preference for playmates of the other sex

Adults with this disorder state that they were born the wrong sex and wish to be or be treated as a person of the other sex. They may request surgery to change. Symptoms may include self-loathing or a disgust with their genitals. There is marked preoccupation with:

- Being the wrong sex
- A feeling of being in the wrong body
- A deep and abiding preoccupation of being of the other sex (sex role identification)

TAKING ANOTHER LOOK

You are now ready to respond in more depth to the two situations that were presented in Gaining a Perspective at the beginning of this chapter. After you have written or thought about your responses, you may wish to look at the Suggested Responses on page 328.

22 EATING DISORDERS

TERMS TO DEFINE

anorexia nervosa

binge eating disorder

bulimia nervosa

bulimic anorexia

nonpurging bulimia

obesity

purging

purging bulimia

restricting anorexia

GAINING A PERSPECTIVE

Think about the questions below, and after you have read the Key Concepts for this chapter reconsider the questions and respond in more depth.

1. Why do you think the incidence of eating disorders seems to be increasing?

2. How would you, as a nurse, deal with the following situation?

   A 17-year-old female patient has a diagnosis of bulimia. The patient is permitted to eat in a group dining room on the unit. After dinner, however, the patient is not permitted to return to her room, but is expected to remain in the dayroom for at least one hour, where staff members are able to see her. The patient insists she must return to her room.

Key Concepts

- **AN IMPORTANT ETIOLOGIC FACTOR IN EATING DISORDERS** is believed to be this society's emphasis on beauty and fashion. During the past 25 years, about 8% of the U.S. population, predominately women, has experienced an eating disorder. (These disorders were first described in the 1870s but not commonly diagnosed until the 1970s.) Women often feel pressured to mirror today's image of the ideal woman who is thin. This stereotype creates stressors that can lead to guilt, shame, and for some, a pattern of behavior that is harmful to the self. Given these and many other stressors women experience, a few women develop eating disorders to gain control of their lives.

  Primary symptoms are preoccupation with weight and a strong desire to be thinner; generally a psychological struggle to maintain a sense of personal autonomy and self-control is involved. Considerable morbidity and mortality can arise from consequent physical problems, many of which can not be diagnosed in isolation. Two eating disorders, anorexia nervosa and bulimia nervosa, are classified in the DSM-IV. Binge eating and obesity have also gained considerable attention.

  Epidemiology. Eating disorders are more common in women than men; 95% of persons with eating disorders are women; 1% to 5% suffer from anorexia nervosa and 6% to 18% from bulimia nervosa. Athletic women are more likely to suffer from one of these disorders (ballet dancers, gymnasts, and runners).

  Etiologic factors and family patterns. The multidimensional nature of the disorders makes it difficult to determine precise etiologic factors. Assessment and treatment require that the interrelationship of biologic, psychologic, and sociologic factors be understood.

  Biologic theories

  - Hypothalamic abnormality. This theory accounts for low serum-estrogen levels; disturbances in secretion of follicle-stimulating hormone, luteinizing hormone, and cortisol; and deviations in opioid and catecholamine metabolism (one problem is that data are based on patients with severe eating disorders).

- Genetic basis. There is division over the theory. A familial pattern is seen, but studies have not shown whether the influence is genetic or environmental.
- Relationship to mood disorder. The resemblances in neuroendocrine dysfunction, neurotransmitter dysregulation, and patient response to antidepressant medication have shown a link between mood and eating disorders, especially the bulimic syndromes. Major depression frequently occurs prior to the onset of an eating disorder. There is recurrent co-morbidity of affective disturbance and eating disorders.
- Autointoxication. Exercising and dieting may cause autointoxication with endogenous opioids. Opioids can initially produce pleasurable feelings.

Psychologic theories

- Cognitive distortion. Socially awkward adolescents misperceive what others think of their physical appearance. The adolescent especially tends cognitively to overgeneralize, take things too personally, magnify events, and view the world in absolutes.
- Perceived distortion. One's perception of body width is distorted, which may create the sense of being fat. Other perceptive problems deal with identifying emotional states and hunger/satiety.
- Maladaptive stress response.
- Developmental conflict. Adolescent discord over "growing up" can lead to regression and inability to deal with developmental issues.
- Low self-esteem.
- Familial factors. Family characteristics such as being overinvolved with the child's life/activities, overprotective, having rigid communication patterns, and avoiding conflict tend to be present, as is a family history of depression, alcoholism, or chronic dieting.

Sociological theories

- Maturational differences between the sexes.
- Societal ideals and values.

Age of onset and course. Onset is generally in adolescence or young adulthood and may be triggered by a stressful life event. About 30% to 50% of anorexics recover fully in a few years. For bulimics, however, the disorder is usually chronic and can last for decades. Periods of remission occur and about 40% recover.

Nursing assessment and diagnosis. Key is to recognize the psychophysiological impact of associated medical and psychological conditions. Assessment is through history taking, asking about patterns of daily living (e.g., exercise, menstruation, meals), physical examination, and laboratory studies.

- **ANOREXIA NERVOSA** is a complex disorder involving behavioral, physiological, and psychological changes related to an obsession with thinness. In children and adolescents, body weight is 15% below expected. Weight loss results in significant problems, which if left untreated could lead to death. Eating behavior becomes bizarre in an effort to loss weight.
  - Tendency to eat alone
  - Use of unusual spices and food flavorings
  - Low caloric intake (300 to 600 calories per day)
  - Excessive compulsive exercise
  - Avoidance of certain groups of foods

Anorexics are obsessed with thinking about food and preparing it, with little actual eating. Low self-esteem is common. Other psychological problems, often compounded by drug and alcohol abuse, include depression, emotional lability, erratic behavior, and an irritable mood. There are two subgroups:

Restricting anorexic limits food intake, is socially withdrawn, and exhibits obsessive and ritualistic behaviors not related to food.

Bulimic anorexic experiences food binges and/or purges by self-induced vomiting or misuse of laxatives, enemas, or diuretics.

Impairments and complications. Five to ten percent die within 10 years from starvation, suicide, and electrolyte imbalances; 20% die within 20 years of onset. Harmful effects include muscle wasting, arrhythmias, fat depletion, constipation, lethargy, osteoporosis, and in severe cases, cachexia and lanugo. All females stop menstruating and experience alterations in thyroid and reproductive functioning. Anorexics have a higher incidence (50%) of major depressive disorders; 25% have obsessive-compulsive disorder. Other psychological impairments include social withdrawal, irritability, insomnia, and decreased interest in sex. These symptoms may be secondary to the effects of starvation.

Treatment. A multidisciplinary approach is needed (see Study Guide Table 22-1). How well a patient complies with the treatment plan is closely connected with the degree of trust developed between the psychiatric nurse and patient. Because of the illness, the early nurse-patient relationship will involve some secretive patient behaviors. The following measures may help create an environment that discourages such behaviors:

- Have the patient eat meals with other people.
- Carefully check the eating tray and record what is eaten.
- Have the patient remain in a public area for at least one hour after eating.
- Check the patient's room regularly.

Nursing care is individualized to meet the patient's needs (see Study Guide Figure 22-1).

- **PATIENTS WITH BULIMIA NERVOSA** are females who are preoccupied with their weight and who have eating binges when they will consume from 5,000 to 10,000 calories and purging episodes at least two times a week for three consecutive months. Prior to binging, the individual has a dysphoric mood, interpersonal stress, and intense hunger. After binging, the depressed mood returns along with feelings of guilt and shame. Two types of bulimics are:

Binging bulimics who use self-induced vomiting or laxatives (18 pills a day) and/or diuretics.

Nonpurging bulimics who exercise excessively or fast.

Typical behavior involves avoiding social eating situations, secretive eating, compulsive exercise, disappearance after meals, and unrelenting overconcern expressed about weight and body shape.

Impairments and complications. Seventy-five percent of bulimics have a concurrent major depressive or anxiety disorder and higher rates of chemical dependency and personality disorders. Several physical problems may develop.

- Fluid and electrolyte abnormalities may in-

TABLE 22–1.

TREATMENT APPROACH TO ANOREXIA NERVOSA

1. Assess and treat the medical complications of starvation. Determine whether purging is present, and treat for dehydration and electrolyte imbalance as necessary.
2. Decide whether hospitalization is necessary. If dizziness, lightheadedness, or fainting from bradycardia or hypotension is reported, if any sign of congestive heart failure is present (including reports of dyspnea on exertion), fluid and electrolyte balance cannot be maintained, excessive exercise presents a risk of congestive heart failure and cannot be monitored safely on an outpatient basis, cognitive impairment from starvation precludes the utility of outpatient psychotherapy, or the patient reports mental exhaustion from battling food and eating issues, hospitalization is essential. Hospitalization is also indicated when reasonable outpatient efforts have failed.
3. Complete laboratory investigation. This includes a full electrolyte profile including potassium, magnesium, calcium and phosphates, glucose, complete blood count (CBC), erythrocyte sedimentation rate (ESR), total protein, albumin, liver function tests, renal function tests, thyroid function tests, iron, folate, B12, electrocardiogram (ECG), chest X-ray, and bone-density studies.
4. Restore nutritional balance through normal eating, and encourage weight gain. This often involves setting up a behavior-modification protocol. Low-dose neuroleptics or benzodiazepine-class anxiolytics may be used if fear of weight gain is excessive. Cyproheptadine may be useful to encourage weight gain in cases where weight loss is extreme.
5. Diagnose and treat psychiatric co-morbidity. The presence of affective disorder may warrant the use of antidepressant medications. These medications may not be especially effective when patients are significantly underweight, but may be very effective when weight gain has occurred. Issues stemming from personality disorders should be addressed in psychotherapy.
6. Identify and treat underlying ideas, attitudes, and psychological conflicts. Treat with cognitive and/or psychodynamically based psychotherapy.
7. Assess the family. Utilize family therapy to facilitate support for the patient and to address family dynamics that may be contributing to the patient's development of illness.
8. Provide ongoing support. Support healthy diet and exercise habits, constructive approaches to self, family, and interpersonal problems, enhanced self-esteem, and a sense of autonomy with ongoing psychotherapy.

From: Norman, K: Eating disorders, in Goldman HH (ed): Review of General Psychiatry, ed. 4. Stamford, CT; Appleton & Lange, 1995.

Figure 22-1
Nursing Pathway Plan of Care

DSM-IV Diagnoses: ANOREXIA NERVOSA

Nursing Diagnosis: DISTURBANCE IN SELF-CONCEPT (LOW SELF-ESTEEM)

Related to: (check at least one)

☐ Lack of positive feedback.
☐ Preoccupation with appearance and how others perceive them.
☐ Unmet dependency needs.
☐ Perceived failures.
☐ Threat to security secondary to dysfunctional family dynamics.

Short-term outcome: Patient will verbalize three positive aspects of self and exhibit decreased preoccupation with own appearance.

Long-term outcome:
1. Patient will verbalize five positive aspects of self.
2. Patient will express interest in welfare of others and decreased preoccupation with own appearance.

Interventions: _____

Day:_____**Date :** _____

Initiated   **Discontinued**

_____   _____   1. Assist patient to recognize his or her positive attributes

_____   _____   2. Offer positive reinforcement for independent decision making (i.e., verbal praise, encouragement, increased privileges).

_____   _____   3. Offer positive reinforcement when honest feelings related to autonomy/dependency issues remain separated from maladaptive eating behaviors (i.e., verbal praise, encouragement, increased privileges).

_____   _____   4. Assist patient to develop a realistic perception of body image and relationship with food.

_____   _____   5. Promote feelings of control within the environment through participation, independent decision making, and offering reasonable choices whenever possible.

_____   _____   6. Help patient realize that perfection is unrealistic and explore this need.

_____   _____   7. Teach patient to claim angry feelings and to recognize that expressing them is acceptable if done in an appropriate manner.

Source: Adapted from nursing care plans developed by nursing staff at 1st Hospital Wyoming Valley, Wilkes Barre, PA, under the direction of Theresa Croushore.

clude fluid volume depletion, metabolic acidosis, and bicarbonate imbalance leading to a lower seizure threshold.

- Gastrointestinal tract problems may include cathartic colitis and bleeding.
- Dental enamel erosion and decay may result from acidic vomitus.
- Parotid and salivary glands may become enlarged.

Many bulimics deny their physical problems to avoid detection. Bulimia is an insidious disorder and often goes undetected. Therefore, health care professionals must be knowledgeable about the nature of the disorder.

Treatment. Medical complications are treated first, as with anorexia nervosa. Psychoeducation and psychotherapy follow to help change attitudes (see Study Guide Table 22-2). Antidepressants and cognitive behavior thera-

TABLE 22–2.
TREATMENT APPROACHES TO BULIMIA NERVOSA

1. Evaluate and treat the medical complications associated with bulimia nervosa. Replace fluid and electrolytes as necessary. Monitor electrolytes on a regular basis. Refer for dental evaluation.
2. Ascertain the mechanism of purging. Educate patients about the medical dangers of chemical purgatives such as ipecac and baking soda, as well as of diuretic and laxative abuse.
3. Hospitalize when necessary. If fluid and electrolyte balance cannot be maintained, episodes of fainting occur, concentration impairment makes employment or schoolwork impossible to perform, or binge eating and purging behavior are the dominant activities in the patient's life, a brief hospitalization is necessary to break the cycle and initiate treatment.
4. Diagnose and treat co-morbidity. The presence of an affective disorder is an indication for treatment with an antidepressant medication if such treatment has not already been initiated on the basis of bulimic symptoms alone. Indeed, a trial of antidepressant medication is generally indicated for bulimia nervosa and is often effective even in the absence of concurrent affective disorder. Issues pertaining to personality disorders, when present, should be addressed in psychotherapy.
5. Identify and address psychological and cognitive underpinnings of bulimic behavior. Psychodynamically oriented and cognitive behavior therapy that addresses attitudes and feelings related to self and body images are effective treatment modalities. Such treatments may be especially effective for many patients when combined with antidepressant medications. Support groups are also often helpful in the treatment of bulimia nervosa.

From: Norman, K: Eating disorders, In Goldman HH (ed): Review of General Psychiatry, ed. 4. Stamford, CT; Appleton & Lange, 1995.

py are often successful. Keeping a food diary helps to keep track of what has been eaten and what feelings were present prior to, during, and after eating. The patient learns to identify what triggers eating behaviors and eventually to cope with them. Nursing care is individualized. (See Study Guide Figures 22-2 and 22-3.)

- **OBESITY** is a disorder in which the person weighs 20% more than ideal weight. One subgroup of obesity is defined by emotionally based patterns of overeating. For these individuals, dieting creates substantial biologic and psychosocial stress.

Epidemiology. Estimates are that 15% to 50% of the U.S. population is obese; more women then men and 25% of children are significantly overweight. People in lower socioeconomic classes tend to have a greater likelihood of being obese. Certain ethnic groups — Hungarian and Italian — and religious groups — Jews — have a higher prevalence of obesity.

Etiologic factors and family patterns. High rates of obesity are seen among adolescents with obese parents. Weight studies show a biologic "set point" for body weight. For obese individuals who are dieting, weight loss efforts are working against this natural process. The number of fat cells cannot be reduced; however, the size of the cell can be reduced. In juvenile onset obesity, a larger than normal number of fat cells exist. In adult onset obesity, there is usually a normal number of larger-sized fat cells. Other factors include anomalies in triglyceride metabolism, disturbances in the central nervous system's chemical regulators of appetite, and unresolved dependency issues (fixated at the oral stage).

Age of onset and course. Obesity can develop anytime during childhood to adulthood. The course of obesity is usually chronic and progressive. The odds of a person's losing weight and keeping it off are not good. Increased mortality, up to 90%, occurs among severely obese individuals, more than 50% higher than ideal weight.

Impairments and complications. Psychological problems are major depression, anxiety disorders, social phobias, and drug and alco-

Figure 22-2
Nursing Pathway Plan of Care

DSM-IV Diagnoses: BULIMIA NERVOSA

Nuring Diagnosis: INEFFECTIVE INDIVIDUAL COPING

Related to: (check at least one)

- ☐ Unfulfilled tasks of trust.
- ☐ Excessive overeating.
- ☐ Self-induced vomiting.
- ☐ Dysfunctional family situation.
- ☐ Laxatives and diuretics.
- ☐ Refusal to eat.
- ☐ Obsession with food.
- ☐ Feelings of helplessness and lack of control.
- ☐ Low self-esteem.
- ☐ Chronic depression.

Short-term outcome: Patient will verbalize three adaptive coping mechanisms that can be realistically used in his or her life by discharge.

Long-term outcome:
1. Patient will assess three maladaptive coping behaviors accurately.
2. Patient will be able to utilize five adaptive coping strategies that can be utilized in home environment.

Interventions: _____

Day:_____**Date :** _____

Initiated   **Discontinued**

_____   _____   1. Establish a trusting relationship with patient by being honest and accepting.

_____   _____   2. Acknowledge patient's anger and feelings of loss of control.

_____   _____   3. When nutritional status has improved, explore feelings associated with gaining weight.

_____   _____   4. Explore family dynamics (i.e., assist patient to identify specific concerns within family structure and ways to relieve those concerns).

_____   _____   5. Discuss with patient the importance of patient's separation of self as an individual within the family situation.

_____   _____   6. Initially, allow patient to maintain dependent role.

_____   _____   7. Encourage independence in self-care activities as trust is developed and physical condition improves.

_____   _____   8. Offer positive reinforcement for independent behavior and problem solving/decision making (i.e., increased privileges, verbal praise, encouragement).

_____   _____   9. Explore with patient ways in which he or she may feel control within the environment without resorting to maladaptive eating behaviors.

_____   _____   10. Other: _____.

Source: Adapted from nursing care plans developed by nursing staff at 1st Hospital Wyoming Valley, Wilkes-Barre, PA, under the direction of Theresa Croushore.

Figure 22-3
Nursing Pathway Plan of Care

DSM-IV Diagnosis: BULIMIA NERVOSA

Nursing Diagnosis: ALTERATION IN NUTRITION: LESS THAN BODY REQUIREMENTS

Related to: (check at least one)

- ☐ Refusal to eat.
- ☐ Ingestion of large amounts of food, followed by self-induced vomiting.
- ☐ Abuse of laxatives, diuretics, and diet pills.
- ☐ Physical exertion in excess of energy produced through caloric intake.
- ☐ Loss of 15% expected body weight.

Short-term outcome: Patient will exhibit no signs or symptoms of malnutrition by discharge.

Long-term outcome:
1. Patient verbalizes importance of adequate nutrition.
2. BP, VS, lab serum studies are within normal limits.
3. Patient has achieved and maintained at least 90% of expected body weight.

Interventions: _____

Day: _____ **Date :** _____

Initiated	Discontinued	
_____	_____	1. In collaboration with dietician, determine number of calories required to provide adequate nutrition and realistic weight gain.
_____	_____	2. Prescribe behavior modification program as outlined by treatment team; explain details to patient (i.e., contingencies, rewards, consequences). (Identify_____.)
_____	_____	3. Sit with patient during mealtime for support and to observe amount ingested.
_____	_____	4. Reasonably limit time allotted for meals (i.e., 30 minutes).
_____	_____	5. Observe patient for at least 1 hour after meals.
_____	_____	6. Input and output.
_____	_____	7. Daily weights immediately upon arising and following first voiding.
_____	_____	8. Once protocol has been established, do not discuss food/eating with patient.
_____	_____	9. Offer support and additional reinforcement for improvements in eating behaviors (i.e., verbal praise, encouragement, increased privileges).
_____	_____	10. Explore the feelings of fear associated with gaining weight, until nutritional status improves and eating habits are established.
_____	_____	11. If patient is unable or unwilling to maintain adequate intake, notify physician of patient's status and carry out physician's orders (i.e., transfer to medical facility).

Source: Adapted from nursing care plans developed by nursing staff at 1st Hospital Wyoming Valley, Wilkes-Barre, PA, under the direction of Theresa Croushore.

hol abuse. These problems result from or precede obesity. Physical problems include low back pain, huge calluses on feet, aggravated osteoarthritis, amenorrhea, increased sweating, impaired heat loss, edema in the hands and feet, reduced respiratory capacity, and dyspnea. Other associated medical conditions are diabetes mellitus, hypertension, renal dysfunction, pulmonary disorder, and cardiovascular disease. Surgery, anesthesia, and pregnancy pose additional risks for the obese.

Nursing assessment and diagnosis. Assessment includes measuring weight and body fat. Hypothyroidism and other medical conditions must be ruled out.

Treatment. Treatment for obesity is similar to that for eating disorders. Medical conditions must be assessed and treated. Diet and exercise programs are established. Any psychiatric co-morbid conditions, such as binge eating and anxiety disorder, should be treated with antidepressants and cognitive therapy. Appetite suppressants may be given. Surgery is a last resort and may involve intestinal bypass or stapling.

• **BINGE EATING** is a newly recognized medical condition that involves recurrent episodes of uncontrolled eating; inappropriate compensatory behaviors characteristic of bulimia are usually absent. Binge eating entails eating rapidly (20,000 calories in less than two hours) even when not hungry, being uncomfortably full, and then experiencing shame and guilt after the binge.

Epidemiology. Twenty-three to forty-six percent of persons in weight control programs have a binge problem. Approximately 36% of young adults engage in some sort of binge eating.

Etiologic factors and family patterns. Etiology has not been determined; often triggered by dysmorphic mood, depression, and anxiety. Some bingers do not have any precipitant feelings, but find some tension relief from the binge activity.

Impairments and complications. People with this eating pattern reach varying degrees of obesity. They have a long history of dieting without success. Eating problems tend to interfere with relationships, work, and feeling good about themselves. Other impairments include weight gain, and increased risk of high blood pressure, heart attack, stroke, diabetes, and bone and joint problems.

Nursing assessment and diagnosis. This condition is difficult to assess, as binge eaters can easily hide the problem. A thorough interview of the patient's daily patterns and an examination to identify medical conditions may aid in diagnosis.

Treatment. Cognitive behavioral therapy, in which regular eating habits and food diaries are used, and, for some patients, antidepressants have proven to be the best approach. Comorbid conditions need to be treated.

TAKING ANOTHER LOOK

You are now ready to respond to the two questions that were raised in Gaining a Perspective at the beginning of this chapter. After you have written or thought about your responses, you may wish to look at the Suggested Responses on page 328.

23 SLEEP DISORDERS

TERMS TO DEFINE

bruxism

cataplexy

dyssomnias

hypnic myoclonia

hypnogogic hallucination

hypnopompic hallucinations

insomnia

narcolepsy

nightmares

parasomnias

polysonogram

somnambulism

GAINING A PERSPECTIVE

Consider the topics listed below, and after you have read the Key Concepts for this chapter respond to the situations in more detail.

1. What suggestions might you, as the nurse, give a colleague who is having trouble sleeping?

2. What are some of the reasons that a patient in the hospital might have for experiencing problems with sleep?

3. What problems do you foresee in dealing with psychiatric patients who have difficulty with sleep?

Key Concepts

- **SLEEP IS A HUMAN BEHAVIOR, BOTH CONSCIOUSLY AND AUTONOMICALLY CONTROLLED**, and it is sensitive to physiological, pathological, behavioral, and environmental changes. Sleep is affected in most psychiatric disorders and in numerous medical conditions. It may be compromised by the effects of medications or environmental conditions. In many health care settings, nurses are able to observe, assess, intervene, and educate patients about sleep.

- **SLEEP IS DEFINED BEHAVIORALLY** as a reversible behavioral state of perceptual disengagement from and unresponsiveness to the environment. **Physiologically**, sleep is a state of active heterogeneous, neurophysiological functioning, synchronized with the light-dark cycle of the environment and characterized by the cycling of the stages of sleep throughout the sleep period.

Stages of Sleep

- Non-rapid eye movement (NREM) sleep. Described as a relatively inactive, yet actively regulating, brain in a movable body. NREM is itself divided into four stages, representing the depth of sleep along a continuum from Stage 1, the lowest arousal threshold or lightest sleep, to Stage 4, the highest arousal threshold or deepest sleep.

- Rapid eye movement (REM) sleep. Described as a highly active brain in a paralyzed body, and mental activity is associated with dreaming.

Sleep Cycle

- Sleep is entered through NREM.
- NREM sleep and REM sleep alternate within a period of approximately 90 minutes.
- Slow wave sleep predominates in the first third of the night and is linked to the initiation of sleep.

- REM sleep predominates in the last third of the night and is linked to the circadian rhythm of body temperature.
- Wakefulness within sleep usually accounts for less than 5% of sleep time.
- NREM sleep is usually 75% to 85% of sleep.
- REM sleep is usually 15% to 25% of sleep, occurring in four to six discrete episodes.

Sleep and Aging

- The capacity to initiate sleep at any time of the day is greatly diminished after 25 years of age.
- The number and length of awakenings during the night increase with age, dramatically so after age 45. This is true of both conscious and transient arousals.
- It is a myth that older people need less sleep; however, with age, changes may occur in the sleep-wake pattern or sleep architecture. Some of the changes may reflect an age-related change in circadian rhythms.
- The incidence of sleep apnea increases in men during middle age, and in women after menopause.
- A progressive reduction and sometimes disappearance of NREM sleep Stages 3 and 4 occurs during old age, especially among men.
- The percentage of NREM Stage 1 sleep increases greatly during old age.
- Periodic leg movements during sleep may be more frequent among the elderly.
- Napping is common among the elderly, and may be beneficial.

Measuring Sleep

- Polysomnographic recordings are used to objectively measure human sleep, and monitor and record brain wave activity as well as eye movements, chin movements, leg movements, breathing, and heart rate. As with any procedure, the patient must be thoroughly informed about what will be done and must give consent. Conductive paste and electrodes are placed on the patient's head. After the polysomnogram is recorded, it must be scored and staged. Sleep continuity is measured including total time, time from

lights out to onset of the first cycle of Stage 2 sleep, and the awake percentage. Sleep architecture is measured (percentage of time spent in each of the five stages of sleep). REM measures include REM latency (period of time from sleep onset to the start of the first REM period), number of REM periods, percentage of REM sleep, REM activity, density, average REM period duration, and average REM cycle period.
- Sleep histogram is a visual summary of polysomnographic data; a graphic display of sleep stages and transitions throughout the sleep recording period.
- Multiple sleep latency test (MSLT) is a polysomnographic test for daytime sleepiness.
- Sleep history assessment (see Study Guide Figure 23-1).

- ### SLEEP-RELATED SYMPTOMS AND PHENOMENA

Bruxism, the forcible grinding or gnashing of teeth, begins in late childhood or adolescence. Etiology is unknown, but bruxism runs in families, suggesting a genetic component. Psychotherapy may be helpful in some cases where suppressed anger and conflict are present. The most common treatment, however, is the use of mouthguards to prevent dental damage.

Headaches are triggered by sleep; the three types are migraine, cluster, and chronic paroxysmal hemicrania (one-sided headache that occurs more frequently than cluster headaches and is without periods of remission). Morning headaches are associated with several sleep disorders. The symptom of headache should be assessed, not merely medicated and ignored.

Hypnic myoclonia (hypnic jerking) occurs at the onset of sleep. People may report a sensation of falling and then of suddenly being jerked or startled into full wakefulness; may be associated with stress or irregular sleep schedules.

Insomnia as a symptom is a perception of patients that their sleep is inadequate or abnormal. It is a common subjective complaint associated with a variety of medical disorders, psychiatric disorders, and specific sleep dis-

Figure 23-1
Sleep History Assessment

Patient Name: _____

Date:_____

Time:_____

Interviewed by: _____

1. ENVIRONMENT: Usual sleeping arrangements, setting, bed, pillow(s), room temperature, noise level, presence of pets.

2. USUAL BEDTIME

3. PRESLEEP RITUALS/HABITS

4. SLEEP AIDS: Medication, alcoholic beverage, how successful, how often needed.

5. LENGTH OF TIME NEEDED TO FALL ASLEEP

6. UNUSUAL SLEEP ONSET EXPERIENCES: Sleep paralysis, hypnic jerks, hypnogogic hallucinations, how frequent.

7. NOCTURNAL AWAKENINGS: Frequency, duration, precipitants, ease of falling back to sleep.

8. USUAL WAKING TIME: With/without alarm clock.

9. WAKING EXPERIENCES: Condition of bed, rested/refreshed, tired, dry mouth, sleep drunkenness, hypnopompic hallucinations.

10. HISTORY/FAMILY HISTORY OF SLEEP SYMPTOMS OR PHENOMENA:

    Snoring

    Bruxism

    Sleep apnea syndrome

    Narcolepsy

    Cataplexy

    Excessive daytime sleepiness/fatigue

    Sleep attacks

    Restless legs/kicking

    REM behavior syndrome

    Sleepwalking

    Sleeptalking

    Sleep terrors

    Automatic behavior

    Headbanging (jactatio capitus nocturna)

11. DREAMS: Recall, recurrent, nightmares, vividness, traumatic.

12. NAPS: Frequency, environment, duration, effect on nocturnal sleep.

13. PAIN, DISCOMFORT, STIFFNESS, HEADACHE, TMJ DISEASE

14. CAFFEINE/NICOTINE INTAKE

15. ALCOHOL INTAKE: How much, how often, what type, time of last drink, how long

16. MEDICATIONS, OVER-THE-COUNTER DRUGS: dosage, timing, when last taken, how long taking, for what condition, history of side effects, allergies.

17. PSYCHIATRIC HISTORY

18. MEDICAL HISTORY

19. PSYCHOSOCIAL & LIFESTYLE HISTORY: Resources/supports, how reliable, stress reduction & coping strategies, how successful, current sources of stress.

20. IS THERE ANYTHING ELSE THE PATIENT (OR FAMILY) THINKS IS IMPORTANT TO MENTION OR WOULD LIKE TO DISCUSS?

orders. It is important to know whether patients have difficulty falling asleep, staying asleep, or awakening early.

Jactatio capitis nocturna (head banging) is more common among infants and children than adults. The nurses's concern is to prevent injury.

Narcolepsy is a sleep disorder that tends to run in families. Cardinal symptoms are excessive daytime sleepiness with sleep attacks and either cataplexy or recurrent intrusions of REM sleep during the waking state. Narcolepsy is usually treated with central nervous system stimulants and tricyclic antidepressants.

Cataplexy, a cardinal symptom of narcolepsy, is the sudden loss of muscle tone triggered by intense emotional stimuli (e.g., fright, surprise). Patient remains fully conscious during the attack, although if the episode lasts longer then one minute, REM sleep may occur.

Nightmares are long, frightening dreams that awaken a person from REM sleep; common among children. Women report more frequent nightmares than men. A sudden increase in the frequency of nightmares along with insomnia over a period of a few weeks may be a precursor to a psychotic episode. Nightmares do not always require treatment, but psychotherapy and behavioral interventions can be used. Discussion of nightmare content and menacing may be useful in the psychotherapeutic process. Nursing care for a patient who awakens from a nightmare includes gentle reassurance and a willingness to listen and assist the patient to process and integrate the nightmare experience.

Sleep terrors and confusional arousals typically occur during Stages 3 and 4 of NREM sleep and are characterized by signs of increased sympathetic activity (e.g., increased heart and respiratory rates). The patient typically screams and appears terrified, is inconsolable for a few minutes, then relaxes and falls back to sleep. In the morning the patient has no recall of the event. Mild episodes, called confusional arousals, involve moaning, thrashing, muttered verbalization.

Sleep-talking is common at all ages, although more frequent among women. Occurs during NREM Stages 1 and 2. Not abnormal unless it occurs with other abnormal sleep behaviors or with excessive daytime sleepiness.

Sleepwalking, or somnambulism, is more common among children and occurs during the first third of the night. The individual will not respond to commands, but can be led back to bed. The episode is not remembered. Sleepwalking can cause injury; doors should be locked, windows closed, stairways protected.

Sleep apneas are episodes in which breathing ceases for at least 10 seconds. There are three types:

- OBSTRUCTIVE SLEEP APNEA is caused by upper airway obstruction; treatment involves a device that prevents obstruction.
- CENTRAL SLEEP APNEA is associated with cardiac or neurological problems affecting ventilation.
- MIXED SLEEP APNEA is a combination of obstructive and central sleep apnea.

Apnea should be reported to the physician. Patients should be carefully observed and episodes documented.

Snoring is common, although more common among men. Loud snoring is not a benign symptom; an increase in volume or character strongly suggests sleep apnea, which needs to be reported.

Hypnogogic hallucinations may be visual, auditory, or tactile and appear at the onset of sleep; they may be pleasant or frightening. If coupled with excessive daytime sleepiness they may suggest narcolepsy. May occur in anyone with a disrupted sleep schedule. Hypnogogic hallucinations differ from psychotic hallucinations in that the person does not confuse hypnogogic hallucinations with reality and is aware that he or she is hallucinating.

Hypnopompic hallucinations are similar to hypnogogoic hallucinations, but occur at the termination of sleep.

Sleep paralysis is when an individual feels partially or fully awake but is unable to move. The person may describe struggling to move or wake up. It starts suddenly and lasts a few minutes. Common in narcolepsy, but can occur in anyone, especially when sleep and circadian rhythms are disrupted.

Automatic behavior consists of seemingly purposeful, repetitive activity performed by sleepy persons. The person generally has no memory of the episode.

Sleep drunkenness is an inability to attain full alertness for some time after awakening. The person may report deep sleep with difficulty awakening. Often associated with sleep apnea or central nervous system disorders, but can occur in anyone following sleep deprivation.

Restless leg syndrome consists of unpleasant, crawling, pulling, or painful sensations in the legs, especially in the calfs while sitting or lying down, and an almost irresistible urge to move the legs. Symptoms commonly appear at bedtime and walking relieves them. Insomnia may occur.

In **REM behavior syndrome, or REM without atonia**, muscle tone, and therefore movement, is preserved during REM sleep, allowing patients to act out their dreams. Behaviors are complex, vigorous, and sometimes violent. About one third of patients also have a neurological disorder. Nursing responsibilities include documenting the disorder and notifying the physician for appropriate evaluation and referral.

Excessive daytime sleepiness (EDS), widespread in sleep disorders, reflects poor quality of nocturnal sleep and/or a disturbed sleep-wake cycle. Persistent EDS should not be ignored. Patients should be evaluated for the presence of a medical, psychiatric, or sleep disorder.

- **PRINCIPLES OF SLEEP HYGIENE** are behavioral interventions that promote sleep and decrease awakenings.

  A regular bedtime and awakening time should be established and maintained.

  Sleep only as much as needed to feel refreshed. The amount of sleep varies.

  Reserve the bedroom for sleep; don't, for example, use the room as an office.

  Do not go to bed hungry, but do not eat a large meal before bedtime.

  Avoid caffeine in the evening.

  Avoid alcohol intake prior to sleep.

  Regular moderate exercise is healthy and may deepen sleep over time.

  Naps can disrupt sleep if taken at the wrong time. The elderly may benefit from periodic naps.

  Clear the mind prior to sleep. Relax with a book, music, or relaxation exercises.

  Do not struggle to fall asleep. If unable to sleep after five minutes, turn on the light, get up, and do something relaxing.

  Bedroom environment should be kept dark, quiet, and at a moderate temperature.

  Pets allowed to sleep in the bedroom or on the bed can disrupt sleep.

- **THE NURSING DIAGNOSIS FOR SLEEP DISTURBANCES IS "SLEEP PATTERN DISTURBANCES RELATED TO" A SPECIFIC CAUSE OR ASSOCIATED FACTORS.** Sleep pattern disturbances must be differentiated from sleep disorders (e.g., sleep apnea and narcolepsy), which are usually not treated by a nurse generalist. To make a diagnosis, the nurse must gather information about the patient's lifestyle, environment, fears, and circadian rhythms.

- **NURSING INTERVENTIONS** are based on the principles of good sleep hygiene, and the care plan is individualized.

  The environment should be kept as quiet as possible in an inpatient environment to minimize disruption and promote sleep.

  A plan for effective pain control should be collaboratively developed by the nurse and physician, as pain is a major cause of disturbed sleep.

  A regular toileting schedule may minimize nighttime bathroom trips.

  The patient's presleep habits and rituals should be learned by the nurse, and the patient allowed to follow them as much as possible.

  A moderate temperature should be maintained in the patient's room.

  Extra pillows should be provided if requested.

  Try to plan nursing assessments, routine treatments, and medication administration so that patients get a minimum of four hours uninterrupted sleep at night.

Make sure the call bell is within the patient's easy reach.

Spend some time with patients who awaken during the night; use relaxation techniques and provide warm milk, or use other calming approaches.

The need for and effectiveness of hypnotic and other medications is evaluated.

- **PRIMARY SLEEP DISORDERS ARE THOSE IN WHICH THE ETIOLOGY CANNOT BE ACCOUNTED FOR BY A MENTAL DISORDER, THE PHYSIOLOGICAL EFFECTS OF A MEDICAL DISORDER, OR A SUBSTANCE.** The diagnostic criteria for sleep disorder is that the sleep disturbance causes clinically significant distress and impairment in social, occupational, or other important functioning.

  Dyssomnias are characterized by abnormalities in the amount, quality, or timing of sleep.

  - PRIMARY INSOMNIA is difficulty initiating or maintaining sleep or nonrestorative sleep, lasts for at least one month, and causes clinically significant distress or impairment in social, occupational, or other important areas of functioning. Prevalence is unknown. Onset is usually sudden and associated with psychological, social, or medical stress. The patient gradually develops negative associations related to unsuccessful attempts to sleep and becomes negatively conditioned.

  - PRIMARY HYPERSOMNIA is excessive sleepiness for at least one month as evidenced by prolonged sleep (at least 8 to 12 hours per night) or daytime sleep episodes almost every day. True prevalence is unknown. Onset is between 15 and 30 years of age. Hypersomnia is considered recurrent if periods of excessive sleepiness last at least three days and occur several times a year for at least two years.

  - NARCOLEPSY is repeated, irresistible attacks of refreshing sleep occurring daily for at least three months. In addition, the patient experiences either cataplexy or, during the transition between sleep and wakefulness, recurrent intrusions of elements of REM sleep. Attacks typically last 10 to 20 minutes, but

can persist for up to an hour. They can occur any time and if untreated can be dangerous. Narcolepsy is equally frequent among males and females. The adult prevalence rate ranges from 0.027% to 0.16%. Daytime sleepiness is the first symptom usually noted in adolescence; there may be a genetic component.

- BREATHING-RELATED SLEEP DISORDERS are sleep disruptions caused by abnormalities in ventilation. Three forms of this disorder are briefly described below.

  - Obstructive sleep apnea syndrome. Most common form; repeated episodes of upper airway obstruction. Associated with overweight and loud snoring, alternating with episodes of silence.

  - Central sleep apnea syndrome. Patient with no airway obstruction, episodically stops breathing. More common in the elderly as a result of cardiac or neurological conditions.

  - Central alveolar hypoventilation syndrome. Impaired ventilation that results in abnormally low oxygen levels further worsened by sleep. It occurs in very overweight people.

  People with sleep-related breathing disorders often awaken feeling more tired then they did before going to sleep. Memory disturbances, poor concentration, irritability, and personality changes may result from excessive sleepiness. Mood disorders, anxiety disorders, and dementia are associated with sleep-related breathing disorders, and each type of disorder is associated with specific polysomnographic and physiological findings. The disorders usually have a gradual onset, gradual progression, and a chronic course. Obstructive sleep apnea may lead to death.

- CIRCADIAN RHYTHM SLEEP DISORDER is a persistent or recurrent pattern of sleep disruption that results from a mismatch between the individual's circadian sleep-wake system and exogenous demands on the timing and duration of sleep. Diagnosis is primarily based on clinical history. Four subtypes are briefly described below.

- Delayed sleep phase type. Internal sleep-wake cycle is delayed relative to social norms (a night owl). The patient becomes sleep deprived because of need to rise early.
- Jet lag type. Internal clock is normal, but conflict occurs between the individual's sleep-wake cycle and the pattern demanded by a different time zone.
- Shift work type. Internal sleep-wake cycle is normal, but there is conflict between the internal cycle and the pattern of sleep and wakefulness required by shift work.
- Unspecified type. Encompasses sleep-wake patterns that vary from normal.

Individuals with circadian rhythm sleep disorders are at risk for substance-related disorders, as they may use alcohol, sedatives, hypnotics, or stimulants to control symptoms.

- DYSSOMNIA NOT OTHERWISE SPECIFIED is reserved for insomnias, hypersomnias, and circadian rhythm disturbances that do not meet criteria for any specific dyssomnia.

Parasomnias are characterized by abnormal or physiological events that occur in association with sleep, specific sleep stages, or sleep-wake transitions.

- NIGHTMARE DISORDER involves repeated frightening dreams that lead to awakening fully alert. Nightmares typically involve physical danger, and less commonly, personal failure or embarrassment. Polysomnograms show abrupt awakening from REM sleep, which correlates with patient's report of nightmares. Frequent in childhood; more frequently reported by women; prevalence rate unknown.

- SLEEP TERROR DISORDER involves recurrent abrupt awakenings in the first third of the night, beginning with a panic scream and accompanied by intense fear and autonomic arousal. The person is difficult to awaken or comfort, no detailed dream is recalled, and there is amnesia for the episode. Among adults, sleep terror disorder occurs frequently in people with post-traumatic stress disorder and generalized anxiety disorder, as well as in persons with dependent, schizoid, and borderline personality disorders. Among children, the disorder begins between 4 and 12 years of age and resolves during adolescence. Among adults, onset is between 20 and 30 years of age; the course is chronic.

- SLEEPWALKING DISORDER involves repeated episodes of complex motor behavior initiated during sleep, including arising from bed and walking about. The patient is unresponsive during the episode; little recall after the episode. Frequency of episodes can increase with sleep deprivation or fever. Migraines and obstructive sleep apnea are associated with this disorder. True prevalence is not known. Up to 30% of children have had at least one episode. Sleepwalking rarely begins in adulthood without prior childhood episodes. Among adults, the disorder is chronic and up to 80% have a familial history.

- PARASOMNIA NOT OTHERWISE SPECIFIED is characterized by abnormal behavioral or physiological events during sleep or sleep-wake transitions that do not meet criteria for more specific parasomnia, e.g., REM sleep behavior disorder and sleep paralysis.

- **DISTURBED SLEEP IS A SYMPTOM OF VIRTUALLY ALL PSYCHIATRIC DISORDERS.** Understanding the related sleep disturbance enhances the nurse's ability to observe, assess, plan, and evaluate nursing care and collaborate with others in the overall treatment of mentally ill patients.

Mood Disorders. Disturbed sleep (insomnia or hypersomnia) is part of the diagnostic criteria for all mood disorders.

- MAJOR DEPRESSIVE DISORDER. Approximately 90% of depressed patients show some form of EEG-verified sleep disorder. The change is seen even when the depressive illness is in remission. EEG studies confirm a depressed patient's reports of difficulty getting to sleep, waking up frequently, early morning awakening, and a reduction of total sleep time. Symptoms should be of concern to the nurse.

- BIPOLAR DISORDER. During depressive cycle most patients report insomnia, but some report hypersomnia. During manic phase, patients report reduced amounts of sleep and a sense of needing less sleep. A manic phase may be preceded by periods of sleeplessness.

Anxiety Disorders

- POST-TRAUMATIC STRESS DISORDER (PTSD). Victims of psychic trauma, including rape, commonly report sleep disturbances, nightmares, and/or repetitive dreams. PTSD, at least in males, is associated with more insomnia, less efficient sleep, and shorter total sleep time than normal.

- PANIC DISORDER. Recent research verifies the existence of so-called panic attacks. Insomnia and sleep panic attacks are reported by a majority of patients with panic disorder. Patients with sleep panic attacks develop bizarre sleep habits and try to hide their illness. Careful nursing assessment is necessary.

- GENERALIZED ANXIETY DISORDER (GAD). The major problems associated with GADs are difficulty initiating or maintaining sleep and restless, fragmented sleep.

Schizophrenia. Sleep patterns indicate that the problem is that the patient takes longer to get to sleep after going to bed. REM sleep is reduced early in the course of an acute exacerbation, with a return to normal as illness improves.

Dementia. Moderate to severe sleep disturbances occur; may be that these disturbances are an exaggeration of the sleep deterioration seen in normal aging. Wandering at night is common and may lead to the older person being institutionalized.

TAKING ANOTHER LOOK

You are now ready to respond in greater detail to the situations described in Gaining a Perspective at the beginning of this chapter. After you have written or thought about your responses, you may wish to look at the Suggested Responses on page 329.

24 TREATING CHILD SEXUAL TRAUMA

TERMS TO DEFINE

integration of trauma

limbic system

post-traumatic stress disorder

aggressive pattern

anxious pattern

avoidant pattern

trauma learning

displacement

reenactment

repetition

traumatic event

GAINING A PERSPECTIVE

Think about the question posed below, and after you have read the Key Concepts for this chapter respond more specifically to the question.

1. What do you think will be your major role as a nurse in dealing with a child who has been sexually traumatized?

Key Concepts

- **INCREASING CONCERN IS EXPRESSED ABOUT THE OCCURRENCE OF CHILD SEXUAL TRAUMA;** its emotional impact on the victim has become a major social issue. Childhood traumatic memories are important, as is their relationship to acting-out behavior, such as aggressive sexual behaviors among teenagers.

- **THE INFORMATION PROCESSING OF TRAUMA MODEL** assumes the basic constructs of information processing in a living system. Experiences are processed on three levels: sensory (basic registering of the experience), perceptual (beginning classification of the sensory processing), and cognitive (organizing experience into a meaning system). (See Chapter 5).

  In researching the impact of trauma and the response to stressful stimuli, a general response syndrome was identified by noting a clustering of disturbing psychological phenomena of intrusive imagery associated with memories of the traumatic event. Avoidant strategies keep memories and associations out of awareness until placed in distant memory. Trauma resolution occurs when processing is sufficient for the information to be stored. The event is remembered, attendant feelings are neutralized, and anxiety is controlled. When the traumatic event is not resolved, the diagnosis becomes post-traumatic stress disorder (PTSD). The unresolved event is either kept in memory or becomes defended by cognitive mechanisms, such as denial, dissociation, or splitting; the individual reexperiences the original trauma both unconsciously and consciously.

  The four major phases of the Information Processing of Trauma Model give a rationale to response patterns identified in child victims.

  Pretrauma phase identifies the child's makeup and social context which might affect how the child manages and resolves the sexual abuse. These factors mediate that which is particular to the general stress-response syndrome.

Trauma encapsulating phase focuses on the mechanisms used by the child to regulate the ongoing sexual activities and responses.

- INPUT is derived from the offender's behavior.

- THRUPUT includes the coping and defensive mechanisms employed by the child to deal with anxiety, fear, and danger evoked by the abuse. The defense mechanisms shape the primary meaning of the event as well as the structure of how the abuse information is processed, stored, and represented through affect and nonverbal behavior.

- OUTPUT is the primary trauma learning which charges the sensory, perceptual, and cognitive memory base of the event and is an important anxiety management mechanism. The information associated with trauma learning results in an important feedback loop of intermediate outputs and includes trauma replay, reenactment, repetition, and displacement. (Key Concepts below define these mechanisms.) The feedback loop also contains the dynamic individual meaning that the trauma holds for the child. Nondisclosure presumes encapsulation of the primary trauma learning. To the degree that the event produces anxiety and remains charged (non-neutralized), relationships, social and academic achievement, and a sense of right and wrong and of self can be distorted. Within the child, self-comforting and caring are disturbed, as are the protective functions.

In the output phase, the emphasis is on the looping-back principle in an active system. Continued abuse is registered and modified in the process.

Figure 24-1
Patterns of Trauma Learning and Memory Presentations

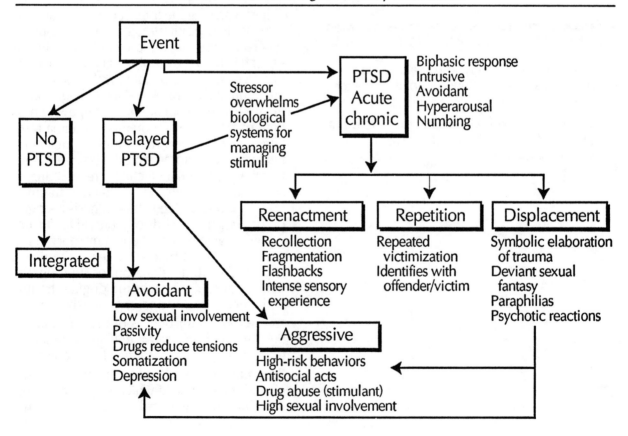

Disclosure phase contains the secondary and social meaning. By revealing the abuse, the child has to field the reactions of his or her social network. This learning can result in reformulation of the trauma.

Post-traumatic outcome phase sees the victim of the traumatic event exhibit a progression of symptomatology (see Study Guide Figure 24-1).

- INTEGRATION OF TRAUMA is the optimal response. The patient is able to relate to the sexual abuse experience, but does not dwell on it or avoid it through psychological defenses.

- POST-TRAUMATIC STRESS DISORDER (PTSD) may be the response. The victim may display intrusive and/or avoidant behaviors. Exposure to stimuli can induce a state of hyperarousal and numbing, which may cause the victim to experience highly emotional states with lower levels of thinking. Visual and motoric reliving of the traumatic event may occur through nightmares and flashbacks that are generally preceded by physiological arousal. Disruption can impact sensory, perceptual/cognitive, and interpersonal performance. Symptoms of sensory disruption may include hyperactivity, headaches, stomachaches, backaches, genitourinary distress, and nightmares. Perceptual/cognitive disruption may produce intrusion of information (images, auditory, and kinesthetic) associated with the trauma and may be related to future concerns about repeated danger. Interpersonal disruption may include excessive fear of others, inability to assert and/or defend oneself, as well as aggressive behaviors, such as agitation, aggression toward peers/family/pets, and potential sexualized behaviors toward others. Several patterns of PTSD symptoms are noted below:

  - Anxious pattern. It is characterized by generalized fears that have to do with developmental tasks as well as the abusive situation. Anxiety disorders, eating disorders, phobias, and obsessive compulsive disorders may be present.

  - Avoidant pattern. Denial that the abuse has occurred. Patient appears distant and alienated, lacks energy for living or learning. Youth may have a substance abuse history, de-

pression, suicidal thoughts, phobic behavior, adjustment problems, and/or conduct disorder.

  - Aggressive pattern. Characterized by sexual and/or aggressive behavior. Acting out may be bold or secret. Minimal acknowledgement or frank denial of prior abuse is typical.

- DELAYED PTSD may be experienced by some victims who do not initially develop PTSD and who display no sequelae. These sufferers may continue to live in the emotional atmosphere of the traumatic event, with an enduring vigilance for and sensitivity to environmental threat. Avoidant behavior includes infrequent sexual involvement, substance use to reduce tension and depression, or aggressive patterns including participating in high-risk behaviors and antisocial acts.

  Delayed PTSD becomes active and moves to the third pattern (aggressive) of acute PTSD when the event overwhelms both psychological and biological mechanisms for managing stimuli.

- **TRAUMA LEARNING EMPHASIZES THE REPETITION OF BEHAVIOR** and can be observed in traumatized children as reenactment of the trauma, repetition of the trauma as victim or aggressor, or displacement of the aggression.

Reenactment

The patient recollects the traumatic event in flashbacks. In young children, repetitive play may occur in which themes of the trauma are expressed. Verbal play or behaviors demonstrate that the child is acting as if the trauma were happening again and identification with the role of victim continues. Nursing interventions may include teaching children to self-soothe and calm themselves. The environment must be free of abuse. Focus of the treatment may be the alteration of response patterns to the initially overwhelming, fearful experience.

Repetition

The behavioral repetition, noted in victim's play with others, may be played out in the role of the victim or victimizer. It is suggested that the trauma replay through repetition of sexual acts upon younger, weaker children gives the child a sense of mastery and superiority. The child may be at high risk for prostitution, drug abuse, and suicide.

Children can be helped through play that links aggressive acting-out behavior to the abuse the child received. The task is for the child to acknowledge that the behavior was wrong or hateful, although the context may have made its appearance understandable.

Displacement

During this stage of the trauma learning process, behaviors and thoughts of the trauma are symbolically elaborated, which may manifest itself as a restorative dream or fantasy (doll play, dreams, deviant sexual fantasies, paraphilias, or psychotic reactions). A child's denial of his or her own position of vulnerability and helplessness as a victim or a child's dissociation from the terror of vulnerability enhances identification with the aggressor, thereby creating the link from abused to abuser. The child may become very aggressive and act out. Work usually needs to be directed toward the child's destructive behavior, which is usually a reflection of the child's defensiveness caused by the overwhelming anxiety the child has experienced.

• **NURSES MUST HELP VICTIMIZED CHILDREN STRENGTHEN PERSONAL RESOURCES** so that the children are able to begin to process traumatic memories.

TAKING ANOTHER LOOK

You are now ready to respond in greater depth to the question posed in Gaining a Perspective at the beginning of this chapter. After you have written or thought about your response, you may wish to look at the Suggested Responses on page 329.

25 VICTIMS OF SEXUAL TRAUMA

GAINING A PERSPECTIVE

Think about the problem described briefly below, and after you have read the Key Concepts for this chapter describe with more insight what your feelings might be in such a situation.

1. How would you, as a nurse, feel when doing an initial interview with a young teenager who had been raped by a man in his mid-thirties?

Key Concepts

- **SEXUAL VICTIMIZATION — RAPE, INCEST, AND SEXUAL HARASSMENT —** disrupts the lives of thousands of people each year. Sexual victimization includes direct and indirect physical and sexual contact. Psychological trauma (an indirect act) is a major component of the psychological impact. Rape implies that the offender is a stranger or an acquaintance; incest implies that the offender is a family member; and harassment implies that the offender is in the victim's workplace. The symptoms of stress response to victimization vary. Nurses are key health care professionals to provide early intervention and care to victims.

- **RAPE** is forced, violent, sexual penetration of a body orifice without the victim's consent. Rape trauma describes a cluster of bio-psycho-social and cognitive symptoms exhibited by the victim following a rape.

  The acute phase of rape trauma syndrome, which lasts a few days to several weeks, may include many physical symptoms, especially skeletal-muscle tension, gastrointestinal irritability, and genitourinary disturbance. Disturbances may occur in sleeping or eating. The reorganization phase includes increased motor activity (many times the victim changes his or her address, etc.); increased need for family and social network; and development of fears and phobic reactions, including nightmares.

- **INCEST,** a social issue throughout civilization, refers to sexual intimacies between two persons so closely related that they are forbidden to marry. Two major dilemmas are role/identity confusion and divided loyalty (family and victimizer).

- **SEXUAL HARASSMENT** is a new and serious offense. Its methods include sexual language, discrimination for jobs, and physical contact.

- **TWO TYPES OF SEXUAL TRAUMA** are described below.

CHAPTER 25

Rape Trauma

No consent. The offender achieves power and control over his victim through intimidation by means of a weapon, physical force, or threat of bodily harm.

Pressured Sex

Victim unable to make responsible decision of consent. Victims, many are children and young adolescents, are pressured into sexual activity by a person who stands in a power position, for example, through age or authority. An incest victim is of this type; the victim's emotional reaction results from his or her being pressured into sexual activity and the tension to keep the act secret. The offender gains access by offering material reward (e.g., candy) or psychological reward (e.g., affection) or by misrepresenting moral standards ("It's okay, your mother and I do it."). The victim over time may gradually withdraw socially and psychologically from usual life activities, especially if the sexual activity is repeated and the victim is pressured into secrecy.

- **FOUR TYPES OF OFFENDERS** have been identified.

Compensatory Offender

Assault is primarily an expression of the offender's rape fantasies. Motivation is that he is so inadequate that no woman would voluntarily have sex with him.

Exploitative Offender

Sexual behavior is expressed as an impulsive, predatory act; a distinctive "macho" style; cannot believe that a woman could or would say "no" to sexual advances.

Displaced Anger Offender

Sexual behavior is an expression of anger and rage; the victim represents a hated individual; persistent, angry, negative attitude toward women.

Sadistic Offender

Sexual behavior is an expression of sadistic fantasies. Sadistic violence is directed at parts of the body having sexual significance; death may be the victim's outcome.

- **THE INITIAL INTERVIEW WITH THE VICTIM** is a primary therapeutic tool, an opportunity to assess the amount of psychological distress and to identify the victim's support network. At the time of the interview, consideration is given to the stress that the victim has already experienced, coping with the traumatic event (how the victimizer gained and maintains control over the victim), and disclosing the event (telling someone what happened to oneself).

Of consequence in the victim's adjustment is the family's response to the traumatic event, as well as that of the nurse and others who have contact with the victim. Assessment of sexually traumatized individuals follows the following general principles:

Establish Rapport

Explain the purpose and procedure of what is to be done. Victims must be treated with respect and honesty; they need to be relaxed and comfortable.

Evaluate the Victim's Sense of Self

Assess the victim's recall of what happened and reaction to it. The meanings and beliefs that the victim attributes to a variety of experiences give clues about how the victim coped with the assault. Is the victim developing a sense of total helplessness or self-blame?

Important details to be gathered are:

- MEDICAL ISSUES: Are there physical signs and symptoms of trauma? Is there evidence of sexual intercourse (including laboratory tests)?

- CIRCUMSTANCES OF THE ASSAULT: When and where was the victim approached? Who was the assailant (stranger, acquaintance, relative)? How is the victimizer described? What conversation occurred? What methods of control were used (e.g., weapons, threats, physical force)?

- BEHAVIORAL ISSUES: What types of sex were demanded and obtained? What other degrading acts occurred?

- PSYCHOLOGICAL ISSUES: What coping strategies (behaviors) did the victim use before, after, and during the assault? What signs and symptoms suggest emotional trauma?

When completing the initial assessment, the victim is assessed for self-harm. The nurse also explores in detail the victim's expectations regarding encounters with family and significant others. Who will be immediately available to assist the victim? Referrals, arranging for telephone follow-up, and crisis center services are important in closing the interview.

• **THE TREATMENT AND FOLLOW-UP PHASE**

Physical Health

Review any physical symptoms or alterations in the victim's body systems; do a gynecologic and medical follow-up after the victim completes her first menstrual period after the assault, including blood work for sexually transmitted diseases. Cultures should be done every four to six weeks following the assault.

Social Network

The network may assist victim in strengthening self-confidence. Victim is encouraged to resume normal activity as soon as possible. Victim often needs advice about whether to press charges, quit school or work, and/or to tell people about the incident.

Behavior

Intervention concerning behavior is aimed at desensitizing the victim to the painful aspects of the assault. The victim is encouraged to talk about the event as a way to master fears.

Psychological Issues

Victim is made aware of the relationship between the description of symptoms and the rape trauma. Mental functioning (e.g., impaired attention, poor memory, changes in outlook) must be assessed. Emotional reactions (e.g., irritability, mood changes) should also be reviewed. Talking with the victim as soon as possible after the assault helps repair emotional damage; victim's impulse is to avoid dealing with the experience. The treatment goal is to reestablish normal living style and restore equilibrium.

TAKING ANOTHER LOOK

You are now ready to respond again to the problem presented in Gaining a Perspective at the beginning of this chapter. After you have written or thought about your response, you may wish to look at the Suggested Responses on page 330.

26 PERSONALITY DISORDERS

TERMS TO DEFINE

Cluster A

Paranoid personality disorder

Schizoid personality disorder

Schizotypal personality disorder

Cluster B

Antisocial personality disorder

Borderline personality disorder

Histrionic personality disorder

Narcissistic personality disorder

Cluster C

Avoidant personality disorder

Dependent personality disorder

Obsessive-compulsive personality

GAINING A PERSPECTIVE

Think about the situations described below, and after you have read the Key Concepts for this chapter answer the questions in greater depth.

1. Think of a co-worker or fellow student of yours who is very inflexible. Do you think that that person is personally distressed?

2. How would you, as a nurse, assist the patient described in the Case Example below?

   Mrs. Terry Jamison has been diagnosed as having a borderline personality disorder. She has very severe anxiety when she feels abandoned, for example, when her husband goes on business trips for a few days or when her 23-year-old daughter recently decided to move into an apartment of her own.

Key Concepts

- **PERSONALITY STRUCTURE DETERMINES** how a person thinks and feels about self, evaluates the environment, and interacts with others in the family and community. A patient's personality structure also determines how much information that person will disclose to the nurse providing care, how personal problems are interpreted, and what information can be learned by the patient during intervention. It is important to assess every patient for a personality disorder. Several symptoms of personality disorder are outlined in DSM-IV. Criteria for personality disorder are listed below.

The individual's thought process, emotional reactivity, interpersonal relationships, and impulse control are markedly different from others in his or her culture and peer group.

Different patterns of thought, emotionality, and behavior are enduring and inflexible and are demonstrated consistently in most personal and social situations.

Significant personal distress and/or impairment is evident during interactions within the family and with others in a social or occupational setting.

Patterns of enduring thoughts, emotions, and behavior become evident during adolescence and early adulthood.

The cognitive, emotional, and behavioral patterns are not due to any other psychiatric disorder or the physiological effects of a substance, the side effects of medications, or exposure to toxic chemicals.

- **THEORETICAL PERSPECTIVES** of personality disorder are defined below.

  Freud's tripartite model hypothesizes that a person's internal psychic structures are made up of:

  - ID: an unconscious structure that houses primitive thoughts, feelings, or impulses in the adult and contains intellectual drives where repressed material is stored.

  - EGO: mostly in the conscious realm of thinking, although some is unconscious; "the observer" watches and attempts to understand in the context of earlier experiences; mediates primitive demands of the id and restraints of the superego. The ego keeps primitive impulses, such as sexual desires, aggressive fantasies, and/or unconscious conflict, from coming into conscious awareness.

  - SUPEREGO: the guilt center; a person's conscience based on culturally acquired mores, values, and restrictions; includes conscious and unconscious operations.

  Developmental Theories of Freud and Erickson

  The stages outlined below illustrate Freud's and Erickson's stages of psychosexual development. Freud's definitions extend through puberty and preparation for marriage and family; Erickson viewed development as a life-long process and elaborated Freud's theory by including three additional adult stages of psychic development.

  - FREUD'S ORAL STAGE. Needs are primarily centered around the oral zone. Child learns to give, receive, and trust without an excessive amount of dependence or envy, otherwise narcissism may develop and the individual is self-absorbed, unable to empathize with others; narcissistic traits often seen in patients with Cluster A and Cluster B personality disorders (DSM-IV descriptions of personality disorders, page 172).

  - ERICKSON'S BASIC TRUST VS. BASIC MISTRUST. Infant can sleep peacefully, take nourishment comfortably, and excrete without negative feelings. Infants learn trust and hope by receiving consistent care and satisfying experiences; or, infant can experience a sense of separation and abandonment.

  - FREUD'S ANAL STAGE. From 1 to 3 years of age, neuromuscular control over the anal sphincter matures and control over bowels becomes voluntary; toilet training occurs. The child strives for independence and experiences ambivalent separation from dependence and parental control. The child strives for a level of autonomy without excessive shame and doubt. Conflicts result in character traits of ambivalence, messiness, defiance, rage, frugality, and orderliness; traits often seen in patients in Cluster C. (DSM-IV descriptions of personality disorders are listed below.)

  - ERICKSON'S AUTONOMY VS. SHAME AND DOUBT. Child 1 to 3 years of age learns parental expectations, obligations, and privileges and behavior limitations. Adults assist the child to understand limits by exercising control in a firmly reassuring manner; preventing secretive, sneaky, sly behaviors. Failure of self-control can cause feelings of shame and doubt. The child's gradual acceptance of limit setting shapes the child's later understanding of societal rules; begins to differentiate right and wrong.

  - FREUD'S PHALLIC STAGE. Child 3 to 5 years of age begins genital interest; increase in genital masturbation with unconscious fantasies of sexual involvement with opposite sex parent. (Guilt feelings about this may cause castration anxiety.) Working through these conflicts, child develops superego and begins to lay the foundation for gender identity, which emerges to give child a sense of mastery over people and objects in the environment, as well as internal processes and ultimately adult impulse control. Patients who have antisocial personality disorder exhibit a deficit in this stage of development, as they demonstrate no remorse for behavior that would cause others to feel guilt.

  - ERICKSON'S INITIATIVE VS. GUILT. Child's major activity at this age is playing, which assists the child to achieve goals resulting from play. Mastery and responsibility are involved as initiative combines with autonomy. The threat of this stage is the guilt that may haunt the child for an overzealous contemplation of goals, including aggression and/or manipulation to achieve these goals.

- FREUD'S LATENCY STAGE. From ages 6 or 7 years through puberty, including the first menses or first ejaculation emission. Sexual and aggressive focus is quieted, replaced by learning and play activities mastery. Individuals who have difficulty completing the tasks of this stage have difficulty with impulse control and exhibit diminished capacity to complete tasks. Others, however, become too adept at controlling impulses and develop obsessive character traits.

- ERICKSON'S INDUSTRY VS. INFERIORITY. Through formal education, children control their exuberant imaginations and settle down to a sense of industry; competence emerges. Perseverance and diligence are rewards. Failures may result in a sense of inferiority. Phase continues through puberty. Individuals who have difficulty in this stage may have difficulty with impulse control.

- FREUD'S GENITAL STAGE. During puberty, until adulthood, sexual drives intensify and unresolved conflicts are reopened with the aim being to achieve mature sexual and adult identity (ability to enjoy participating in work and love and to problem-solve). Tasks are to separate from parents and establish relationships that are lasting and satisfy need for affection and dependency. Individuals who are unable to resolve conflicts develop multiple psychological and personality deficits.

- ERICKSON'S IDENTITY VS. IDENTITY CONFUSION. Adolescents become aware of their individual characteristics, anticipate future goals, and realize that they have strength and purpose to control their destiny. Individuals who experience identity or role confusion can feel isolated, empty, anxious, and indecisive. Adolescent behavior is inconsistent and unpredictable during this chaotic state; projection is the most common defense mechanism. Adolescents seek a knowledge of self and attempt to formulate a set of values.

- ERICKSON'S INTIMACY VS. ISOLATION. The young adult prepares to unite his or her identity with another; relationships of intimacy, partnership, and affiliation develop. Person may have diffi-culty with intimacy, isolate self, or be unwilling to commit to intimacy.

- ERICKSON'S GENERATIVITY VS. STAGNATION. Concern that the next generation will have access to information, products, and ideas may be expressed through caring (showing concern, wanting to care for those in need, sharing knowledge with others), which is needed for survival of the culture.

- ERICKSON'S INTEGRITY VS. DESPAIR. Virtue in this stage is wisdom, which maintains and conveys the integrity of accumulated experiences from previous years. Feelings of wholeness counteract feelings of despair that life was meaningless.

Object Relations

This theory explores how an individual views self and relationships with others; it is a particularly useful concept when working with patients with severe personality disorders.

Psychiatrist Otto Kernberg's definition of object relations states: "... stability and depth of the patient's relation with significant others as manifested by warmth, dedication, concern, and tactfulness. Other qualitative aspects are empathy, understanding, and the ability to maintain a relationship when it is invaded by conflict or frustration." Theory used by Kernberg to understand borderline personality and narcissistic personality disorders. One symptom of importance is splitting; an individual is unable to integrate "good" and "bad" images of self and others.

- OBJECT CONSTANCY, or the ability to maintain a relationship even during times of frustration and change in a relationship, is evaluated when caring for persons with severe personality disorder.

Margaret Mahler developed a theory of separation and individuation. A child's task in the first three years of life is to develop a separate unique identity, and to learn self-soothing behaviors when comfort is not received from a mother figure. Individuals with severe personality disorders did not fully develop object constancy.

Studies In Personality Disorder Development

- TWO TESTS — SMOOTH-PURSUIT EYE TRACKING AND BACKWARD MASKING — are used to study individuals with schizotypal personality disorder and the role of the brain in abnormal interpersonal relations.

- Smooth-pursuit eye tracking. Important for cognitive interpretation of information in the environment. Impaired tracking is associated with social isolation, detachment, and inability to relate to others.

- Backward masking. A visual stimulus is shown, immediately followed by a different visual stimulus; this can indicate cognitive-perceptual difficulties, often in patients with schizotypal personality disorder.

• AN INCREASE IN CEREBROSPINAL FLUID HO-MOVANILLIC ACID has been indicated in studies of schizotypal patients.

• THE ROLE OF NEUROTRANSMITTERS, ESPECIALLY SEROTONIN, has been studied and implicated in the etiology of suicidal, aggressive, and impulsive behaviors.

• A DYSFUNCTION IN THE BRAIN SYSTEM'S ABILITY TO MODULATE AND INHIBIT AGGRESSIVE RESPONSES TO ENVIRONMENTAL STIMULI has been suggested by some studies.

• **A VARIETY OF CRISES HAVE OCCURRED IN THE LIVES OF INDIVIDUALS WITH PERSONALITY DISORDER,** particularly those in Clusters A (paranoid, schizoid, and schizotypal disorders) and B (antisocial, borderline, histrionic, and narcissistic disorders). To plan care for these individuals (persons with Cluster C disorders tend not to seek help from mental health care providers), it is helpful to consider levels of the stress-crisis continuum (Burgess, Roberts, 1995). Individuals with personality disorder due to only partial mastery of a developmental task or stage can be classified under level 2: transition stress. Other individuals, depending on their degree of stress, may be classified at other levels, for example, level 5 if there is an ongoing psychotic process, or level 6 if suicidal or if psychiatric emergencies arise.

• **DSM-IV (1994) CLASSIFIES PERSONALITY DISORDERS IN THREE CLUSTERS.**

Cluster A: Personality disorders in which the behavior of the individual appears odd or eccentric.

• PARANOID PERSONALITY DISORDER involves a pattern of distrust and suspiciousness such that

others' motives are interpreted as malevolent.

• SCHIZOID PERSONALITY DISORDER involves a pattern of detachment from social relationships and a restricted range of emotional expression.

• SCHIZOTYPAL PERSONALITY DISORDER involves a pattern of acute discomfort in close relationships, cognitive or perceptual distortions, and eccentricities of behavior.

Cluster B: Personality disorders in which the behavior of the individual appears dramatic, emotional, or erratic.

• ANTISOCIAL PERSONALITY DISORDER involves a pattern of disregard for and violation of the rights of others.

• BORDERLINE PERSONALITY DISORDER involves a pattern of instability in interpersonal relationships, self-image, and affects, and marked impulsivity.

• HISTRIONIC PERSONALITY DISORDER involves a pattern of excessive emotionality and attention seeking.

• NARCISSISTIC PERSONALITY DISORDER involves a pattern of grandiosity, need for admiration, and lack of empathy.

Cluster C: Personality disorders in which the behavior of the individual appears anxious or fearful.

• AVOIDANT PERSONALITY DISORDER involves a pattern of social inhibition, feelings of inadequacy, and hypersensitivity to negative evaluation.

• DEPENDENT PERSONALITY DISORDER involves a pattern of submissive and clinging behavior related to excessive need to be taken care of.

• OBSESSIVE-COMPULSIVE PERSONALITY involves a pattern of preoccupation with orderliness, perfectionism, and control.

• **AN INTERDISCIPLINARY APPROACH TO PROVIDING CARE** is built around assessment, nursing diagnosis, planning and determining patient outcomes, intervention, and evaluating outcomes.

Assessment
Basis for determining diagnoses and expected outcomes. To determine what questions to ask,

review the characteristics of an individual with a personality disorder.

- IDENTIFICATION OF SELF is assessed in a patient by considering several questions.

How does the patient take care of physical needs? Is he or she clean, appropriately dressed, and getting sufficient sleep, nourishment, and exercise?

Does the patient exhibit an inappropriate facial expression or have a flat, constricted affect?

Ask the patient to describe self, elaborating on strengths and weaknesses. (This assesses self-esteem and view of self.)

How anxious is the patient? What is he or she worrying about?

Ask the patient to describe what calming measures are used when feeling anxious, upset, or sad. Does he or she use alcohol or drugs, engage in sex with multiple partners, overeat, or harm self in anyway?

Ask patient if he or she has ever tried to mutilate self. Ask patient to describe these episodes in detail.

Does the patient deny strong emotions, such as anger and joy?

- INTERPERSONAL RELATIONSHIPS in the patient's life are assessed by considering several questions.

How does the patient interact with family? Does the patient have friends? How does the patient react to frustrations and disappointments in a relationship?

How does the patient function in the work place? Does he or she need constant supervision, or complain about the boss? Are the complaints centered around resenting assignments and accountability for work? (These questions can assist in understanding the patient's view of authority figures.)

Can the patient identify with others? Does he or she show empathy, or need to be the center of attention? Is patient critical of others, concerned about how others will evaluate him or her?

Does the patient demonstrate a low tolerance for frustration? How?

Does the patient identify self in the context of a relationship?

Does the patient have friends and or an intimate relationship or multiple sexual relationships? Ask patient to describe these relationships. (These questions will assist the nurse to assess the ability of the patient to form friendships and the nature of the relationships — stormy, intense, supportive, and/or reciprocal.)

- BEHAVIORAL PATTERNS of the patient may be assessed by considering the following questions.

How does the patient describe the problem areas that provoked the need for help? Can he or she identify the problem and discuss possible options to solve the problem?

Does the patient engage in illegal activities? If so, how does the patient view these activities? Is there a history of arrest(s)?

Has the patient experienced a lack of consensual validation, ideas of reference? Does the patient discuss odd beliefs, magical thinking?

Does the patient read hidden meanings into benign remarks of others? Is he or she suspicious? Does the patient question the fidelity of others?

Is the patient impulsive? Can he or she learn from mistakes?

Does the patient have a history of failing to honor financial obligations?

How does the patient view parenting responsibilities? Is there a history of child abuse or neglect?

Does the patient use drugs or alcohol?

Nursing Diagnosis

Diagnoses label the patient's problems from a behavioral perspective, which requires nursing interventions.

CLUSTER A

- ALTERED THOUGHT PROCESS related to inability to trust

- IMPAIRED SOCIAL INTERACTION related to inability to establish a relationship with others due to disruption in interpersonal skills

- PANIC LEVEL OF ANXIETY AND STRESS SUFFICIENTLY SEVERE to threaten work performance

- SELF-ESTEEM DISTURBANCE related to perceived threat to self-concept

CLUSTER B

- RISK FOR VIOLENCE: DIRECTED AT OTHERS related

to overt and aggressive acts

- RISK FOR VIOLENCE: SELF-DIRECTED related to marital conflict
- INEFFECTIVE INDIVIDUAL COPING related to threat of abandonment
- SELF-ESTEEM DISTURBANCE related to perceived occupational and/or relationship problem
- DEFENSIVE COPING related to unrealistic expectations of self and others

CLUSTER C

- SELF-ESTEEM DISTURBANCE related to negative feedback resulting in diminished self-worth
- INEFFECTIVE INDIVIDUAL COPING related to inadequate psychological resources due to an immature developmental level
- IMPAIRED SOCIAL INTERACTIONS related to unmet dependency need and a knowledge deficit about ways to enhance mutuality

Planning

The collaborative process of planning is done after expected outcome criteria are determined, based on diagnoses. The plan is integrated within critical pathways and identifies expected length of treatment. Patient is presented with plan, and feedback is carefully evaluated. Because symptoms are chronic, interview focuses on repeated problem areas and new options for problem solving.

Expected Outcome Criteria

Criteria are expressed as measurable statements to facilitate evaluating patient outcomes.

Interventions

Discussion within the context of the therapeutic relationship promotes patient's problem solving by asking strategic questions. Individuals with personality disorder have difficulty relating to others and often distort information; patient should be helped to discover his or her pattern of thought and behavior. Interventions focus on the patient's developing new coping skills. Patient teaching can incorporate books, movies, and television to broaden the patient's experiences to learn skills. Patient should also be taught about psychotropic medications.

Nurses have an important role in case management (Chapter 44). Milieu therapy, usually group therapy, is used to explore universal issues.

Evaluation

Patient's current symptoms are evaluated with reference to expected outcome statements. If criteria have not been met, consider if outcome statements are at an inappropriate level. (Patient may have enduring problems of maladaptive behavior.) The nurse needs to verify that the patient feels he or she has been active in care.

- **PERSONAL AND PROFESSIONAL BOUNDARIES** are an essential consideration in therapeutic relationships. Patients with personality disorder have difficulty identifying self and understanding the concept of personal boundaries. Professional boundaries help the nurse prevent "overhelping" and becoming too controlling, or focusing on the patient's negative symptoms, excluding his or her strengths. Setting limits is important with impulsive patients; discussing inappropriate behavior with the patient and contracting with the patient can prevent this type of conduct. In addition, nurses must monitor themselves to determine whether they are becoming too emotionally invested in patients, especially patients with borderline personality disorder. This investment can take the form of anger, withdrawing from interactions with the patient, as well as protecting or defending the patient in the care setting with other care providers. Clinical supervision for the nurse may be helpful.

TAKING ANOTHER LOOK

You are now ready to respond to situations described in Gaining a Perspective at the beginning of this chapter. After you have written or thought about your responses, you may wish to look at the Suggested Responses on page 330.

27 CHILD MALTREATMENT

GAINING A PERSPECTIVE

Consider the issues alluded to below, and after you have read the Key Concepts for this chapter describe your thoughts in greater detail.

1. How would you, as a nurse, feel about dealing with a parent who had physically abused a child?

2. Why do you think a nurse must be aware of physical signs of maltreatment?

Key Concepts

- **CHILD MALTREATMENT IS ONE OF THE MOST SERIOUS MENTAL HEALTH PROBLEMS IN THE UNITED STATES.** In 1962, Dr. C. Henry Kempe and his colleagues introduced the concept of battered child syndrome, but not until 1967 did all states pass laws that address reporting child abuse. Reported cases of child maltreatment, however, represent only the tip of the iceberg, as many maltreated children remain unidentified. Nurses need to be aware that child abuse occurs frequently. The increase in reported cases is due to public awareness and an actual increase in maltreatment, which is often provoked by poor economic conditions and fewer resources for parents.

  In 1994, 3,140,000 children were reported to child protective services. Statistics by type of maltreatment were: 45% neglect, 26% physical abuse, 11% sexual abuse, 3% psychological, and 16% other. Father's and mother's partners are frequent perpetrators, but the majority of child maltreatment is committed by mothers. Mothers spend more time with children and are often a single parent (risk factor).

- **FOUR MAJOR CATEGORIES OF CHILD MALTREATMENT** have been identified.

  Physical Abuse: physical injury intentionally inflicted on a child by a parent or caretaker through the use of excessive and inappropriate physical force.

  Sexual Abuse: any sexual contact between a child and an adult (or considerably older child) whether by physical force, persuasion, or coercion; can also include such acts as exhibitionism, sexually explicit language or materials, and voyeurism.

  Neglect: failure to meet a child's basic needs, including food, shelter, clothing, health care, education, and safety. Neglect involves acts of omission, rather than commission as in physical abuse.

Psychological Abuse: parental behaviors that are spurning, degrading, terrorizing, isolating, or rejecting.

Different types of child abuse often occur together.

• **MANY THEORETICAL FRAMEWORKS** have been used to explain child maltreatment. In recently devised models, multifactorial etiology takes into account parental, child, and ecological variables. The ecological perspective (Belsky, 1993) conceptualizes child maltreatment as a social and psychological phenomenon determined by multiple forces in the individual, family, community, and culture. What determines whether child maltreatment occurs is the balance of stressors and supports — the balance of potentiating (risk) and compensatory (protective) factors. There is, therefore, no single cause of child abuse and no single solution.

Another comprehensive approach to child maltreatment is the stress and coping model (Hillson and Kurper, 1994). The model (Study Guide Figure 27-1) explains the need for continuous monitoring of parental, child, and ecological factors. The stressful or nonstressful nature of these factors is determined by primary cognitive appraisal. If a stressor is present, then secondary appraisals are used to determine the internal and external resources the caregiver has to cope. Coping strategies may be facilitative and not result in maltreatment or may be less facilitative and result in child neglect.

• **INDIVIDUAL, FAMILIAL, AND SOCIAL FACTORS ALL CONTRIBUTE** to the likelihood that a caregiver will abuse a child: Enhancing parents' potential for abuse are stress factors, such as economic difficulty and unemployment; parenting factors, such as unrealistic expectations of children; and psychological factors, such as poor impulse control or substance abuse. Children whose mothers are physically abused by husbands/partners are at increased risk for physical abuse. Physical abuse may also be the result of excessive corporal punishment "to teach

Figure 27-1
A Stress and Coping Model of Child Maltreatment

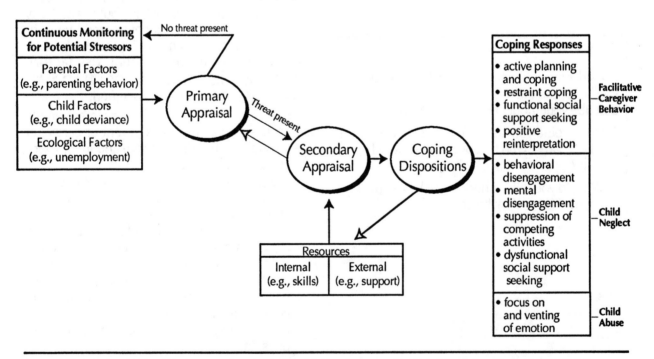

Source: Hillson JMC and Kuiper NA. A stress and coping model of child maltreatment. IN *Clinical Psychology Review* 14:270 (1994).

the child a lesson." The type of parenting one received as a child is another major factor that may influence parenting; parents may relate as their parents related to them, with rejecting and mistreating behaviors. It is estimated that 30% of abused children become abusive parents. Subsequent involvement in emotionally supporting relationships decreases the likelihood that a maltreated child will become a maltreating parent.

Substance-abusing caregivers are at risk for maltreating their children. Characteristics of substance-abusing women that interfere with parenting include depression, increased parenting stress, inadequate social support, and low educational attainment. Because substance abuse is a common problem, all parents should be screened for substance abuse histories. Parental risk factors for physical abuse are listed below:

Nonbiologic parent present in the home
Single parent
Lower level of education
Social isolation
Negative social support
Child health problems
Parent health problems
Parental anxiety, depression, anger, distress
Substance abuse
Reliance on corporal punishment for discipline
Negative parent-child interactions
Parental history of child abuse
Lack of economic resources
Inadequate living conditions
Spousal/partner abuse

- **SEVERAL CHILD CHARACTERISTICS ARE BELIEVED TO PLACE CHILDREN AT RISK FOR MALTREATMENT.**
Premature birth
Congenital defect
Product of multiple birth
Developmental disability
Physical disability
Chronic illness

These factors do not cause the parent to abuse the child, but may increase stress in the family system. Many children who are maltreated do not possess any of these characteristics.

- **THE COGNITIVE, EMOTIONAL, SOCIAL, AND SOMETIMES PHYSICAL DEVELOPMENT OF CHILDREN IS NEGATIVELY AFFECTED BY MALTREATMENT.** It often has serious immediate and long-term consequences. Child maltreatment is associated with lower intelligence, developmental delays, poor academic performance, aggressive and/or antisocial behaviors, lower self-esteem, family dysfunction, withdrawn and/or submissive behaviors, fear of new situations, and chronic anger and anxiety. Long-term effects include depression, psychopathology, sexual difficulties, and in severe cases post-traumatic stress disorder and dissociation.

- **NEGLECT IS THE MOST PREVALENT FORM OF CHILD MALTREATMENT.** Physical neglect tends to be chronic. Neglect is often not obvious, as it is difficult to distinguish it from poverty. Recognition involves skilled clinical judgement.

Physical Indicators of Neglect
- Malnourishment, poor hygiene, and inappropriate dress, including very soiled clothing.
- Inadequate medical care, including dental problems and lack of immunization.
- Numerous accidental injuries due to inadequate supervision.
- Educational neglect, history of truancy, and avoidance.

Behavioral Indicators of Neglect
- Developmental delays particularly in the language area.
- Poor school performance, inability to concentrate, and inadequate sleep at home.
- Infants appear dull, inactive, and excessively passive.

Failure to thrive (FTT) is a diagnosis that describes growth that is below expected norms for age and sex. It typically appears in the first two years of life. Diagnostic criterion is an infant's/child's weight falling below the fifth percentile. Poverty is considered the greatest single risk factor for FTT.

- **PSYCHOLOGICAL MALTREATMENT** is often part of other types of maltreatment, but can occur independently. It is usually a chronic impediment to normal development. It is difficult to define.

  Effects of psychological maltreatment may include:

  Failure to thrive syndrome

  Developmental delays

  Speech disorders

  Poor appetite

  Enuresis

  Encopresis

  Sleep disorders

  Low self-esteem

  Aggressive behavior

  Depression

  Suicidal behavior

  Five Types of Psychological Maltreatment

  - SPURNING: verbal battering combining rejection and hostile degradation, e.g., belittling, shaming, ridiculing normal emotions, singling out to criticize and punish, and humiliating publicly.

  - TERRORIZING: threatening to physically hurt, kill, or abandon the child, e.g., placing a child in chaotic circumstances or recognizably dangerous situations, setting unrealistic standards, exploiting the child's fears, or threatening violence against the child's objects or loved ones.

  - ISOLATING: confining or placing unreasonable limitations on the child's freedom or environment.

  - EXPLOITING AND CORRUPTING: modeling antisocial acts, or unrealistic roles, or encouraging deviant standards or beliefs, e.g., encouraging prostitution or pornographic performances or substance abuse.

  - DENYING EMOTIONAL RESPONSIVENESS: ignoring a child's attempts to interact or interacting with a child in a mechanical way devoid of affection or touch.

Factitious Disorder By Proxy (FDBP), Also Called Munchausen Syndrome By Proxy (MS-BP)

A form of child abuse where the parent falsifies an illness in a child by lying or creating symptoms and then seeks medical care. Victim is usually between infancy and 6 years of age. Parents may also induce physical findings in their children, for example by suffocation, administration of drugs or toxic substances, or putting blood in the urine or feces.

- CLINICAL INDICATORS of FDBP are listed below.

  Recurrent illnesses for which no cause is identified.

  Unusual symptoms that do not make clinical sense.

  Symptoms that are observed only by the parent.

  Frequent visits to hospitals and findings reported normal.

  Presence of drugs that induced symptoms in a toxic screen.

  Discrepancies between the history and physical findings.

  Numerous hospitalizations at different locations.

The mother, who is usually the perpetrator, seems truly concerned and may have Munchausen's syndrome herself.

- **THE DEATH OF A CHILD CAUSED BY ABUSE OR NEGLECT** is a tragic clinical situation encountered by nurses. An estimated 1271 children died of neglect in 1994. The high rate of homicide among children younger than 5 years is due to caretaker abuse and neglect. (Homicide is the second leading cause of death among children.) Children are at the greatest risk for being killed during the first month of life; children at this age are biologically vulnerable to assault, and their dependency (behavior) may annoy some adults. The victims of abuse are usually the youngest or second youngest in the family. Boys are at great risk after the first year of life. Mothers who begin childbearing at an early age are considered at increased risk for fatally maltreating their children. Most children experience maltreatment before the fatal incident. This finding speaks to the importance of early detection and reporting. Most states have an interagency, multidisciplinary child death review team at a local level to systematically evaluate and manage cases. The teams improve communication and cooperation among agencies, increase knowledge of risk factors for child homicide, systematically evaluate agency actions and interactions, and identify surviving siblings at risk for maltreatment.

- **INDICATORS OF PHYSICAL ABUSE MUST BE RECOGNIZED BY NURSES DURING THEIR ASSESSMENTS OF CHILDREN** so that early intervention can prevent subsequent abuse.

  History. A careful, detailed history is done of all injuries, including an explanation of how they occurred. Abusive parents may give implausible explanations for the injury or deny knowledge. Parent and child should be interviewed separately whenever feasible. Characteristic histories of child abuse include:

  History inconsistent with injury.

  Denial of any knowledge of cause or mechanism of injury.

  Parent reluctant to give information.

  Parent blames sibling for injury.

  Child developmentally incapable of specific self-injury.

  Delay in seeking medical attention or unnecessarily traveling long distances for medical care that is available at a closer location.

  Inconsistencies in history.

  History of repeated injuries or hospitalizations.

  Inappropriate response to severity of injury.

  Previous placement of a child in foster care.

  Previous involvement with child protective services agency.

  Physical examination. The child may be receiving treatment for a condition other than the injury caused by abuse. Indicators of abuse may be recognized at that time (see Study Guide Table 27-1).

  Bruises change color with time as blood is absorbed (see Study Guide Table 27-2).

- **SEXUAL ABUSE ENCOMPASSES A WIDE RANGE OF BEHAVIORS,** and most sexually abused children experience multiple types of abusive acts. The legal definition of sexual abuse varies by state jurisdiction. In general, most state statues define abuse as any sexual contact or activity between a child and an adult whether by force or coercion.

  Sexual activity between adult and child is generally progressive, and the severity of the sexual act usually escalates. Most adults who sexually abuse children are relatives, friends of the family, or others that the child knows and trusts. There are generally two prerequisites for sexual abuse: sexual arousal of children and willingness to act on the arousal. Most offenders are men (10% are women) and many offenders commit the first act during adolescence. Sexual abuse is common in our society.

  Risk factors for sexual abuse

  Presence of stepfather.

  Children who are living without one or both biological parents.

  Poor parenting.

  Mother who is disabled, ill, or out of the home.

  Paternal violence.

  It is important to note that race, social class, and ethnicity are not risk factors for sexual abuse.

  Impact of sexual abuse

  - IMMEDIATE IMPACT ON THE CHILD depends on frequency and duration of the abuse, use of force, penetration, and family reaction. Changes are seen in the following areas.
    – Behavior problems
    – Low self-esteem
    – Anxiety and depression
    – Increased fears
    –- Increased sexualized behaviors
  - LONG-TERM IMPACT is strongly associated with the following problems in adulthood: anxiety, anger, depression, revictimization, self-mutilation, sexual problems, substance abuse, suicidality, impairment of self-image, interpersonal problems, obsession and compulsion, dissociation, post-traumatic stress syndrome, and somatization.

TABLE 27–1.
INDICATORS OF PHYSICAL ABUSE

Cutaneous injuries
Bruises
In various states of healing
Bilateral, linear, or geometric injuries
In configuration of object
Pinch marks, pair of crescent bruises
Located on face, neck, thighs, genitals, back, inner upper arms, thorax
Grip marks on upper arms
Human bite marks
Oval shape pattern of teeth marks

Traction alopecia
Irregular areas of hair loss
Broken hair
Subgaleal hematoma

Abrasions, lacerations
Circumferential abrasions or friction burns from ropes at neck, wrist, ankles, torso
Chain imprints
Linear puncture marks from fork

Burns
Immersion burns
Uniform in depth, sharp lines of demarcation
Bilateral burns of feet, hands, and buttocks
Flexion creases spared because child flexes extremities
Contact burns
Resemble configuration of object In various stages of healing
Circular crater the diameter of a cigarette
Commonly located on face and dorsum of hands and feet

Head trauma and central nervous system injuries
Bilateral skull fractures
Multiple skull fractures
Skull fractures with widths greater than 5 mm
Subdural hematomas

Separation of sutures due to chronic subdural hematoma
Subgaleal hematoma
Decreased level of consciousness
Grip marks on upper arms
Spinal cord injury

Ophthalmic injuries
Hyphema
Retinal detachment
Dislocated lens
Retinal hemorrhage
Subconjunctival bleeding
Periorbital ecchymosis

Neck trauma
Subluxation or dislocation

Skeletal injuries
Multiple fractures, especially bilateral
Fractures of various ages
Spiral fractures of humerus (forcible twisting)
Transverse fractures (blunt trauma)
Rib fractures, especially if multiple, bilateral, or posterior
Fractures of the sternum, spinous processes, scapula
Fractures of femur in children younger than 3 years
Fractures of the epiphyseal–metaphyseal junction
Digital fractures

Blunt abdominal trauma
Abdominal distention, tenderness, bruising
Absent bowel sounds
Peritoneal or mesenteric bleeding
Persistent vomiting or abdominal pain
Bilious vomiting
Hypovolemic shock
Injury to liver, spleen, pancreas, duodenum, jejunum, kidneys
Signs of peritonitis

Adapted from Kelley SJ (ed): Pediatric Emergency Nursing, ed. 2. Norwalk, CT, Appleton & Lange, 1994.

Traumagenic Dynamics Model

In this frequently used conceptual model the effects of abuse depend on the characteristics of the abuse and on four areas of child development: sexuality, ability to trust, self-esteem, and the sense of being able to affect the world. Four mechanisms account for differences in the effects of sexual abuse:

- TRAUMATIC SEXUALIZATION refers to how the sexual abuse is done, e.g., fondling, penetration.
- BETRAYAL refers to the discovery that someone trusted has harmed — not protected — them.
- STIGMATIZATION refers to negative messages about self (shamefulness and guilt) that are communicated during the abuse experience.
- POWERLESSNESS refers to the child's sense of control and efficacy being overridden.

Assessment of sexual abuse

- HISTORY-TAKING should involve interviewing the parent and child separately, as both have the need to express feelings as well as provide information. Why does the parent feel the child has been abused, and who is suspected of the abuse?
- PHYSICAL INDICATORS of sexual abuse
  - Trauma to the genitals or rectum.
  - Chafing, abrasions, or bruising of inner thigh.
  - Scarring and tears of the hymen.
  - Decrease in hymenal tissue.
  - Vaginal or rectal bleeding.
  - Vaginal or penile discharge.
  - Foreign body in the urethra, vagina, or rectum.

TABLE 27–2.
GENERAL GUIDE TO ESTIMATION OF AGE OF BRUISES

Color	Age of Bruise
Red-blue	1–2 days
Blue-purple	2–4 days
Greenish yellow	5–7 days
Yellow-brown	7–14 days
Normal skin color	14–21 days

Reproduced with permission from Kelley SJ (ed): Pediatric Emergency Nursing, ed. 2. Norwalk, CT, Appleton & Lange, 1994.

- Pregnancy, especially among young adolescents.
- Complaints of vaginal or rectal pain.
- A sexually transmitted disease.
- BEHAVIORAL CHANGES are more common than physical complaints. Is the child acting out sexually with peers, siblings, and/or adults? The abused child may masturbate frequently and compulsively or make precocious sexual remarks.

- **INTERVENTION** is required for any type of child maltreatment. A child needs to be referred for psychological evaluation. Because abuse usually occurs in a family context, family dysfunction needs to be addressed. Treatment modalities include individual therapy, group therapy, family therapy, and play and art therapies. The treatment should be abused-focused therapy (AFT). AFT is based on the concept that abuse is a form of victimization by the powerful against the powerless; abuse is described and explored in an effort to comprehend it.

A nurse's responsibilities in child maltreatment include:

Knowing the indicators of child abuse and neglect.

Case identification.

Obtaining a careful history and comparing it with existing injuries.

Observing interactions between parent and child.

Collaborating with other members of the health care team.

Carefully documenting all objective data.

Reporting all suspected cases of maltreatment to child protective services.

Assessing child's immediate risk if returned home.

Protectiing child from subsequent abuse through hospitalization or foster placement.

Referring family for services.

Providing emotional support to child and parents.

Preventing child maltreatment.

- **LEGAL ISSUES** are clarifed by careful recording of procedures. Documentation, including photographs, of suspected abuse or neglect is essential. Statements should be recorded whenever possible, and the behavior of parent and child described fully and carefully. Subjective opinions should be omitted. These records are often subpoenaed and used as evidence in a legal proceeding. The disposition of the case has many variables. Will the child be at immediate risk for further abuse if returned home? Alternatives are admission to the hospital, placement with a family member, or in an emergency, placement in a foster home. All states provide a mechanism to protect children in emergencies.

Legislation usually outlines the procedures for reporting suspected child abuse and neglect. Legislation in 50 states mandates reporting by professionals who work with children. Nurses need to be knowledgeable about child abuse laws in the states in which they work so they know the procedures for reporting and the penalties for not reporting. Only a suspicion of abuse is necessary to report a case; actual proof or evidence is not required by law. Reporting is not a punitive action, but rather a referral for further investigation into the child's environment. Parents should always be informed.

• **A MULTIDISCIPLINARY APPROACH TO CHILD MALTREATMENT,** including nurses, physicians, therapists, attorneys, and social workers, is imperative. Nurses can become involved in the American Professional Society on the Abuse of Children which supports research, education, and advocacy.

TAKING ANOTHER LOOK

You are now ready to respond to the questions raised in Gaining a Perspective at the beginning of this chapter. After you have written or thought about your responses, you may wish to look at the Suggested Responses on page 330.

28 VIOLENCE IN FAMILIES

TERMS TO DEFINE

attachment theory

foster care

interpersonal violence

primary prevention programs

GAINING A PERSPECTIVE

Think about the following problems, and after you have read the Key Concepts for this chapter present your responses in greater detail.

1. Why are women more likely to be victims of family violence?

2. What might you, as a nurse, do in the following situation?

> A neighbor comes to your home and tells you that she is very afraid of her husband. He has beaten her on several occasions and is verbally abusive. Her two young children are also afraid of him. He is a heavy drinker and usually is most violent when he is drinking. She has threatened to leave him, but he becomes more abusive when she does this. She does not work out of the home and sees no way to support herself.

KEY CONCEPTS

- **HUNDREDS OF THOUSANDS OF AMERICANS ARE HARMED BY THEIR FAMILIES.** Vicious crimes of violence are committed by or against children, parents or grandparents, spouses, and other close relatives. To be abused by a partner, parent, or child or to witness abuse leaves deeply ingrained memories and has serious consequences. Victims must deal with feelings of fear, loyalty, love, self-blame, guilt, and shame all at the same time. For most people, home represents security; to victims of domestic violence, home is a place of danger.

  Family violence has always existed. Women have been battered by their partners in almost every society in the world. From biblical times, the history of childhood is replete with suffering.

- **AS A LEGAL MATTER,** violence within the family has only recently surfaced. Research into the causes and consequences of family violence is limited. "Family" has no national legal definition. Data on violence are classified by marital status, spousal status, or relationships among members of the household. Trends in family violence must be interpreted against a decline in the percentage of households with exclusively married couples and their biologic children.

  Violence between growing numbers of same-sex and opposite-sex cohabiting partners is increasingly being regarded as family violence, regardless of legal status. Violence between divorced or separated couples is also listed as family violence.

- **FAMILY VIOLENCE IS DISTINGUISHED FROM INTERPERSONAL VIOLENCE,** interpersonal violence being behavior by persons against persons that intentionally threatens, attempts, or actually inflicts harm. Within families, however, daily interaction and a shared domicile usually increase the opportunity for violent encounters. Because family members are bound together in a continuing relationship, it is quite likely the offender within the family will repeat the violation. An unequal power relationship makes one more vulnerable to aggression and violence. Moreover, the offender often threatens additional violence if the incidents of violence are disclosed. The victim may refrain from disclosure, anticipating stigmatization and denigration. Finally, episodes of violence often occur in private places, invisible to others, and are less likely to be detected.

- **FAMILY VIOLENCE MAY BE VIEWED AS PROGRESSING THROUGH DEVELOPMENTAL STAGES.**

Courtship

Dating violence includes slapping, pushing, beating, and threatening. Recurring and escalating episodes of violence within a relationship are quite common if the relationship is not terminated (about 50% of relationships are terminated). Research indicates that a large number of college students (20% to 50%) experience physical aggression in dating relationships. Problems that lead to violence include jealousy, interference from family and friends outside the relationship, and more fighting and conflict between the couple. Jealousy may be conceptualized as a reaction to the threat of loss and can result in anger. Possessiveness and control can also lead to aggression.

Marriage

Spousal assault is the single most common cause of injury for which women seek emergency medical attention. Women are three times more likely to be injured while they are pregnant. One survey reported that 16 of every 100 couples reported at least one incident of physical aggression during the year preceding data collection. The prevalence of severe violence was four in 100 females, five in 100 males. Factors linked to women's likelihood of being raped or battered are violence in the family of origin (most important factor), passivity, hostility, low self-esteem, alcohol and drug abuse, being more educated than one's partner, and if violence is being used against children.

Children

The incidence of assaults against children has increased greatly. Family violence can escalate to homicide. Newborns, infants, and children aged 1 to 4 years are more vulnerable to homicide than children aged 5 to 9. Infants are more likely to be killed by their mothers. For children younger than 5 years, the risk for males is greater than for females. Compared with men, women face a greater risk of homicide perpetrated by a family member.

Elderly

Little is known about the occurrence of assaults against elderly persons. Studies do not separate elder abuse from neglect, but it is estimated that 2.5% to 3.9% of elderly persons had experienced physical violence, verbal aggression, or neglect.

- **MOST THEORIES ONLY PARTIALLY EXPLAIN THE CAUSES OF FAMILY VIOLENCE.**

Social and Cultural Perspective

Feminist theory asserts that the unequal power distribution between men and women subjects women to male dominance in all spheres of life. Power extends to sexual as well as social relationships. Unequal distribution of power also helps explain physical and sexual abuse of children by parents. Growing up in a patriarchal society, children are socialized into respective sex roles and children learn through family experience or through the media about the "macho" culture.

Recent changes in family organization and structure may account for some family aggression. Foster care, adoption, and informal placement of children with relatives expose children to violence from caretakers for whom the minimal moral constraints of parenting are less salient. Increasing numbers of children are not living with their natural parents.

Social isolation is characteristic of some families that are at high risk of physical and sexual abuse of a spouse or child. Victims of abuse often become isolated from family of origin, neighbors, or anyone who could become acquainted with the abusive events. The transmission of violence from one generation to the next is as much a component of subcultura-tion as any other learned behavior.

Biopsychosocial Perspective

Children's perceptions of and interactions with family members are important in a child's development. Social bonding can fail or become narrow and selective.

Children who lack caretaker protection experience tremendous anxiety and may survive by dissociating themselves from trauma. Dissociations produce feelings of numbness. One early manifestation may be that the child is cruel to animals, siblings, friends, and even parents; the child lacks sensitivity to the pain of others. This cruel and detached behavior may be noted in date abuse or events like gang rapes occurring in junior and senior high school. There is no sense of the impact on the victim.

Family violence has been linked to mental illness and personality disorders. People prone to depression may be prone to violence.

- **ASSAULTIVE AND HOMICIDAL BEHAVIORS ARE DIFFICULT TO EXPLAIN.** In courtship violence, the aggressor may not want the relationship to end; the harasser can not tolerate separation because rejection is an attack on the ego. Rage and aggression inhibit impulse control: "I killed her because I loved her."

Three formative events contribute to the development of hostility in people who murder.

Early childhood trauma in which the distress caused by the physical or sexual abuse is not handled properly

Developmental failure in which the caretaker has no influence over the child/adolescent, probably because of poor attachment

Interpersonal failure in which the adult caretaker is not a role model for the developing child.

- **AGGRESSION TOWARD THE ELDERLY IS MULTIFACETED** and the dynamics differ. Much research is needed.

- **NO CONTINUUM OF FAMILY SUPPORT PROGRAMS ADDRESSES THE DEVELOP-MENTAL PHASES OF FAMILY VIOLENCE.** It is critical to identify families at risk for violence as well as to provide services for abuse victims. Counseling and education must respond to community needs and utilize community resources.

PoliceResponse

Arrest, which is intended to stop domestic violence, may increase the incidence.

Shelters and Other Services

Shelters provide a safe residence and emotional support for battered women and their children. Woman can become self-sufficient. Typical family stays are from 2 days to 3 months; there are approximately 1200 shelters that service more than 300,000 women and children a year. Many times there are services for the children and sometimes even for the batterers.

Primary Prevention Programs

Educational programs and awareness campaigns are available for batterers. Programs teach children and adults nonviolent ways of coping with anger and frustration; they stress that family violence is a crime and help is available. Courts often mandate that batterers attend these programs as well as alcohol and drug rehabilitation programs if necessary.

Medication

Drugs may be used to treat depression and affective disorders; a significant number of abusive caretakers suffer from these conditions.

Foster Care

Foster care is a major intervention in child abuse cases. It is used to stop abuse immediately. One must, however, keep in mind what the long-term effects might be on the child.

Home Nurse Visitation

Visiting the home is a proactive means of detecting maltreatment of infants and children. When abuse is not evident, intervention is appropriate for high-risk groups (poor, unmarried teenagers having their first child). Nurses can be supportive, teach parenting skills, and link families to community and social service agencies.

- **CLASSIFICATION OF FAMILY VIOLENCE CASES** can center on the level of stress/crisis.

Level 1: Somatic Distress

Generally, the patient is seen in primary care facilities for medical presentation of such symptoms as bruises, fractures, bleeding. The patient's response is fear, anxiety, and/or masked depressive symptoms. Etiology of the crisis is physical injury and psychological abuse. Interventions include:

- Treating the injury, and identifying and confirming abuse
- Assessing patient safety may include referral for the following services: a shelter, proper legal/law enforcement assistance, home nursing for assessment and teaching, or support groups for mother and/or children

Level 2: Transitional or Altered Self-Regulatory Pattern

Violence may occur during pregnancy, after delivery of the baby, or during arguments about paternity, infidelity, or custody. Usually a prior contact with a child protective service is involved; nursing staff may be endangered. Interventions may include:

- Referral to family court
- Staff training for critical incident planning (defining roles in advance)
- Debriefing staff after the incident
- Referral of victims to ensure their safety and follow-up to determine that it is continued

Level 3: Traumatic Stress Crisis

Usually precipitated by externally imposed stress that overwhelms the individual, e.g., physical assault, rape. Response is intense fear, helplessness, and behavior disorganization. Interventions include:

- Reporting the assault to law enforcement
- Referring victims of rape or assault for short-term counseling and/or group sessions

Level 4: Family Crises

Violence reflects serious disruption in partner or caregiving relationships. Crises involve failure to master adult developmental issues, such as dependency, value conflicts, emotional intimacy, and power and control. Examples are child abuse, adolescent runaways, homelessness, and domestic homicide. Interventions include:

- Reviewing the case to determine who should assist the abusive family and/or the affected individuals

Level 5: Serious Mental Illness

Violence reflects a preexisting psychiatric problem that interacts with patient's disorganized thinking and behavior. Interventions include:

- Careful case monitoring
- Assessing need for hospitalization or shelter care
- Monitoring compliance with medication and treatment plan

Level 6: Psychiatric Emergencies

Situations in which general functioning has been impaired involve threat of harm to self and/or others, e.g., suicide attempts, stalking, rape, out-of-control behavior. Interventions include:

- Rapidly assessing the patient's psychological and medical condition
- Clarifying the situation
- Mobilizing mental health, medical, and/or legal resources
- Arranging for follow-up and coordination of services

Level 7: Cataclysmic Crises

Interpersonal cataclysmic crises, unlike a mass disaster type crisis, have a Level 3 crisis in combination with a Level 4,5, or 6 stressor. For example, a battered wife is threatened that her children will be harmed.

TAKING ANOTHER LOOK

You are now ready to respond to the problems that were raised in Gaining a Perspective at the beginning of this chapter. After you have written or thought about your responses, you may wish to look at the Suggested Responses on page 331.

29 SCHIZOPHRENIA

TERMS TO DEFINE

catatonia

concreteness

delusions

dopamine

hallucinations

high expressed emotions

loose associations

negative symptoms

positive symptoms

schizophrenia

social skills training

stress-vulnerability model

GAINING A PERSPECTIVE

Think about the following questions, and after you have read the Key Concepts of this chapter respond more comprehensively to the queries.

1. What do you think makes schizophrenia a chronic disease, and why is it so difficult to deal with?

2. As a nurse, what should your first reaction be to a patient who is diagnosed as having schizophrenia and who tells you that he is hearing voices?

KEY CONCEPTS

• **SCHIZOPHRENIA, AN ILLNESS OFTEN SYNONYMOUS WITH MADNESS, CONNOTES BOTH MYSTERY AND FEAR.** The distorted perception of reality that a person with schizophrenia has was historically misunderstood, feared, and regarded as evil or punishment for some wrongdoing. Individuals were not viewed as persons with a chronic mental disease.

Presently, allocation of resources is a low priority, and advocacy groups are trying to encourage proper restoration of funds for needed resources for schizophrenic patients. Nurses have a dual responsibility in caring for these individuals: first, to provide direct care and education to the patients and their families, and second, to advocate for funding and expansion of the nursing role, and to dispell myths about the illness.

Several myths surround schizophrenia.

• Schizophrenia means split personality.
• Schizophrenia is caused by "inadequate mothering."
• Schizophrenia is caused by LSD and street drugs.
• Persons with schizophrenia are mentally retarded.
• Schizophrenia is uncontrollable and disabling.

• **EPIDEMIOLOGY**
The incidence of schizophrenia is 1:100,00, but because of its chronic nature, it affects 0.5% to 1% of the world's population. Median age of onset in males is the early to late twenties, and in females, the late twenties. There is equal frequency of the disease among males and females, but it is more severe in males and they may require hospitalization. With the deinstitutionalization movement, persons previously hospitalized lost their social support network.

TABLE 29–1
DSM-IV KEY FEATURES OF SCHIZOPHRENIA

- Psychotic symptoms (at least two) present for at least a month:
  Hallucinations
  Delusions
  Disorganized speech
  Disorganized or catatonic behavior
  Negative symptoms (flat affect, lack of motivation)
- Impairment in social or occupational functioning
- Duration of the illness for at least 6 months
- Symptoms are not primarily due to a mood disorder; schizoaffective disorder; or medical, neurologic or substance-induced disorder

Approximately, 30% to 50% of homeless Americans have a diagnosis of schizophrenia.

- **THE DIAGOSTIC CRITERIA** in DSM-IV that must be met for the diagnosis of schizophrenia are included in Study Guide Table 29-1. Schizophrenia must be differentiated from other psychiatric illnesses, drug reactions, and medical syndromes (see Study Guide Table 29-2).

- **ETIOLOGY**
  Schizophrenia is a brain disease of unknown etiology. It manifests a variety of symptoms and has a variable course. It is suggested that most explanatory models fall into one of three categories that define the disease:
  A single process leading to diverse manifestations. A medical disease that exemplifies such a process is multiple sclerosis.
  Multiple disease entities leading to the illness (e.g., mental retardation).
  Specific symptom clusters reflecting different disease processes that combine in different ways in different patients.

- **SEVERAL THEORIES HAVE BEEN PROPOSED ABOUT THE CAUSE OF SCHIZOPHRENIA.** In the past, theories reflected the nature versus nurture or biological versus psychological dichotomies; now more integrative models have been proposed.

Psychoanalytic and Family Interaction
- Mostly historical. Psychoanalytic theories explained schizophrenia as caused or precipitated by dysfunctional family interactions and deficient parenting.

Biologic Theories
- Genetic. Schizophrenia runs in families; first-degree relatives of individuals with schizophrenia have a tenfold greater risk of developing the disease.
- Prenatal and environmental. Children born in the winter months are at greater risk. Prenatal factors include nutritional state at delivery, complications during delivery, and postnatal apnea and hypoxia.
- Neurophysiological. Findings from imaging techniques include ventricle enlargement, cerebral asymmetry, and decreased cell density.
- Biochemical. Excessive dopamine in the limbic system may account for psychotic symptoms of schizophrenia; evidence that neuroleptic medications alleviate symptoms by

TABLE 29–2
IMITATORS OF SCHIZOPHRENIA-LIKE PSYCHOSES

Brain disorders	Drug reactions
Embolism	Alcohol withdrawal
Ischemia	Amantadine
Trauma	Amphetamines
Tumor	Atropine
Epilepsy	Bromide
Encephalitis	Bromocriptine
Narcolepsy	Carbon monoxide
Systemic disorders	Cocaine
Vitamin B-12 deficiency	Corticosteroids
Acquired immune deficiency	Dexatrim
syndrome (AIDS)	Ephedrine
Syphilis	Levodopa
Tuberculous meningitis	Lidocaine
Pellagra	LSD
Hypoglycemia	MAO inhibitors
Hepatic encephalopathy	Phencyclidine
Hyperthyroidism	Propranolol
Lead poisoning	Tricyclic antidepressants
Lupus	
Multiple sclerosis	

blocking dopamine receptors supports this view. Dopamine imbalance is also thought to be responsible for many of the cognitive dysfunctions.

Stress Vulnerability Model

The integrative process is clearly circular with multiple feedbacks.

- **Vulnerability**

    DOPAMINE DYSFUNCTION. An individual with schizophrenia has an inherent vulnerability to dopamine dysfunction. Some defect in neurotransmission of dopamine to the prefrontal (learning) area of the brain is present accompanied by decreased blood flow while carrying out challenging cognitive tasks; decreased cognitive performance may be the result of decreased processing capacity. Increased dopamine in the mesolimbic system causes psychotic symptoms. Stress increases dopamine release into mesolimbic system, where dopamine is unmodulated by inhibitors; schizophrenic symptoms thereby increase during stress. Stress also reduces cognitive processing ability.

    COGNITIVE PROCESSING DEFICITS. Understanding cognitive processing deficits helps explain some of the thinking difficulties of persons with schizophrenia. Deficits occur in selective attention, active and long-term memory, and the function responsibile for "switching" information from one perceptual mode to another. Persons with schizophrenia have delays in "switching" (i.e., sight to hearing), lapses in attention when performing complex tasks, difficulty in selectively focusing their attention, and poor response to requests (may respond to a new request by performing an activity previously asked for).

- **Stress**

    Various levels of stress are identified in the vulnerability model of schizophrenia. LIFE EVENTS. Stresses of daily living (e.g., losses or financial problems) often correlate with exacerbation or onset of schizophrenia. ENVIRONMENT. Stimulation (e.g., noise, crowds, or moving objects) demands ability to adequately process and selectively fo-

cus attention; these abilities are decreased or lacking in persons with schizophrenia. FAMILY CONFLICT. A critical or emotionally overinvolved family climate (a high level of expressed emotion) is the third category of stress in the stress-vulnerability model. The problematic behavior exhibited by a person with schizophrenia may provoke negative and stressful reactions among family members which, in turn, exacerbate schizophrenic symptoms.

- **Protectors**

    ANTIPSYCHOTIC MEDICATION AND COPING SKILLS. Medication raises the threshold for psychotic symptoms. To help prevent hospitalization, a patient is taught to monitor symptoms, report early symptoms of relapse, and seek medication adjustment and intensive treatment.

    FAMILY EDUCATION, PROBLEM SOLVING, AND SOCIAL SUPPORT. Family programs provide basic information about schizophrenia, relapse prevention, resource utilization, and stress management techniques. Social support for patients includes intensive case management and drop-in centers.

- **TREATMENT**

    ### Psychopharmacological

    - Use of neuroleptics, such as chlorpromazine. The high-potency agents have greater extrapyramidal side effects; lower-potency agents have higher sedative and anticholinergic effects.
    - An antipsychotic, clozapine, causes no movement disorders and is used to treat resistant patients; it can cause life-threatening blood dyscrasias.

    ### Environmental

    - Crisis intervention

        SHORT-TERM HOSPITALIZATION FOR ACUTELY DISTURBED PATIENTS. Goals of hospitalization include maintenance of safety, and diagnostic assessment and evaluation. Then, movement is to a less intensive treatment environment, e.g., partial hospitalization, assisted-living programs, or home care. Because schizophrenia is a chronic disease, the patient may require intermittent hospitalization for acute exacerbations.

SOCIAL SKILL TRAINING (SST). An effective way to learn to counteract the deficits resulting from isolation and alienation that accompanies schizophrenic symptoms. First, acute symptoms are controlled by medication; then, in a highly structured format, patients engage in conversation, and learn assertiveness, heterosocial, and medication management skills.

- **NURSING ASSESSMENT** is directed toward the patient's responses to an illness that drastically alters his or her experience of the environment and others. The patient's behavior and verbalizations reflect an altered perception of reality and a decreased ability to coordinate and sort information—a compromise in the way he or she functions mentally or socially.

One task of the nurse is to recognize the manifestations of schizophrenia.

Alterations of Thinking

- Altered senses. Patient feels a sensory overload, an acuity of smells, sounds, and colors. Later in the illness, senses are dulled and the world seems flat. When sensory overload is occurring, patient may pace and move about, or be unable to concentrate or remain in a noisy area. Patient may state that he or she is having a mystical experience.
- Inability to interpret incoming sensations. Patients have difficulty understanding meanings of sentences, or connecting individual words or visual and auditory perceptions, or performing simple tasks. Consequently, the patient loses the ability to perform activities of daily living and to function in simple jobs. Patients are unable to make decisions and appear frozen.
- Loose associations. Unable to distinguish concepts by meaning.
- Concreteness. Unable to abstract.
- Hallucination. A sensory perception (sight, sound, smell, taste, or touch) in the absence of an external stimuli to the corresponding sense organ; most hallucinations in persons with schizophrenia are auditory. Patients may be seen mouthing words when no one is there, having conversations, reacting in fear and anger, or taking actions.
- Delusions. Fixed, false beliefs that are maintained despite experience and evidence to the contrary. They may be prosecutory, negative, somatic, or grandiose, or delusions of control. The patient's behaviors are guided by false beliefs, e.g., a patient who thinks he is being poisoned won't eat.

Alterations in Feelings

- Altered sense of self. The sense of body boundaries and personal space is disrupted. Patients with schizophrenia frequently need increased personal space or none at all.
- Changes in emotion. Patients may have inappropriate flat or exaggerated affect. They report fear and excessive guilt. In the later stage of schizophrenia, there is no observable affect.

Alterations in Movement and Behavior

Catatonia is the most dramatic change in movement. Patient remains motionless and demonstrates "waxy flexibility" (remains in the new position that he or she is placed in). Neuroleptic medications may account for many of the movement alterations and these must be differentiated from the illness. Brain involvement can result in repetitive movements, tics, and general awkwardness or clumsiness.

- **NURSING INTERVENTIONS,** both verbal and environmental, are initiated to decrease a patient's need to function beyond his or her capacities. Support must be provided during an acute episode, and education follows the cessation of symptoms.

General principles of intervention have been established.

- Maintain a nonjudgmental attitude. Be aware of your own fears and biases and beliefs about individuals with odd or eccentric speech or behavior.
- Maintain a serious attitude. Attempt to understand the speech or behavior of patients

from the perspective of their world.

- Develop the patient's trust by being honest and keeping agreements.
- Present your reality without challenging the patient. Acknowledge the patient's experience and ask him or her to consider the possibility of distortion caused by the disease.
- Promote and create structure for the patient.
- Carefully assess for side effects of neuroleptic medication and distinguish bizarre behavior, mannerisms, flatness, and catatonia from dystonic (slowed) movements and muscular rigidity caused by medication.
- Maintain awareness of patient's personal space and body boundaries.
- Advocate increased or reduced medication doses as appropriate, and treatment of medication side effects.

Interventions for Alteration of Senses

- Environmental interventions. Decrease stimuli; monitor noise level.
- Verbal interventions. Speak slowly and softly; express one thought at a time; assess whether patient is able to focus on the sound of your voice.

Interventions for Inability to Synthesize and Respond

- Environmental interventions. Simplify environment; perform tasks with patient to assess level of functioning; make a schedule and assign a team member to ensure that patient follows schedule.
- Verbal interventions. Simplify sentences to one complete thought; interact in a quiet environment; use restatement and reflection.

Interventions for Loose Association

Attempt to clarify what you hear; emphasize most relevant theme; let patient know when you see the connection and when you do not.

Interventions for Delusions

- Environmental interventions. Assess patient's response to environment; be alert for suspiciousness. If patient is paranoid, be aware of spatial distances in groups; be aware of potentially dangerous objects if patient feels threatened, and allow for an appropriate degree of choice.
- Verbal interventions. Do not challenge the delusion, but acknowledge it and respond to the patient's expressed feelings.

Interventions for Altered Sense of Self

Assess patient's use of personal space; set limits if patient is intrusive and maintain distance if patient is fearful. Use touch judiciously; ask permission to touch, as touch can be therapeutic for these isolated individuals.

Interventions for Changes in Emotion

Recognize that patients may not be able to express emotions appropriately; limit environmental stimulation, and monitor and manage others' inappropriate responses to the patient.

Interventions for Changes in Movement and Behavior

Provide opportunities for movement and exercise; assess rituals and set time limits or promote privacy for inappropriate sexual behavior (public masturbation); explore meaning of behavior; assess for medication side effects.

TAKING ANOTHER LOOK

You are now ready to respond more comprehensively to the questions that were raised in Gaining a Perspective at the beginning of this chapter. After you have written or thought about your responses, you may wish to look at the Suggested Responses on page 331.

30 THE SERIOUSLY MENTALLY ILL, HOMELESS POPULATION

TERMS TO DEFINE

assertive community treatment

Critical Time Intervention Model (CTI)

homelessness

National Alliance for the Mentally Ill (NAMI)

nurse case manager

recidivism

seriously mentally ill (SMI)

GAINING A PERSPECTIVE

Think about the issues presented below, and after you have read the Key Concepts of this chapter address the problems in greater detail.

1. Why do you think the deinstitutionalization movement has lead to increased homelessness for the seriously mentally ill?

2. Why do you think you could or could not work as a nurse dealing with the seriously mentally ill, homeless population?

KEY CONCEPTS

• **SERIOUSLY MENTALLY ILL PATIENTS, ABOUT 500,000, WERE DISCHARGED FROM LONG-TERM STATE HOSPITALS** over a period of 20 years as a result of the Community Mental Health Centers Act of 1963. The act promoted mental health care in the least restrictive environment, emphasizing comprehensive services at the local level. Early intervention and comprehensive services were intended to reduce hospitalization and hence costs.

The mental health care delivery system was not prepared and monies were not available for the necessary reorganization. The result was a loss of focus on services for seriously mentally ill persons. At the beginning of the community mental health movement, it was suggested that the role of the psychiatric nurse be expanded to include individual and group therapies, as well as to work with nonpsychiatric nurses so that they could understand and help families understand the nature of serious mental illness among deinstitutionalized patients. Nurses could assist in maximizing these individuals' capacities to function, an essential component of caring for patients with incurable illness.

Community mental health centers (CMHCs) overestimated the seriously mentally ill patient's ability to function in the community. The predictable outcome for these difficulties was often homelessness.

Persons with severe, persistent mental illness are often described in terms similar to those used to describe homeless people: unemployed, physically disabled, victimized, substance abusers, severe social disaffiliation, frequent contact with the criminal justice system, and subsistence-level incomes. Homelessness poses a considerable additional burden on the lives of the seriously mentally ill.

- **CONTINUOUS SCHIZOPHRENIA IS A CONDITION OF MANY SERIOUSLY MENTALLY ILL PATIENTS.** "Continuous" means there has been no remission of symptoms during the period described. Schizophrenia can be a seriously disabling disease (see Chapter 29). These seriously mentally ill patients usually have enduring (over a year) self-care deficits in all biopsychosocial spheres. Although the causes are multifactorial, the neurobiological changes have been confirmed by technology.

- **THE CONCEPT OF MANAGED CARE** has developed from models of health maintenance organizations (HMOs), conceived to provide comprehensive health care services at reduced cost. The principles of care are based on prevention, early intervention, and continuity of care, similar to those promoted as part of the community mental health centers and deinstitutionalization. To avoid managed care pitfalls similar to those experienced with deinstitutionalization, the following actions are suggested:
  - Programs be developed to educate the health team in interdisciplinary collaboration.
  - Safeguards be in place in the system to prevent usurping mental health dollars in favor of other health care services.
  - Strategies be developed for supporting and maintaining patients in the community.

Case Management
In this multidisciplinary strategy for intervention, case managers, who are public health advocates, act as agents for the seriously mentally ill. Managers find and secure appropriate resources in the community. As community mental health workers they make assessments, home visits, and referrals. They participate in crisis intervention and assist with social skills training and family support (see Chapter 44, Case Management).

Nurse case managers, who represent about 10% of all case managers, are trained in psychiatric and community mental health nursing. In addition to the activities mentioned above, the nurse case manager is also involved in mental health education and is usually responsible for medication activities, such as ordering stock supplies for patients (particularly those on long-acting antipsychotic injections), keeping records, and monitoring side effects and adverse reactions. The nurse case manager may also assist the patient in obtaining Medicaid benefits, enabling the patient to obtain medications from the pharmacy.

- **THE PROGRAM OF ASSERTIVENESS COMMUNITY TREATMENT (PACT) EMPHASIZES STRONG COLLABORATION** among service providers for the seriously mentally ill (SMI). Whether the program, which is a model, will be effective with the homeless SMI remains to be seen. Complicating factors in homelessness are an individual's distrust of authority and disenchantment with mental health care providers; the staff must be empathetic. Collaboration is multifaceted: it is a vital ingredient in the nurse-patient relationship, and an essential characteristic of the interactions among team members and in team interactions with the numerous community organizations. This model does not replace the case management model, but rather is adapted to complement and enhance it. Its effectiveness is measured in the reduced rates of recidivism and psychiatric emergencies and in increased compliance with medication and socialization regimens.

- **THE MENTAL HEALTH SYSTEM IS HAUNTED BY RECIDIVISM (THE "REVOLVING DOOR SYNDROME")** in which the seriously mentally ill have short discharges into the community and repeated hospitalizations. This happens for a variety of reasons, including noncompliance with medications; lack of insight into their own illness; lack of careful discharge planning and limited resources, especially housing; and accessibility to street drugs.

Medication Issues
- The patient's compliance is enhanced when peers counsel and teach seriously mentally ill persons.
- Seriously mentally ill individuals associate medications with control issues.
  -They do not like the side effects.
  -They do not like to be told that they must

take the medications for a long time. Titration of doses is ideally done in a mutually agreeable way; the nurse may have more success teaching on an individual basis.

- When medication is not effective and symptoms become such that the patient is dangerous to self or others, then involuntary admission may be advisable. Psychiatric emergency services, homeless outreach, and mobile crisis teams assess the person for homicidal or suicidal ideation, history of physical violence to self, others, or property, and other key factors in the mental health status of the patient.

Crisis Intervention

- SMI patients may not have the communication skills to ask for the help they need. Their self-esteem is often too low to admit vulnerable feelings of inner weakness.
- Stresses in the environment build and if lines of communication are not kept open, crises may occur. Approaching the patient in a sensitive manner in the early stages of a perceived problem usually helps reduce emotional intensity.
- If a gentle approach fails and the patient perceives no allies, a "show of force" (uniformed police) may help to enlist cooperation. Once the patient is calm, the nurse judges what should be the course of action. Usually the SMI person is not as dangerous as the uninformed public thinks; invariably there is a trigger that can be identified and avoided before emotions escalate to rage.

Substance Abuse

Seriously mentally ill patients have a high incidence of alcohol and drug abuse. The nurse needs to understand the motivating factors behind the patient's use of the substance. If the reason for the abuse can be identified, then, perhaps, alternative options can be identified to satisfy the need. With nowhere to go and nothing to loose but profound feelings of loneliness and sadness, substance abuse is a temptation that is difficult to overcome. Later in treatment, when the patient is engaged in service programs, the nurse can set firm limits. High expectations are not imposed; rather an attitude of confidence in the patient to eventually help himself or herself is necessary.

Statistically speaking, the Twelve-Step Program (Chapter 31, Substance Abuse) has achieved the best results for those willing and able to try it. Many SMI patients, however, do not have the communication skills to use this method. Inpatient detoxification programs are also available.

- **FAMILIES OF SERIOUSLY MENTALLY ILL INDIVIDUALS** suffer enormously in trying to cope with the patient; the persistent nature of the illness often overwhelms a family's frustration level. The National Alliance for the Mentally Ill (NAMI), a patient advocacy organization, supports family members. NAMI members (140,000) lobby to prevent budget cuts and to promote mental health. NAMI is committed to decreasing the stigma of mental illness research.

  The emotional cost of having a family member with a serious mental illness is incalculable, but support groups and family therapy are recommended.

- **HOMELESSNESS IS DEFINED AS SLEEPING IN PUBLIC PLACES, BUS OR TRAIN STATIONS, STREETS, ABANDONED BUILDINGS, PARKS, BEACHES, OR SHELTERS FOR ANY NUMBER OF NIGHTS; HOMELESSNESS MAY ALSO BE VIEWED AS DISAFFILIATION.** Disaffiliation refers to a lack of social support or friends to whom one can turn in time of need. This does not mean that the homeless do not feel emotional attachments; most people do not choose to be homeless.

  It is argued that there is a false dichotomy between the mentally ill homeless and other homeless persons. Socioeconomic data and political groups view homelessness among all groups with or without mental illness.

  The number of homeless persons grew dramatically in the 1980s and continues to increase; the number could be as high as 3 million. It would seem reasonable to assume that the prevalence of mental illness among the homeless will also continue to increase, especially if funding for services continues to decline. The estimate is that approximately 30% of the homeless have mental illness, but this figure may not be accurate.

Epidemiology

The epidemiology of homeless people has changed from a stereotyped skid row male to younger people of both genders, and families. Physical health problems, such as tuberculosis and AIDS, are increasing in shelters. Statistics about the SMI homeless population have been collected in Baltimore, New York, and San Diego, and they indicate that 33% of the population had not finished high school, 75% had been homeless one year or longer, almost 33% had been homeless 10 years or longer, and 23% were homeless before the age of 18. About 72% were male; 30 % were female. Approximately 30% had been been placed out of their homes before the age of 18, and 63% reported that they had been incarcerated at least once.

- **HOMELESSNESS, HOUSING INSTABILITY, AND INADEQUATE HOUSING** are common problems for the SMI population, especially those with substance abuse problems. Factors such as deinstitutionalization, the loss of low-cost housing units, fragmentation of responsibility among health care providers, and limited resources contribute to homelessness.

Models for Housing

Two models — residential and supported — are described for organizing housing for persons with severe and persistent mental illness. One is the residential model in which persons are assigned to residences for the mentally ill. A residence is linked to treatment facilities and the patient progresses within the facility until he or she is able to live independently. The second model is supported housing in which housing is generally independent and not linked to services. Support services are provided as needed.

The Critical Time Intervention (CTI) Model emerged as a result of research in New York. The critical time of adjustment from shelter to community housing includes the first months when new relationships have to be forged. As this is an obvious time of stress for the seriously

mentally ill individual, extra services are provided. CTI specialists are case managers who know the community's resources, information which allows them to provide a stable linkage between the shelter and the small community agencies. A manager follows the patient for 9 months after the patient leaves a shelter.

Programs, such as the Fort Washinhgton's Men's Shelter in New York, use the CTI model. They take the patient from the street to the shelter, and provide medical, nursing, and psychiatric services as well as group education in medication, money management, housing, and substance abuse. Most referrals start with a well structured community residence.

It has been written that winning the confidence of the seriously mentally ill patient is vital; it is often facilitated by identifying one positive attribute of the patient. The time of intervention is also important; when a patient enters a shelter, it is a time when he or she feels demoralized and consequently may be most receptive to outreach. For the nurse to engage SMI patients, warmth is required in the interaction. A positive impression must be evoked. The nurse must initiate contact and establish communication. Residents in shelters, like all people, value being respected. The nurse's role is to facilitate an emotional connection with the seriously mentally ill person without violating professional boundaries or institutional policies.

TAKING ANOTHER LOOK

You are now ready to respond again to the issues presented in Gaining a Perspective at the beginning of this chapter. After you have written or thought about your responses, you may wish to look at the Suggested Responses on page 332.

31 SUBSTANCE ABUSE

TERMS TO DEFINE

addiction

alcoholic hepatitis

chemical dependence

denial

depressant drugs

dual diagnosis

hallucinogenic drugs

hypnotic drugs

impairment

intoxication

narcotic-analgesic

peripheral anesthesia

rationalization

sedative drugs

stimulant drugs

substance abuse

tolerance

withdrawal

GAINING A PERSPECTIVE

Think about the situations described below, and after you have read the Key Concepts of this chapter express your thoughts in greater detail.

1. How would you, as a nurse, feel in the following situation?

   A 36-year-old man is suspected of abusing alcohol and is admitted to the hospital. You are asked to do an admission interview. The first statement the man makes is, "I drink, but I'm not an alcoholic."

2. What are your concerns likely to be on a postoperative unit when a patient, who is admitted from emergency surgery, has a history of drug abuse?

KEY CONCEPTS

- **HUMAN BEINGS SEEM TO HAVE A NEED TO PERIODICALLY ALTER THEIR STATES OF CONSCIOUSNESS;** sometimes drugs or alcohol is used. Substance abuse and dependence tend to provoke strong emotional reactions from health care providers as well as the general public. One's emotional reaction is influenced by whether addiction is seen as a physical illness, learned behavior, genetic manifestation, or moral failing.

- **ADDICTION** is a process of proactive substance use resulting in the user's physical and/or emotional dependence on the substance (see Study Guide Table 31-1). Five phases are involved in the addiction process.

  Experimentation: a trial to assess the drug's effects.

  Recreation: using the drug expressly for entertainment and/or relaxation.

  Habituation: using the drug routinely, not for diversion or recreation.

  Abuse: using the drug of choice becomes more central to daily activities; more time is spent seeking and using the drug.

  Dependence: using a psychoactive chemical. This phase incorporates:
  - Tolerance of the substance
  - Continued use despite the life problems caused by the substance
  - Withdrawal symptoms when the substance is discontinued

  The drugs used, in addition to alcohol, are generally depressants, stimulants, or hallucinogens. Impairment refers to the alteration of judgment and/or physical response due to the ingestion of a psychoactive substance. Intoxication is the elated, excited, or exhilarated physical and emotional states that follow ingestion of the chemical. Tolerance is the need to increase the amounts of the chemical to pro-

TABLE 31–1
SUBSTANCE ABUSE AND DEPENDENCE

DSM-IV Criteria: Substance Abuse
The person must have experienced one or more of these in the past 12 months:
- failure to fulfill role obligations at home, school, or work
- recurrent drug or alcohol use in physically dangerous settings
- recurring drug-related legal problems
- continued use despite recurring interpersonal problems

DSM-IV Criteria: Substance Dependence
The person must have experienced three or more of these in the past 12 months:
- drug tolerance
- drug withdrawal
- drug use is greater in amount and frequency of use than intended (i.e., loss of control)
- persistent desire and unsuccessful attempts to stop or control drug use
- increasing time and energy spent in obtaining the drug
- lifestyle changes (social, recreational, or occupational) due to drug use
- drug use is continued despite knowledge of life problems

American Psychiatric Association (1994). Diagnostic and Statistical Manual of Mental Disorders, 4th Edition: Washington, D.C.: American Psychiatric Association.

duce consistent results. Withdrawal refers to the cluster of signs and symptoms that are experienced when the chemical upon which one is dependent is removed. The cluster reflects hyperactivity of the system that is in opposition to the one affected by the chemical of dependence; i.e., when heroin (a parasympathetic stimulator) is withdrawn, an individual experiences symptoms of sympathetic stimulation.

- **SUBSTANCE ABUSE IS AT EPIDEMIC LEVELS.** There is a 13% prevalence of alcohol dependence; approximately 18 million Americans have significant life problems due to alcohol. The use of cocaine has steadily been dropping since the mid1980s; the number of regular users in 1990 was approximately 800,000. Although use has declined, mortality has remained stable since the 1980s.

Opiate addiction includes the use of heroin and morphine as well as synthetic derivatives. Among cocaine users are people in poor urban areas and men who became addicted in Vietnam during the conflict there. Another group of opiate-dependent persons are those who had narcotics prescribed inappropriately for medical problems. Prevalence figures are not readily available because of the focus on cocaine abuse. New users have developed because of the use of "black tar" (a pure form of heroin) and "China white" (a synthetic narcotic).

Hallucinogens have changed. Lysergic acid diethylamide (LSD) was popular in the 1960s and early 1970s; now phencyclidine (PCP) is used.

- **THE USE OF PSYCHOACTIVE AGENTS IS COMMON TO ALL CULTURES AND ETHNIC GROUPS; HOWEVER, ATTITUDES TOWARD THEIR USE VARY WITHIN CULTURES AND ETHNIC GROUPS.** Specific drug use may be geographically defined. Research has shown significant differences in the way genetically similar groups metabolize specific drugs.

Women constitute 25% to 30% of the addicted population. The following information, based on research, describes some of what we know about women addicts:

- Women tend to begin using drugs and alcohol when with partners/mates; men tend to start using with other men.
- Fewer women enter into treatment than do men.
- Women tend to have more physical health problems as a result of using drugs than do men.
- Women tend to have stronger cravings for drugs and to relapse in the week before their menstrual periods.
- Up to 79% of women addicts were sexually abused as children.
- Pregnant addicts do not seek drug treatment because they fear being jailed and having their children removed by Child Protective Services.
- Women become drunk more rapidly than men do because they have proportionately less body fluid.
- Alcohol use has always been common

among adolescents as they experiment with adult behavior. Statistics on high school seniors indicate a decline in adolescent drug use; however, young people who dropped out of school were not included (the overall drop-out rate in the U.S. is 29.6%; black and Latino drop-out rate is 50%).

- The health care professional is in no way immune from substance abuse and dependence. Previously there was a very punitive attitude toward these professionals. Now, most state boards of nursing have moved toward rehabilitation.

Individuals may also have a dual diagnosis, both psychiatric and substance abuse disorders. These people have a cluster of problems (e.g., employment, financial, relationships) produced by the interaction of mental illness with substance abuse. Dual diagnosis is thought by some to be the mentally ill person's self-medication; e.g., hallucinations may lose their intensity when dulled by chemicals. Some propose that such common factors as trauma and genetics produce both substance abuse and mental illness. Others believe that substance abuse may produce mental illness. Persons with a dual diagnosis have great difficulty finding treatment.

TABLE 31–2
BLOOD ALCOHOL CONCENTRATIONS (BAC) AND BEHAVIORS

BAC	Behaviors
0.05	Impaired judgment, reduced alertness, loss of inhibitions, euphoria
0.10	Slower reaction times, decreased caution in risk-taking behavior, impaired fine-motor control
0.15	Significant and consistent losses in reaction time
0.20	Gross impairment in sensory and motor function
0.25	Severe sensory and motor impairment
0.30	Stuporous
0.35	Surgical anesthesia
0.40	Respiratory depression, lethal in approximately half of population

• THEORETICAL FRAMEWORKS
Medical Model

- To produce dependence, a drug must inhibit or stimulate cerebral neurotransmitters. Specific neurotransmitters have been identified for most common drugs.

- All addicting drugs act to eventually stimulate the release of or inhibit the reabsorption of dopamine.

- No evidence has been identified of a specific gene dysfunction common to all chemically dependent persons.

- In terms of alcohol metabolism, four variants of aldehyde dehydrogenase have been found. The fourth variant permits copious alcohol metabolism (greater alcohol intake) and is found in persons with severe addiction and concomitant physical illness.

Psychosocial Model

- Social learning theory holds that people learn to use specific drugs in specific settings. Teachers may be peers or family. Learning of addiction as a way of coping may occur if feelings of low self-esteem and/or effects of poverty and hopelessness are blunted by the drug.

- People use drugs to relieve anxiety. Use of drugs or alcohol becomes maladaptive coping.

- No specific personality disorder can be ascribed to addicted persons.

Family Systems Theory

The family systems theory views use of drugs and alcohol as a response to increased anxiety within the family. The person with the least power displays the symptoms (uses the substance) when anxiety in the family increases. The more powerful person(s) acts to protect the weak member and preserve the family (see Chapter 8, Systems Theory as a Model for Understanding Families).

• SUBSTANCES OF ABUSE
Alcohol

- Universal appeal; all cultures have used alcohol in some form. Acceptance of alcohol while condemning its effects is the prevailing attitude in the United States.

- Pharmacokinetics. Metabolism begins in the stomach; most goes unchanged into the small intestine and is absorbed into the circulatory system. It is disseminated to all body tissues, including cerebral. About 10% is excreted unchanged via perspiration and respiration; the remainder is metabolized by the liver and converted to acetic acid and water. Alcohol bathing the cerebral tissue acts similarly to narcotics and endorphins; the dopamine pathway is stimulated. An average-sized adult male can metabolize 1/2 ounce of alcohol per hour (four ounces of wine, 12 ounces of beer, one shot of whisky). Blood alcohol levels represent concentration of alcohol in the blood, usually measurable 20 minutes after ingestion; it peaks in one and a half hours (see Study Guide Table 31-2).

  As a drug that produces dependence, alcohol leads to tolerance. It takes a greater amount of alcohol to produce the effect. When the liver becomes less functional, less alcohol is needed for intoxication.

- Assessment of the alcoholic patient

  NURSE MUST ASSESS HIS OR HER OWN UNDERLYING ATTITUDES TOWARD ALCOHOL and must not have a punitive attitude. Patients may be frightened, fearful of rejection, and dependent.

  DEFENSE MECHANISMS frequently used by patients include:

  –Denial. If challenged, the patient becomes anxious and hostile, and it is difficult to establish a therapeutic relationship.

  –Rationalization. The patient minimizes the problem; the reasons sound plausible until one examines the outcomes of behavior.

  MANIPULATIVE BEHAVIORS may be used.

  USE DSM-IV CRITERIA TO GUIDE QUESTIONING. For example: Are you having problems with work? Is your family concerned about your drinking?

  PHYSICAL FACTORS. Breath odor, unsteady gait, or slurred speech may be detected. Tremors, irritability, increase in vital signs could signal lack of alcohol in a dependent person. Check nutritional status. Check for symptoms of alcoholic liver disease (cirrhosis): pain in right upper quadrant, anorexia, jaundice, elevated temperature, leukocytosis, and enlarged liver mass. The patient may have a history of

esophageal bleeding, cardiomyopathy, and heart failure. A CT scan may reveal cerebral atrophy; cognitive losses do not return with abstinence from alcohol.

Withdrawal from alcohol

-A potentially lethal phenomenon.

-Initially symptoms of central nervous system irritability: restlessness, anxiety, tachycardia,

TABLE 31-3
DRUGS OF ABUSE AND SYMPTOMS

DRUG CLASS	SYMPTOMS
Depressants	
Narcotic-Analgesics	
Opium	Constricted pupils,
Heroin	respiratory depression,
Morphine	hypotension, bradycardia,
Codeine	nausea, drowsiness,
Methadone	euphoria
Demerol	
Fentanyl	
Dilaudid	
Percodan	
Talwin	
Benzodiazepines	
Valium	Slurred speech,
Ativan	disorientation,
Halcion	staggering, relief from
Xanax	anxiety
Dalmane	
Librium	
Alcohol	Slurred speech,
	disorientation,
	staggering
Barbiturates	
Seconal	Slurred speech,
Tuinal	disorientation,
Phenobarbital	staggering
Amytal	
Stimulants	
Cocaine	Hypervigilance,
Amphetamine	euphoria, excitation,
Desoxyn	insomnia, anorexia,
Dexedrine	hypertension, tachycardia
Biphetamine	
Ritalin	
Hallucinogens	Visual, tactile,
Lysergic acid	auditory, or olfactory
diethylamide	hallucinations;
Phencyclidine	delusions; labile
Psilocybin	emotions
Mescaline	

nausea (symptoms are relieved by a drink).

–Restlessness progresses to visible tremors, diaphoresis, anorexia, insomnia, confusion, and transient hallucinations; convulsions may begin. Treatment is with a sedative.

–If not treated, within 72 hours the patient will experience delirium tremens with uncontrollable, severe shaking, restlessness, and agitation; the patient may experience dry heaves. Disorientation, confusion, and hallucinations may occur. All vital signs are elevated. Grand mal seizures are common. Treatment focuses on rehydration (oral or intravenous fluids) and decreasing autonomic reactivity (benzodiazepines used with CAUTION; if alcohol is taken with drug the effects may be lethal).

Depressants

Depressants are drugs that have a depressing effect on the central nervous system or that stimulate the parasympathetic nervous system. Depressants include sedatives, used to calm or relax; hypnotics, to promote sleep; and narcotic-analgesics, to relieve pain. The Harrison Act (1914) made it possible to secure narcotics only from a physician. In the U.S., narcotics are seen as appropriate for medical purposes; however, recreational or abusive narcotic users are individuals outside the law.

• Pharmacokinetics

DEPRESSANTS suppress the sympathetic nervous system by altering neurotransmitter levels.

OPIATE DRUGS (morphine, codeine, heroin, and the synthetic opiates such as meperidine) load the endorphin receptor sites, producing euphoria and analgesia; in overdose, can cause respiratory depression and death. Chronic users of narcotics deplete serotonin which regulates pain perception and anxiety. Tolerance is produced in the individual. Health care providers ascribe drug-seeking motivation to the addicted person, even when he or she is having pain.

– Withdrawal. Six to eight hours after use of the opiate the addict begins to feel nervous and edgy and begins to experience a runny nose, tearing, and piloerection. Muscles, joints, and bones begin to ache. Nausea, vomiting, and diarrhea start. These symptoms last 4 to 7 days and are uncomfortable but not lethal. Relief comes with ingestion of opiates or central nervous system depressants.

SEDATIVE-HYPNOTICS enhance the effects of gamma-aminobutyric acid (GABA), which inhibits synaptic activity in the central nervous system, producing a sense of calm and relaxation. Drugs produce tolerance. The most commonly used drugs are the benzodiazepines: diazepam (Valium), lorazepem (Ativan), alprazolam (Xanax), chlordiazepoxide (Librium), oxazepam (Serax), and triazolam (Halcion). These drugs are relatively safe compared with opiates. It is almost impossible to digest a lethal dose, but they are lethal with alcohol; the respiratory center becomes depressed and breathing stops.

–Withdrawal. As individuals become tolerant, the seizure threshold of the brain is raised; abrupt cessation of benzodiazepene lowers the threshold and causes seizures, frequently status epilepticus. Individuals are best tapered off the drug in an inpatient setting.

• **Nursing Assessment**

Persons addicted to depressant drugs may or may not fit the common stereotype of the addict. Users of intravenous heroin may indeed be emaciated with large inflamed areas from recurrent cellulitis. If, however, the person uses heroin intranasally, there will be few obvious signs of addiction.

HISTORY TAKING should include questions about all medications, including over-the-counter drugs. Ask about recreational use of drugs, as well as injuries and illness.

NUTRITIONAL DEFICITS are strongly correlated with drug dependence.

INFECTION STATUS is important to evaluate. Intravenous drug users and their partners have high rates of newly diagnosed HIV infection. The tuberculosis rate is also high. Cellulitis is common among needle users and pneumonia among heroin addicts. Sexually transmitted diseases are frequent because of impaired sexual judgment and the high rate of prostitution. Prostitution is a way of getting money for drugs.

A GENOGRAM is helpful. It is essentially a nonthreatening way to determine transmission of addiction and the availability of a potential

TABLE 31–4
WITHDRAWAL AND OVERDOSE SYMPTOMS

DRUG CATEGORY	WITHDRAWAL	OVERDOSE
Alcohol	Hypertension, tachycardia, tremors, nausea, anxiety, delirium, vomiting, seizures, death	Respiratory depression, bradycardia, hypotension
Depressants		
Narcotics	Anorexia, nausea, vomiting, chills, diaphoresis, panic, muscle cramps, watery eyes, runny nose	Shallow respirations, constricted pupils, shock, coma, death
Benzodiazepines	Anxiety, nausea, seizures	Respiratory depression
Stimulants		
Cocaine	Depression, hypersomnia, apathy, anhedonia, irritability	Seizures, hyperthermia, agitation, hallucinations
Amphetamines	Depression, hypersomnia, apathy, anhedonia, irritability	Paranoia, hyperthermia, agitation, seizures
Hallucinogens	None	Psychosis

support system.

Stimulants

Caffeine does not meet the criteria for tolerance, but withdrawal symptoms may be experienced and it can be addictive. Nicotine is also addictive and has strong withdrawal symptoms; it creates strong urges to relapse in its users. Only cocaine and amphetamines (illegal drugs) will be considered in this chapter.

• Historical Perspective. Cocaine could be purchased in over-the-counter tonics (Coca Cola) until the passage of the Harrison Act (1914). During the 1920s, cocaine was popular among entertainers and gangsters. In the 1980s, middle-class young, ambitious people found that cocaine produced euphoria and boundless energy. In the mid-1980s, crack-cocaine was introduced. People smoking crack receive an immediate euphoria which lasts 15 to 20 minutes. After this, a profound crash occurs with immediate dysphoria. Strong motivation exists to use more of the drug.

Amphetamines, methamphetamine, and dexedrine, known for years as "speed," have long histories of use. Amphetamine was used during World War II in the military. Dexedrine

was used by people who needed to stay awake for long periods. The anorexic effects of amphetamine were noted, and in a culture beginning to be obsessed with slenderness, diet pills were produced using the drug. In 1970, the FDA restricted the use of amphetamines to attention deficit/hyperactivity disorders, short-term weight loss, and narcolepsy. A smokeable form of methamphetamime, "ice," has the same general effect as crack, but lasts up to 14 hours.

• Pharmacokinetics. Cocaine blocks reuptake of norepinephrine, dopamine, and serotonin and the accumulations stimulate the sympathetic nervous system and produce a sense of well-being, energy, and euphoria. Cocaine is metabolized by the liver and is assessed by measuring its metabolites (usually in urine).

• Nursing assessment. An overview is gained of the psychiatric/psychological sequelae of drug use; assessment is the same as discussed for alcohol and depressants. The stimulant addict in withdrawal is dysphoric and anhedonic, incapable of feeling pleasure. Mood and affect may be difficult to assess as a function of withdrawal; even after the last dose of drug has been detoxified, neurotransmitter levels may be so unbalanced as to produce signs of clinical depression. Physical effects of stimulant addiction include tachycardia, hypertension, increased respiratory and metabolic rates, anorexia, restlessness, and pupillary constriction. Cocaine use causes massive systemic vasoconstriction, which can produce myocardial infarction with coronary artery spasm, cerebral accident with cerebral vessel constriction, and spontaneous abortion with uterine artery constriction. Epistaxis from snorting cocaine, trauma due to lifestyle, and infections are prevalent in cocaine-addicted populations, as is malnutrition. The addict may crave high-sugar foods, but has marked anorexia.

- Withdrawal. The overwhelming symptom is fatigue; during withdrawal the person may spend innumerable hours sleeping.

Hallucinogens

Deliberate use of hallucinogens has its roots in religious practice. Accidental ingestion occurred in the laboratory creation of LSD in 1938, and later it was used in the 1960s for recreational purposes. Phencyclidine (PCP) was developed by Parke-Davis (1956) for use as a general anesthetic. At low doses, PCP produces euphoria; at higher doses, hallucinations are produced and the PCP user becomes delusional and peripherally anesthetized.

There is no withdrawal. When these hallucinogenic drugs are insufficiently metabolized, they are stored in fat tissue; when fat tissue is metabolized, drugs may be released into circulation, producing hallucinations.

Users of hallucinogenic drugs have sympathomimetic signs, dilated pupils, salivation, hypertension, and hyperthermia. They are at risk for trauma due to an altered state of consciousness.

- **DRUG TESTING** may be required by companies as a condition of employment. A danger associated with drug testing is false negatives (drinking large quantities of water may produce a false negative) or false positives. Some false positives include:

alcohol	cough syrup or any medication in tincture
opiates	poppy seeds (large quantities), ibuprofen
amphetamines	decongestants containing ephedrine or pseudoephedrine

- **CARE OF THE DRUG-ABUSING CLIENT**
Planning
- Clear goals must be set by the nurse. Is the patient presenting for treatment of the addiction? The nurse must be aware that the patient being treated for other health problems may begin to have withdrawal symptoms (see Study Guide Table 31-4).
- A holistic approach is needed that takes into account the stage of the patient's addiction or recovery. Regardless of the staff's assessment of a patient's readiness, an addicted person requesting help must be given assistance and information.

Implementation
- The first priority is physiological stability and detoxification. A nurse's responsibility is to monitor physiological stability and insure adequate fluid and nutritional intake, emotional support, and education.

Treatment Options To Prevent Relapse
- Medical Model
  MEDICATIONS
  –Disulfiram (Antabuse) is for alcoholic recovery. A person using alcohol when taking Antabuse will have palpitations, nausea and vomiting, facial flushing, and diaphoresis.

  –Nalatrexone is a long-acting narcotic antagonist that acts to block craving. The alcoholic requiring analgesia must use preparations that are non-narcotic.

  –Methadone, a long-acting synthetic opiate, is used for recovery from heroin addiction. Two methods of administering methadone may be used: doses are gradually decreased (tapered withdrawal) and finally discontinued (designed to prevent withdrawal symptoms) or a stable dose may be given to the addict indefinitely.

  –Nursing responsibilities include educating the patient about medication and addiction, and providing emotional support.

  SELF-HELP GROUPS address the problems of addiction and recovery. Nursing responsibilities for patients who are interested include education about the choices of groups that are available.

–Twelve-Step Programs: Alcoholics or Narcotics Anonymous. The programs consider addiction a disease of the body, mind, and spirit. They are self-help groups that use peer support to achieve total abstinence; daily meetings are available. Assistance provided by a "sponsor" (one who has succeeded) prevents isolation of the recovering person.

–Women for Recovery. Group acknowledges the differences in how men and women experience addiction. Women achieve abstinence through building self-esteem and learning new coping skills and ways of thinking (13 Affirmations).

–Rational Recovery. Group rejects spirituality and powerlessness and, instead, members THINK themselves sober. Personal responsibility, choice, and decision making are emphasized.

- Psychosocial Model

  COGNITIVE THERAPY. Therapy attempts to alter thinking and behaviors associated with the person's addiction. Analyzes cognitions and behaviors and builds on new ways of looking at skills and strengths.

  BEHAVIORISM. One looks at specific drug-seeking, drug-using behaviors and teaches alternatives. Another approach deals with extinguishing the conditioned response to the drug.

  HUMANISTIC THERAPY. Therapy seeks to have the individual understand the addiction and teaches new ways of coping.

  NURSING RESPONSIBILITIES in using psychosocial modalities include one-to-one or group therapy, education, emotional support, and coordinating services.

- Family Systems Theory

  The theory views addiction as a function of anxiety. The therapist works with the addicted person and with as many family members as will participate. The family needs to see repeating patterns of its behavior so that blaming the addict can stop. The addicted individual learns new ways of dealing as a healthy person. Alanon for adults and Ala-Teen for adolescents are excellent support groups that teach emotionally nonreactive ways to deal with the addict.

Evaluation

The single most important indicator of success is sobriety or cessation of substance use. In times of great stress, relapse is possible. It may be appropriate to measure periods when the person is sober or not using the addictive substance and periods when the person is intoxicated or using the substance; treatment may be considered successful if periods of intoxication and substance abuse become shorter and increasingly rare and the periods of sobriety and nonsubstance use become longer and more productive.

TAKING ANOTHER LOOK

You are now ready to respond to the situations described in Gaining a Perspective at the beginning of this chapter. After you have written or thought about your responses, you may wish to look at the Suggested Responses on page 332.

32 MANAGEMENT OF SUICIDAL PATIENTS

TERMS TO DEFINE

ambivalence

attempted suicide

completed suicide

crisis

indirect self-destructive behavior

lethality

parasuicide

suicidal ideas

suicide

suicide gesture

GAINING A PERSPECTIVE

Think about the questions presented below, and after you have read the Key Concepts of this chapter describe in more depth how you, as a nurse, would respond in the situations.

1. What should you do initially if you suspect that a patient is suicidal?

2. How might you act in the situation below?

   A suicide has occurred at the high school where you work as the school nurse.

3. How would you feel if a patient on the psychiatric unit where you were working successfully committed suicide?

KEY CONCEPTS

• **SUICIDE IS THE NINTH LEADING CAUSE OF DEATH IN THE U.S. OR 1.4% OF TOTAL DEATHS.** The incidence of suicide has increased greatly since 1950, despite advances in treating mental illness. The increase has occurred especially among young black males (ages 10 to 19) and elderly men. Self-inflicted death annually claims approximately 30,000 individuals in the U.S. Among elderly men, one in four attempts end in death. Youth suicide is contagious; "copycat" suicides may be triggered by media events or other suicides.

• **SUICIDAL BEHAVIOR IS TYPICALLY A CRY FOR HELP.** When possible, nurses should strive to relieve conditions that produce a patient's suffering and to carry out a broad range of measures to prevent suicide. Successful management of suicidal patients depends on accurate assessment, interdisciplinary collaboration, and examination of attitudes toward suicide. To meet standards of practice, nurses need to detect and evaluate a patient's suicidal risk, provide adequate safety, inform the health care team, and document ongoing assessments.

• **A PATIENT'S SUICIDE RISK IS INFLUENCED BY THE PROFESSIONAL'S ATTITUDE** and assumptions about suicide; personal beliefs must be distinguished from professional attitudes. When patients feel devalued or feel that the nurse considers suicide wrong or immoral, they may hesitate to disclose suicidal risk or to follow the nurse's prescription for safety. For nurses who are novices or experts, suicidal patients tend to elicit feelings of inadequacy and anxiety and a fear of failing. The nurse's capacity for empathy and expertise will be enhanced by exploring and understanding his or her own feelings.

• **TERMS AND DEFINITIONS MUST CLEARLY DESCRIBE A PATIENT'S SUICIDAL BEHAVIORS** to avoid the staff's missing serious clues, a cry for help, and opportunities for prevention. Suicide may be defined as killing oneself on purpose by a direct or indirect method. Parasuicide includes all nonfatal suicidal thought, acts, attempts, or wishes. Lethality is the potential to cause death.

- **WIDE VARIATIONS OF SUICIDAL IDEAS, BEHAVIORS, AND ATTEMPTS OCCUR IN DIVERSE SETTINGS.** The frequency, intensity, duration, and goals of behaviors differ. Some patients do not share suicidal ideas unless asked about suicidal attempts; some have vague fleeting thoughts, others a chronic history of attempts.

  Suicidal behaviors vary greatly. A person may be someone who is covertly suicidal and complains of distress, or overtly suicidal and reports suicidal thoughts. Another type of suicidal behavior is seen in someone who denies suicide and is brought for medical attention by loved ones. An individual may periodically attempt suicide, perhaps by engaging in self-mutilation. Patient behavior suggesting the risk for suicide may be identified by other staff; a terminally ill patient may request assistance in dying.

  The patient's loved ones and friends, as well as different members of the health care staff, often provide important observations about suicidal behavior.

  Most patients who mutilate themselves (any form of self-injury) fear criticism or rejection. Self-mutilation occurs in 24% to 40% of psychiatric patients. Chronic self-mutilators typically alienate staff whose therapeutic efforts have been ineffective. Nurses must monitor self-mutilation acts and suicidal clues (see Study Guide Table 32-1).

TABLE 32-1
COMMON RISK FACTORS FOR SUICIDE

Risk Factor	Illustration
Psychiatric disorder,* depressive disorder, chemical dependency	Major depression (40% to 60%); chronic alcoholism (20%), schizophrenia (10%), phobias, post-traumatic stress disorders, borderline and narcissistic personality
Age, race, sex, being an older white male*	Male gender (70%); young adult, adult and older age caucasians > other groups Black, hispanic men (high risk ages 15 to 40)
Physical illness (higher risk if unrelieved pain or symptoms, advanced disease, or depression.)*	AIDS, cancer (head and neck, gastrointestinal neoplasms), Huntington's chorea, temporal lobe epilepsy, multiple sclerosis, peptic ulcer disease, spinal cord injuries, anorexia nervosa, head injury, Cushing's disease and hemodialysis
Prior suicide attempts*	About 15% of nonfatal attempters die by suicide
Suicide ideas, talk,* preparation	Verbal or written messages of suicide, "I want to die"; "I'd be better off dead"; jokes and diaries
Lethal suicide methods*	Firearms used by >60% males; hanging, poisoning by >40% females
Isolated, lives alone, loss of support*	40% to 50% of suicides lived alone or had no close friends vs. 20% nonfatal attempts
Hopelessness	No alternatives to suicide, rigid (either/or) thinking, tunnel vision. "Suicide is the only thing I can do."
Modeling of suicide in the family genetics*	Suicides and depressive illnesses tend to run in families; modeling or imitation predicts suicide among adolescents
Marital problems, family pathology*	Divorced/widowed >married, early separation from parents, physical/sexual abuse
Aggression/anger*	Murderous revenge, dissatisfied with life
Problems at work or school	Unemployment, retirement, no productive activities
Stress, life events*	Stress that erodes self-esteem and raises guilt, fear, interpersonal problems

*Single-variable predictors of suicide that experts agree are present in most suicides (excluding problem of comorbidity or interactions).

- **BECAUSE A UNIFIED, INTEGRATED THEORY OF SUICIDE IS LACKING, NURSES MAY NEED MANY THEORIES** to understand and treat patients.

Psychological Theories
Suicide may arise from diverse intrapersonal, interpersonal, and developmental sources.

- CRISIS THEORY. Crisis is a normal, time-limited response to a distressing event that overwhelms one's coping strategies. What is most important is the patient's perspective of the precipitating event. Nurses must guard against any impulse to discount or belittle a patient's perception of crisis. Crisis intervention focuses on the current situation and includes evaluating the patient's distress. Action is taken to improve the patient's safety, coping, and interaction with others and to reduce powerlessness. Crisis intervention is not as helpful with chronically suicidal patients, who require extensive treatment, and does not explain or evaluate the chronic or multiple suicidal crises that occur in patients with psychiatric disorders.

- COGNITIVE THEORY. Depression arises from distortions in cognitive processes (thinking, knowing, and perceiving). A cognitive triad has identified depression: the self is worthless; the world is barren; and the future is bleak. Depressed people alienate themselves by rejecting help, asking to be alone, and behaving in an "uncooperative manner." They rarely recognize the impact of these negative, isolating behaviors on their mood or self-esteem. Cognitive distortions and irrational beliefs guide thoughts and shape emotions. These beliefs can lead to depression.

  The nurse intervenes by increasing the patient's awareness of his or her negative focus and its influence on coping and depression. The nurse helps the patient examine unrealistic goals, set practical goals, and take pride in reaching a goal. Suicide risk declines as negative thought patterns and depression decline and problem solving improves.

TABLE 32-2
SCREENING INSTRUMENTS FOR ADULTS

Instrument	Characteristics	Scoring
Beck Depression Inventory (BDI)	Patients rate cognitive, affective, and somatic symptoms on a brief 21-item self-report scale. Easily administered.	≤10 = normal. Cognitive/affective items best indicators of depression in medically ill. Valuable measure for medically ill (Cavanaugh; Schwab)
Hamilton Rating Scale (HRS)	Interviewer-scored. Somatic symptoms = 52% of total score.	Gives more credit to somatic symptoms than BDI and can give false positives and low specificity. Measures different components of depression than BDI.
Hospital Anxiety and Depression (HADS) Scale	Easily administered self-report questionnaire. Reported the best measure of stable patients free of disease and effective for patients in treatment	Score ≤ 8 warrants psychiatric evaluation. Score ≤ 11 likely to have Anxiety or Depression (DSM IV criteria)
Hopelessness Scale (HS) (Beck, Weissman, Lester and Trexler, 1974)	A 20-item scale containing true-false self-report statements testing pessimism about the future. The scale differentiates threateners, attempters, and controls. It has three factors and internal consistency of .93 (Kuder Richardson); a 91% sensitivity for inpatients and 94% for outpatients. Some experts argue that HS is a better index of suicidality than depression scales.	One point is given for each item that the respondent marks in the direction of pessimism. The total score is an excellent indicator of suicidality among adults, but not among adolescent minority females.
Center for Epidemiological Studies Depression Scale (CES-D) (Radloff, 1977) for general populations	A 20-question, self-administered tool. The scale has high reliability and discriminant validity. It is unclear whether the scale measures depression or psychological distress.	Myers and Weissman (1980) suggest a cut-off score of 16 or above for major depression. Scale has a low false positive and a high false negative rate.

Beck A, Weissman A, Lester D, Trexler L: Classification of suicidal behaviors: II. Dimensions of suicidal intent. *Arch Gen Psychiatry* 1976; 33, 835-837.

Corcoran K, Fischer J: *Measures for Clinical Practice: A Sourcebook.* New York, Free Press, 1987.

Radloff LS: The CES-D Scale. A self report depression scale for research in general populations. *Appl Psychol Measurement* 1977; 1: 385-401.

Myers J, Weissman MM: Use of a self report symptom scale to detect depression in a community sample. *Am J Psychiatry* 1980; 137.

Psychodynamic Theories

Suicide results from a person's ongoing responses to intolerable psychological distress, frustration, and unmet needs. Suicidal individuals talk of feeling hostile, ashamed, guilty, aggressive, vengeful, afraid, loving, and ambivalent.

Sociological Theories

Alienation, broken relationships and social ties, and loss of status lead to suicide.

- **CLINICAL ASSESSMENT OF SUICIDE VICTIMS RULES OUT TREATABLE DIAGNOSES, SUCH AS DEPRESSION OR CHEMICAL DEPENDENCY.** Comprehensive physical and neurobehavoiral mental status examinations are done.

Screening

Patients in the community and inpatient settings may complete self-report questionnaires that rate depression and/or suicide (see Study Guide Table 32-2).

Tools are available for different age groups; art and play therapy may help to determine problems.

When patients' scores on screening instruments are abnormal, a suicidal assessment interview should be conducted to determine risk.

Evaluating Risk

Systematic examinations of group and individual risk factors are done (see Study Guide Table 32-3).

Essential to individual risk assessment is continuous observation and monitoring of suicidal communication, changes in behavior or mood, and suicidal clues (e.g., giving away prized possessions).

Suicidal messages can be overt (I'm going to kill myself; I should be dead) or covert, less obvious statements suggesting that life is not worthwhile (You won't have to worry about me anymore). People who attempt suicide may tentatively say that they will commit suicide if things become worse; those who complete the act say that suicide is their only choice.

Other clues may come from family or friends. Once risk is detected, evaluating lethality and providing safety are urgent goals.

Evaluating Lethality

A highly lethal rating indicates a clear plan with a deadly method/means (gun, jumping from high places). Moderate ratings reflect moderately lethal methods (barbiturates) or an incomplete or impractical plan. Low-risk methods (wrist cutting) have low risks for death. A patient with a high-risk lethal rating requires immediate intervention and suicidal precautions. The nurse must judge the capability of the staff/setting to provide safety for the patient and then plan accordingly (i.e., 1:1 supervision, transfer or admit patient to a locked unit).

Evaluating Resources and Social Support

Resources are evaluated to determine deficits that could increase risk. Suicidal people may perceive support negatively ("If they loved me, they would know what I need") or they may neglect to ask for support and fail to use internal (humor or coping strategies) or external (family or friends) resources.

- **MANAGEMENT STRATEGIES**

Reducing Lethality

Nurses need to express their concern to a patient, establish an alliance, and formulate a plan to reduce suicidal risk (see Study Guide Table 32-4). Focus on surveillance, safety precautions, communication, documentation, and actions to reduce risk. If the patient asks the nurse to keep his or her suicidal plan confidential, the nurse asserts that anything related to patient safety must be shared with the health team.

Safety Precautions

Protecting suicidal patients is the first priority. Safety precautions include hospitalization (sometimes involuntary) close supervision, and removal of potential suicidal methods or objects. The patient should be in the least restrictive but safe environment. If there is a low lethality, medication, consultation, and other actions to reduce risk may be used. Study Guide Table 32-5 lists guidelines for preventing suicide in a hospital.

Nurses must remain vigilant in all settings; for example, inpatients should be observed to make sure that they swallow and do not hoard medications. Patients often communicate their fear of suicide and hope nurses will take pre-

TABLE 32-3.

ASSESSMENT OF SUICIDE RISK

Detect risk by recognizing risk factors and clues: evaluation of suicide risk requires systematic inquiry about risk factors. Presence of risk factors implies that the nurse should suspect that the patient may have ideas of suicide. Examination of individual risk factors provides information about intensity of suicidal intent and suggests lethality.

Group Risk: Factors indicating individual is in a group at risk for suicide.
1. Psychiatric Diagnosis: Depression, substance abuse, schizophrenia, post-traumatic stress disorder, organic brain syndrome, anxiety
2. Medical Diagnosis: Cancer (head, neck, gastrointestinal tract), AIDS
3. Demographics: age (>18 years, adult or older age), male, single (with no responsibility for children under age 18), unemployed, recent death of spouse. (Note: females have higher rates of attempted suicide; gay men and lesbians have had higher rates of attempted suicide)
4. Personal or Family history of suicide and current risk
5. Mood improvement among depressed patients often precedes suicide
6. Prior suicide attempts (determine intent and pattern of attempts)
7. Hospitalization

Individual Risk Factors
1. Historical — Prior suicide attempts
2. Communication — Verbal suicide messages, jokes, writings, diaries
3. Behavioral — Changes in behavior, saying good-bye (e.g., making a will, giving away prized possessions)
4. Mood — Depressed, hopeless, helpless, ambivalent
5. Social — Social isolation
6. Death Wishes — Themes in art, play, or conversation

Assess for individual risk of suicide and lethality
Determine acuity and lethality/conduct a thorough assessment
1. Ask about, monitor, and continue to assess suicide risk
2. Evaluate pattern, detail, and intensity of suicidal thoughts/behaviors
3. Inquire about suicide plan, method, means and details
4. Estimate immediate and long-term lethality
5. Collect data from colleagues, family or friends

---

cautions. Managing suicidal inpatients requires clinical judgment, ongoing assessment of risk before approving privileges, discharge, and treatment plan. Management is a multidisciplinary effort.

Offering Hope or Help

Risk is decreased when patients believe that help is available and when they are helped to develop realistic goals and hope for realistic outcomes. Patients need regular reminders that the team wants to provide help and believes that the patient can improve or be comfortable.

Informing Others and Seeking Consultation

Nurses need to notify the team when poorly managed pain or depression results in suicidal risk. Consultation with other health care providers is critical and helps resolve the nurses' countertransference issues. A patient's suicide is a significant occupational hazard in psychiatry, and consultation helps nursing staff cope with this occupational stress.

Making No-Suicide Contracts

Contracts are time-limited verbal or written promises not to do anything destructive accidently or intentionally without notifying the primary clinician. They do not guarantee that the suicidal impulse can be controlled. They tend to work better if patients have a relationship with the care provider. They can provide false reassurance with manipulative patients, as promising not to commit suicide will get them privileges or passes.

Reducing Symptom Distress
Adequate pain and symptom (including side effects of medication) management must be a priority in treating medical patients, particularly those with suicidal ideas. Physical symptoms offer clues to suicidal risk and must be evaluated carefully.

Improving Problem-Solving or Coping Strategies
Helping patients to consider options, prioritize problems, and plan constructive strategies can build hope and reduce helplessness; ask about past coping strategies and emphasize effective ones. Helping the patient to cope with grief is an example of a situation that would require management stategy (see Study Guide Table 32-6).

Involving Significant Others and Mobilizing Resources
Patients are empowered by making a list of their skills and of persons who support them. Nurses can assist significant others by encouraging them to express their concerns for the patient and by giving them a list of resources including hotline numbers.

TABLE 32-4

PLAN OF CARE FOR SUICIDAL PATIENT

DSM-IV Diagnosis: Major Depression
Nursing diagnosis: Potential for self-harm due to depression, suicidal thoughts, low self-esteem

Assessment	Outcomes/Goals	Nursing Actions
High risk for suicide due to: depression, alcoholism, isolation	Patient will not physically harm self during treatment or hospitalization.	Notify physician and team of risk. Assign one to one close nursing observation, suicide precautions, place on locked unit near nurse's station.
Concrete, immediate, lethal suicide plan; may have prior lethal attempts; Monitor mood	Patient will not elope from hospital unit or endanger self or others	Staff will: Remove harmful objects. Assist patient with activities of daily living Help patient ventilate feelings and use constructive physical outlets for anger
Inconsistent impulse control	Patient will inform staff promptly of thoughts/feelings of wanting to harm self	Observe closely and ask patient to report any suicidal ideas/feelings Advise and monitor participation in activities Teach alternate coping strategies
Feels hopeless, helpless, ambivalent about life/death	Patient will identify constructive alternatives to self harm	Encourage patient to begin forming or using social support system and to expand resources Reassess and document Set realistic goals
High risk due to being elderly, diagnosis, substance abuse, AIDS, cancer		Advise participation in activities Evaluate/improve pain or symptom management Build self esteem
History: suicidal ideas/feelings, or acts, social isolation, anger or homicidal impulses		Evaluate goal of suicidal behavior and desired outcome and desired outcome Evaluate plans for rescue Investigate how patient handles anger and frustration Help patient establish relationship with nurse, then others Help patient begin to socialize

TABLE 32-5 GUIDELINES FOR SUICIDE PREVENTION IN THE HOSPITAL

Identification

AT ADMISSION

Inquire about current suicidal behavior
Inquire about prior suicidal behavior
(two or more previous events indicate high risk)
Record presence or absence of above (if present, obtain details of method, place, motivation)

AFTER ADMISSION

Watch for suspect behavior
 Refusing food, medication
 Saving medication
 Asking about suicidal methods
 Talking of death, futility
 Giving away possessions
 Checking locks, windows, layout of the ward
 Loosening bolts, tearing sheets into strips
Watch for suspect mood
 Hopelessness, helplessness, worthlessness
 Depression with agitation, restlessness
 Depression with apathy, withdrawal
 Unrelieved anxiety
 Excessive guilt and self-blame
 Severe frustration
 Bitter anger
Observe personality characteristics
 Severe personal disorganization
 Dependent-satisfied behavior
 Dependent-dissatisfied behavior
 Diagnosis of schizophrenia
 Recent object loss
 Negative feelings about hospital
 Feeling of no future

Safeguards

ENVIRONMENTAL

Install safety glass in windows
Restrict window openings with stops
Block off stair wells, access to roof
Use breakaway shower curtain rods, breakaway clothes
hooks in bathrooms and clothes lockers
Cover exposed pipes
Avoid grilles over ventilators, porch screens, and railings

Procedure

Remove from vicinity of suicidal patients all articles easily used in self-harm such as belt, suspenders, bathrobe cord, light cords, shoelaces, glass, ashtrays, vases, razor, pocketknife, nail file, nail clippers
Be alert when suicidal patients are using sharp objects, such as scissors, needles, pins, bottle opener, can opener, dining room utensils, occupational therapy tools
Be alert when suicidal patients are using the bathroom (to prevent hanging, jumping, cutting)
Be alert when giving suicidal patients medication (patients may save or discard medicine)
Observe acutely suicidal patients on a one-to-one basis
Check suicidal patients at least every 15 minutes at night
Be alert to whereabouts of suicidal patients during shift changes
Room suicidal patients with others close to nurses' station; do not room alone if avoidable
Warn visitors about bringing or leaving anything with lethal potential
Apprise off-ward escort of suicide concern
Keep suicidal patient in escorted group; examine anything patient picks up
Define staff responsibility thoroughly
Ensure continuous availability of help

Communication

Document records completely to show that:
 Risk is recognized and evaluated
 Reasonable measures are ordered
 Orders are followed (if not, indicate why not)
Ensure that all staff record pertinent observations
Write orders specifically to show:
 Plan and rationale
 Specific restrictions
 Specific staff responsible for observation or escort
 Specific frequency of night observation
Obtain frequent consultation

Attitudes

Avoid preoccupation and fear
Avoid harsh, repressive measures
Use positive interest and build mutual trust
Restore and strengthen hope
Rebuild self-esteem to overcome helplessness
Accept the reality that mistakes occur; aim for minimum

The Guidelines are reprinted by permission of Norman L. Farberow, Ph.D., and *HOSPITAL AND COMMUNITY PSYCHIATRY.* Dr. Farberow is clinical professor of psychiatry (psychology) at the University of Southern California School of Medicine, and principal investigator at the Central Research Unit of the Veteran's Administration Wadsworth Medical Center, Los Angeles, California. The Guidelines appeared as part of a copyrighted article on *Suicide Prevention in the Hospital,* published in *HOSPITAL & COMMUNITY PSYCHIATRY,* February, 1981 (Volume 32, Number 2).

Developing A Plan for Living

Nurses should encourage a plan that stresses pleasurable activities and supportive relationships. Timing is crucial; if it is premature, the plan may be overwhelming or cause further depression.

Seeking Consultation and Psychiatric Evaluation

- **EFFECTIVE PRIMARY PREVENTION STRATEGIES** include gun control, medication control, barriers within the environment (bridge railings, etc.), and educational campaigns. A serious issue in prevention is that reports of suicide in the media may increase the risk of suicide among some individuals. A suicide prevention educational campaign in the mass media would include information about:

  Effective responses to depression and substance abuse

  Treatment of emotional problems and depression

  Resources for psychiatric treatment

  Friends' and relatives' roles in bringing a patient for treatment

  The inappropriate stigma often attached to seeking psychiatric help; asking for help does not mean that one is crazy or disturbed

- **EUTHANASIA, ASSISTED DYING,** is a current controversial ethical issue. Nurses anguish over responding to patients' requests for help in dying, and few guidelines for responding exist for the practice area. Traditionally, values guiding practice are to preserve life. Consequently, clinicians struggle with how to respond to requests that touch the heart of professional and personal values. Clinicians encounter conflicts between their duties to prevent suicide and respect a patient's autonomy. Many patients, however, who wish to commit suicide may have a severe psychiatric disorder, such as depression, which undermines their ability to think clearly and thus their autonomy. Although some nurses believe that they have a duty to sound the alarm at the first hint of suicide, they also feel a conflicting responsibility to protect a rational patient's confidentiality. Rational suicide is a controversial issue (see Study Guide Table 32-7).

  When the pain of living is greater than the idea of dying, people consider suicide, perhaps as an impulsive response to persistent pain, depression, dementia, or an unacceptable quality of life. When a patient says, "I

TABLE 32-6

DO'S AND DON'TS OF GRIEF SUPPORT

HELPFUL RESPONSES: DO	DON'T
Understand the survivor's perspective of this loss and its meaning.	Impose your meaning or values; avoid mentioning the decreased, or act as if nothing happened.
Use therapeutic communication: listen, accept emotions, invite sharing of thoughts and feelings; there are no right/wrong feelings.	Blame the bereaved survivor for the deceased's mental problems or suicide or criticize the family's actions or omissions.
Give permission to grieve; establish a safe environment. Encourage feelings, confusion, and questions (e.g., "Why did this happen?").	Insist the bereaved "get on with life," find a new love, have a stiff upper lip or stop brooding.
	Expect them to be the life of the party.
Educate clients about normal grief responses. Patterns of grief vary.	Imply that a "one size of grief fits all" (e.g., you should be . . . sad, etc.)
Encourage use of available support and resources (e.g., bereavement groups). Volunteer to offer support.	Expect the person to have the energy and skills to seek help and support when they fear rejection.
Monitor physical health, symptoms, and coping (e.g., sleep, alcohol, suicide, exercise, diet). Advise safety and health (e.g., seatbelts).	Ignore potentially dangerous behaviors (e.g., excessive alcohol, pills or sexual behavior).
Invite talk of practical problems and solutions (e.g., how to tell children, should they attend the funeral, handling tough questions).	Assume you know the best solutions (e.g., "Tell everyone the truth about the suicide" or when to sort through the deceased's belongings).
Respect the survivor's need for time to experience sad, angry, or other feelings. Expect some personal discomfort as you listen to painful, sad, guilty or angry feelings.	Diminish grief by a cheery, positive focus; justify the death as "God's will" or encourage replacement of the deceased (e.g., "Just have another child!")

TABLE 32-7.
ASSESSMENT OF RATIONAL SUICIDE

1. The purpose and motives of the person considering suicide
   Is the person making a request for help?
   Why is the person consulting a health professional?
   Is the request for help in suicide a request for someone else to decide?
   Is the suicide plan financially motivated?
   What has kept the person from committing suicide so far?
   Does the person fear becoming a burden?
2. Stability of request
   How stable is the request?
   Has suicide been planned for a long time or is it a response to a recent event?
3. Is the request consistent with the person's basic values?
4. Are the medical and nonmedical facts cited in the request accurate?
5. Has the person considered the effects of suicide on others?
6. Suicide plan and options
   How far in the future would this take place?
   Has the person picked a method of suicide?
   Would the person be willing to tell others about his or her suicide plan?
   Does the person see suicide as the only way out?
7. What cultural influences are shaping a person's choices?
8. Are the person's affairs in order? Have arrangements been made for a funeral or durable power of attorney? In most states a health professional's relationship with a patient implies a legal and professional duty to refrain from assisting suicide. Terminally ill patients with suicide plans, however, deserve thoughtful evaluation of their rational and irrational requests and appropriate treatment options for their depression, pain, or symptom distress. Clinicians need to understand the ethical issues and criteria for evaluating rational suicide.

Adapted from Battin MP: Rational suicide: How can we respond to a request for help? *Crisis* 1991; 2:73-80.

would be better off dead," clinicians may believe that the patient is right. Only a thorough assessment of suicidal intent will identify distressing symptoms that require and sometimes respond to treatment.

TAKING ANOTHER LOOK

You are now ready to respond to the questions that were raised in Gaining a Perspective at the beginning of this chapter. After you have written or thought about your responses, you may wish to look at the Suggested Responses on page 333.

33 MANAGING ASSAULTIVE PATIENTS

TERMS TO DEFINE

acute crisis phase

aggressive behavior

assessment of dangerousness

behavioral warning signs (of aggression)

crisis (aggression) management

deescalation techniques

mechanical restraint

milieu therapy

GAINING A PERSPECTIVE

Think about the following two questions, and after you have read the Key Concepts for this chapter respond to the situations in greater depth.

1. How would you, as a nurse, feel if a patient threatened to hit you?

2. What would you, as a nurse, think a patient-nurse contract should contain — a contract in which the patient states that he or she will not be violent or aggressive?

KEY CONCEPTS

- **INTERPERSONAL VIOLENCE HAS BEEN CONSIDERED AN IMPORTANT PUBLIC HEALTH ISSUE** since 1985, when violent crime was declared a national public health emergency by Surgeon General C. Everett Koop. Between 1960 and 1987, the rate of violent crime increased almost 400% in the U.S. This increase of violence is evident in general hospitals, emergency rooms, psychiatric settings, and prisons.

- **AGGRESSIVE BEHAVIOR IS DEFINED** as an event of actual or threatened contact (e.g., hitting striking, spitting, throwing objects) where the target is a person or an object in the environment. This definition includes verbal threats and/or physical acts.

- **THEORIES OF THE ORIGINS OF AGGRESSIVE OR VIOLENT BEHAVIOR ARE BASED ON MULTICAUSALITY,** including biological, interpersonal, family systems, socioeconomic, cultural, and environmental factors (see Study Guide Table 33-1). Mental illness, a predisposing factor, has been explored without a causal relationship.

  Patterns of violence are amenable to understanding, intervention, and ultimate recovery. Communicating the belief, overtly or covertly, that the behavior is predetermined promotes a hopeless, helpless response by patients and staff, and thus efforts to promote learning and recovery are impaired. Before they can intervene, nurses must confront the myths, fear, anxiety, and stigma associated with interactions with people who display violence.

  The multifaceted nature of human behavior is also reflected in the variable, diverse nosology contained in the DSM-IV. Violent behavior might be considered a symptom of other psychiatric disorders.

- **RESEARCH** is only beginning to address the potential for violence in persons with mental disorders. Some research indicates that patient assault upon nurses is a much larger problem than has been recognized. Nurses can experience intense physical and emotional reactions when they are victims of a patient's assault.

At-risk factors related to the occurrence of violence include:
- a history of violent behavior
- psychological, physical, or sexual abuse in childhood or witnessing family violence
- alcohol and substance abuse
- rigid, controlling, exploitative family systems

- **THE EXPECTATION THAT VIOLENCE SHOULD NOT OCCUR MUST BE COMMUNICATED** to patients and their families. Violence inside or outside the hospital or home setting is not acceptable. The belief that everyone has a right to work and live in a safe and humane environment must be communicated by the health care team and enacted consistently within the treatment environment. An early show of authority may prevent injuries and property damage.

- **A CALM SYSTEMATIC APPROACH IS CRITICAL** in working with an aggressive, violent, or acutely excited patient, regardless of the setting. A patient's aggressive behavior, viewed as a symptom of an illness, is to be taken seriously. Aggressive patients should not be kept waiting; they view this as a sign they are not important. Assistance should be available to help manage patients who are obviously overtly aggressive or psychotic. The environment should be free of objects that could be used as weapons. If a violent patient escapes, security is notified immediately. Threatening calls or letters should not be ignored; ignoring them may escalate aggressive activity.

Interviewing

When interviewing a potentially violent patient the following steps should be taken:
- Be aware of one's own anxiety.
- Maintain adequate distance to avoid or deflect blows.
- Do not attempt to deal with a violent patient unaided.
- Talk in a calm, soothing voice.
- Use restraints and medications if necessary.

- **ASSESSMENT OF AN AGGRESSIVE PATIENT** requires a careful evaluation of the individual's history and behavior and the person's capacity to employ nonviolent strategies. Patient assessment requires a quiet setting without objects accessible that could be used as weapons.

History of Aggression or Abuse

- Assess history of criminal behavior. Questions should include the following:

  Have you ever caused physical injury to another person?

  What is the closest you have come to being violent?

  Have you ever been harmed? How? When?

  How would you describe what occurred just before you were violent?

TABLE 33–1
THEORIES OF AGGRESSION AND VIOLENCE

THEORY	FOCUS	DIRECTIONS FOR TREATMENT
Neurobiological theory	Violence has a biological basis (i.e., genes, biochemistry)	Address the biological imbalance and control symptoms Pharmacologic therapy Seclusion and restraint
Psychodynamic theory	Aggression is the result of the effects of the unconscious; unresolved issues motivate behavior	Uncover patient's unconscious instincts through talking therapies Performance of expressive, nondestructive acts
Frustration–aggression hypothesis	Aggression is a result of the build-up of frustration (e.g., drive theory) External stimuli affect frustration level	Release of frustration through other activities (sports, punching bag, pillow fights, arts)
Social learning theory	Violence is learned through witness of violence; positive reinforcement (tangible rewards, social reward and approval); negative reinforcement (cycle of violence)	Contingency management (alter the reward system) Emphasize verbal techniques (negotiation and conflict resolution) Problem-solving training

Source: Morrison, 1996. Personal communication.

Have you ever been arrested? What were the charges?

Have you ever been in jail?

When you get excited, what helps to calm you?

What do you believe causes you to be violent?

Do you worry about being violent?

- Compare and contrast the patient's memory and perceptions with other sources, such as hospital records, family interviews.
- Determine if the patient has a vulnerability to behave violently.
- Detail patient's aggression. Obtain specific characteristics of the violent behavior.

Potential for Nonviolence

Assessment is done to determine whether the patient has the capacity to employ nonviolent behavioral strategies. Some questions to ask are listed below:

How has the patient avoided being violent?

What strengths, supports, or resources are available?

How does the patient successfully get along with people?

How has the patient been able to calm himself or herself?

What medication has helped calm the patient?

Does the patient understand his or her violence?

What ability does the patient have to learn?

The above questions may also be asked of the family.

Assessment tools may be used on an ongoing basis.

Behavioral Warning Signs

Specific signs may warn the nurse of potentially aggressive and violent patient behavior. Warning signs include pacing, an angry demeanor, threatening actions, staring, extreme quietness, mumbling, arguing, clenching fists, refusing to talk to staff, or changing usual behavior. Further diagnostic evaluation may be needed.

- Psychological, to assess cognitive and intellectual function.
- Neurological, to detect other disease processes.
- Psychiatric, to determine a differential diagnosis.

Physiological Responses to Aggression/Violence

- The staff's and the patient's responses may include an increase in vital signs, shaky knees, diarrhea, urgency, anger, restlessness, and sweatiness.
- Staff self-assessment seeks answers to the staff's responses to violence. Questions to consider include:

What anxiety or fear do I experience?

How do I cope with being anxious or afraid?

How do I let my peers know about my responses?

Does my response interfere with effective treatment?

What expectations do I have for patients? Are they realistic?

Do I believe the patient will recover?

- **A NURSING DIAGNOSIS IS A STATEMENT THAT REPRESENTS** actual or potential patterns of human functioning in relation to violence.

Some relevant diagnoses related to violence are:

- Defensive coping
- Denial, ineffective
- Fear
- Self-esteem, situational, low
- Thought processes altered
- Violence, risk for: self-directed or directed at others

Outcome Identification

Statements addressing violent behaviors should define what the patient is expected to display as he or she learns to change. Do not use generic or unrealistic statements. Two statements that are examples of outcome identification are:

- The patient will ask the staff to use a quiet room when he has the urge to punch a peer.
- The patient will request PRN medication

when he has an impulse to throw furniture. Behavioral contracts may also be used to clarify outcomes.

- **NURSING INTERVENTIONS** can promote an environment that discourages aggression and violence; crisis intervention deals with the immediate situation. The least restrictive environment is desirable, although this approach may cause a dilemma. Objective of intervention is to help patients cope with their aggressive feelings and behaviors. Intervention also seeks to avoid violence directed to nurses.

  The purposes of crisis intervention techniques are:

  - To assess patient who is losing control of behavior
  - To recognize causes of the violent behavior
  - To provide coordinated team response to patient behavior
  - To teach patient self-calming techniques
  - To reduce the use of restraint and seclusion
  - To reduce the number of patient and staff injuries

Crisis intervention techniques include securing a therapeutic environment, employing verbal intervention, and having a team approach.

- Therapeutic Environment
  - Noise, temperature, lighting, and furniture are controlled.
  - Depersonalization, regimentation, and sensory deprivation must not occur.
  - An inpatient setting should promote interaction, reduce isolation, provide privacy, and not impair staff's ability to observe.
  - Seclusion rooms and private areas should be available where approved restraints may be used.
  - Observation of patients as they interact with family, other patients, or staff is important.
- Verbal Interventions
  - Use immediate feedback: "You're threatening and you must stop."
  - Time Out: a temporary separation of the patient from the social milieu.

- Team Approach During Violent Behavior
  A five-member team, with one member assigned to each limb and one to the head, should be present and ready to act if necessary.
  - Show of concern: conveys to the patient that his or her impulses will be controlled in a safe environment.
  - Team (five members) is visible but non-threatening; acts as a security blanket.
  - If team approach fails, rapidly tranquilize patient, orally or by injection.
  - Defense is physical intervention; actual holding down of the patient.
  - Mechanical restraints are the last resort; never used to threaten patient. A patient in restraints is a psychiatric emergency. Staff must be present. Purpose is to assess patient's reactions and determine when patient can be released from restraints.

Restraints and seclusion are safety interventions, not therapeutic techniques.

- Seclusion is the patient's being in an area/room from which he or she cannot leave at will.
- Restraint is the patient's being placed in a device that interferes with the free movement of arms and legs which the patient is unable to remove easily; restraints are used to prevent imminent harm to the patient and others. Examples of these devices are four-point ankle and wrist, five-point ankle and wrist, and chest strap, camisole, restraint sheets, preventive aggressive devices (wrists attached to waist belt to impede upper body movement).

- **PREVENTING VIOLENCE AND PROMOTING MENTAL HEALTH** in an inpatient setting is usually achieved through milieu therapy, defined as the prevention, structuring, and maintenance of a therapeutic environment by the psychiatric nurse in collaboration with the patient and other health care providers.

Etablishing unit rules should involve patients and staff. It needs to be established that violence and aggression are not acceptable, and how they will be dealt with must be addressed.

A Conceptual Framework to Prevent Aggression

• Contingency Management

Reward appropriate behavior; provide negative consequences, such as removing rewards, should aggression occur.

• Conflict Resolution

• Developing Problem-Solving Skills

Problem Solving

• When attempting to solve problems with a potentially violent patient, the nurse should focus on how to think, not what to think. The several steps involved in the problem-solving process can be taught by staff.

-Stop and think: How do you problem-solve?

-What is the problem?

-What are the different ways the problem can be solved?

-Have you been successful or unsuccessful problem-solving in the past?

-Evaluate alternatives.

-Choose and implement one or more alternatives.

-What resources will you need?

- Plan to implement your chosen solution, and do it.

The patient's efforts to learn should be reinforced by the nurse paying attention to the patient.

• If the patient refuses to examine problem solving and resorts to violence, verbal interactions stop. Effects and consequences are clearly defined. Recognizing and exploring the experience of anxiety and anger without avoidance or denial promotes learning and behavioral change. Unwarranted use of controlling, coercive interventions (medication and restraints) stifles a verbal response and the identification of what is occurring during the uncomfortable situation. Establishing trust between patient and staff is also hindered.

Predictable, Effective Programming

An essential part of violence prevention is the availability of programs that are scheduled, predictable, meaningful, therapeutic, and recreational.

Difficulties of Decision

It is difficult to conclude when an interaction/interpersonal model of nursing is appropriate. How is one to determine when the patient does not have the ability to control behavior or when an impulsive, violent response must be prevented? How does one know when to cease counseling?

Staff Education

Staff must be educated and evaluated in the use of techniques that prevent aggression.

• **OUTCOME EVALUATION** is appraising the effect of nursing interventions. An effective process includes:

-Patient outcome evaluation

-Staff outcome evaluation

-Staff performance evaluation

-Review of outcomes with senior clinical staff

-Patient satisfaction survey

Following an aggressive episode, by examining the patient's responses (debriefing) to the use of interpersonal skills, the nurse is communicating the belief that the patient can understand and recover, that is, reduce and stop violent behavior. The debriefing should investigate: What is the patient's perception and understanding of what caused the behavior? What could the patient have done differently?

Similarly, exploring staff reactions after the episode is also important. Discussion should focus on emotional responses and what did and did not work with the patient and with team members. Regular review of practice and patient outcomes with senior clinical staff is also recommended as a component of an effective outcome evaluation process.

TAKING ANOTHER LOOK

You are now ready to respond to the questions that were raised in Gaining a Perspective at the beginning of this chapter. After you have written or thought about your responses, you may wish to look at the Suggested Responses on page 333.

34 HIV-POSITIVE PERSONS AND THEIR FAMILIES

TERMS TO DEFINE

acquired immune deficiency syndrome (AIDS)

AIDS anxiety syndrome

AIDS dementia complex (ADC)

AIDS-related complex (ARC)

helpless coping

HIV disease

human immunodeficiency virus (HIV)

organic denial

GAINING A PERSPECTIVE

Think about the situations described below, and after you have read the Key Concepts for this chapter respond in greater detail to the questions.

1. What would you expect a patient's reaction to be upon learning that he or she is HIV-positive?

2. What kind of problems might you, as a nurse, expect when dealing with patients who are HIV-positive, have neuropsychiatric problems, and are having pain?

KEY CONCEPTS

- **CARING FOR PSYCHIATRIC PATIENTS WITH HIV INFECTIONS OR AIDS** demands knowledge, compassion, and tolerance; it can be emotionally exhausting. Nurses must be able to accept the limitations of what they can do and, at the same time, help patients and their families to accept and deal with the physical and emotional demands of the disease. The single most important component of nursing care for the HIV-infected patient is optimism. In addition, nurses must address such topics as sex and sexuality, drugs and drug use, AIDS prevention and education, the right to privacy, the right to know, multiple losses, and death and dying issues.

- **AIDS HAS BEEN THE GREATEST HEALTH THREAT OF THE CENTURY; WORLDWIDE, 18 MILLION ADULTS AND 1.5 MILLION CHILDREN** have been infected with HIV. In 1993, the Centers for Disease Control and Prevention (CDC) amended the definition of AIDS to include:

  -Persons with less than 200 T-helper cells

  -HIV-positive persons with any form of tuberculosis

  -Persons with recurrent bacterial pneumonia

  -Infected women who develop cancer of the cervix

  The exapnded definition helps explain the recent increase in reported cases of AIDS among women and the explosion of reported cases of AIDS in the U.S.

  The continuum of HIV disease, the term used to describe the diseases resulting from infection with the human immunodeficiency virus, is divided into three stages. Each stage is associated with distinct physical changes. There are also common psychological issues for the patient, significant others, and caregivers, whether the caregivers are health care professionals, family members, or friends.

TABLE 34-1
NUMBER AND PERCENTAGE OF PERSONS WITH AIDS, UNITED STATES, 1981–OCT. 1995

Characteristic	Cumulative No.	(%)
Sex		
Male	428,480	(85.8)
Female	72,828	(14.5)
Age group (years)		
0–4	5,432	(1.1)
5–12	1,385	(0.3)
13–19	2,300	(0.5)
20–29	91,054	(18.2)
30–39	227,754	(45.4)
40–49	122,569	(24.4)
50–59	36,640	(7.3)
>60	14,176	(2.8)
Race/Ethnicity		
White, non-Hispanic	238,171	(47.5)
Black, non-Hispanic	170,271	(34.0)
Hispanic	87,387	(17.4)
Asian/Pacific Islander	3,457	(0.7)
American Indian/ Alaskan Native	1,283	(0.3)
HIV-exposure category		
Men who have sex with men	254,437	(50.8)
Injecting-drug use	125,440	(25.0)
Men who have sex with men and inject drugs	32,429	(6.5)
Hemophilia	4,258	(0.8)
Heterosexual contact	38,541	(7.7)
Transfusion recipients	7,700	(1.6)
Perinatal transmission	6,124	(1.2)
No risk reported	32,381	(6.4)
Region		
Northeast	156,595	(31.2)
Midwest	49,036	(9.8)
South	165,348	(33.0)
West	113,954	(22.7)
U.S. territories	15,971	(3.2)
Vital status		
Living	189,929	(37.9)
Deceased	311,381	(62.1)
Total	501,310	(100.0)

Adapted from Morbidity and Mortality Weekly Reports (MMWR), Center for Disease Control, Atlanta, Ga, Nov. 24, 1995.

Exposure: first stage

- Lasts 3 to 6 months.
- Exposure is through high-risk sex, needle use, contaminated transfusion, or perinatal transmission (see Study Guide Table 34-1). Each type of exposure entails a different risk (e.g., babies born to HIV-infected mothers become infected only 30% to 50% of the time).
- Infection occurs when the HIV enters the body and incorporates itself into the host cell.
  - A FLU-LIKE ILLNESS a few weeks after exposure sometimes accompanies infection; often there are no physical symptoms, only a positive antibody test.
  - IMMUNE SYSTEM WEAKENS AND THE NUMBER OF T-HELPER CELLS FALLS below the normal range, 800-1200/mm^3 to about 650/mm^3; widely scattered swelling of lymph nodes occurs, persisting for long periods of time.

Latent Infection: second stage

- Lasts 3 to 5 years; the person may remain in this stage 10 years or longer.
- Most individuals feel well and have few indications of infection; some may have swollen glands and fatigue.
- T-helper cell counts continue to fall.
- Psychological distress occurs.

Clinical Disease: third stage

- T-helper cell count falls below 200.
- Opportunistic infections, such as pneumocystic carinii pneumonia (PCP) and Karposi's sarcoma, may occur and affect the patient's body image and self-esteem.
- Neuropsychiatric complications of HIV infection are sometimes misdiagnosed and mistreated.
- Illnesses may occur and resolve themselves over a course of months or years; on average, death occurs in 18 to 36 months.

- **IDENTIFYING PATIENTS AT RISK**

Nurses are in a key position to identify patients with high risk factors.

- Sexual and drug use histories are included in assessment.
- Nurses may have to collect data to differentiate patients exhibiting psychosocial distress

related to HIV, from those whose HIV status exacerbated a preexisting psychiatric diagnosis, from those whose symptoms are a direct result of HIV infection.

- Risk factors include male homosexuality, intravenous drug use, hemophilia, heterosexual contact with an infected partner, transfusion, rape, childhood sexual abuse, and being an adult survivor of childhood sexual abuse.

  The chronically mentally ill are a high-risk population, as poor judgment, hypersexuality, and impulsivity are associated with many chronic mental diseases. The majority of these patients are sexually active and engage in unprotected sex with multiple partners; one-third have sexually transmitted diseases and many exchange sex for money or drugs. The incidence of homosexuality has been reported to be 51% among patients with borderline personality and 14% among patients with mania. A high percentage of patients with affective disorders are intravenous drug users.

- **ASSESSMENT OF PATIENTS WITH HIV DISEASE**

  Physical condition of the patient must be assessed.

  Mental status examination

  - Complete history is done, including sexual preference and history and drug and alcohol use (see Chapter 31, Substance Abuse).

  - Evaluate patient's adjustment and coping skills; patient's personal way of dealing with the disease; psychosocial and environmental problems.

    - ASSESS CAPACITY FOR JUDGMENT, including organization of thoughts and decision making. Patients with difficulty in thought organization may be able to draw, but not write clearly.

    - ORIENTATION AND MEMORY may fluctuate in patients with HIV disease, but can usually be regained with visual or verbal prompting. Patients may distract easily and lose track of what they are saying or doing.

    - AFFECT MAY BE BLANK OR APATHETIC (not to be

confused with depression); may be due to organic causes.

  - LABILITY AND SYMPTOMS OF MANIA may be displayed by patient with HIV disease and organic mental syndrome. Question to ask: Is this typical or is it of recent onset?

  - COGNITIVE SLOWING is the most defining characteristic of the organically impaired patient with HIV disease. Motor skills may also be slowed.

- **THE PSYCHOLOGICAL IMPACT OF HIV INFECTION AMONG DIFFERENT GROUPS** has been shown to be similar in degree both before and after learning the results of HIV testing; 30% of those studied were found to have suicidal thoughts both before and after testing, despite results.

  Reactions when HIV antibody tests are positive

  - Patients may feel relieved, as their position is clarified.

  - If one generalizes that adverse emotional reactions should occur (distraught, depressed, and dysfunctional emotional states), the patient may respond to these cues and feel increased hopelessness, helplessness, and depression.

  - Among gay men, the knowledge of a positive test may result in some behavioral risk reduction or an increase in high-risk activity due to feelings of invulnerability.

  - Patient may experience a reaction similar to post-traumatic stress disorder, i.e., severe anxiety, intrusive ruminative thoughts about failing health and death, and hypervigilance for detecting signs of physical deterioration, insomnia, depression, and guilt.

  - Women may feel isolated and try to cope alone.

  - Loss of physical and cognitive abilities, friends, and certain freedoms contributes to demoralization and grieving.

    The patient's life story can be written or told; the revelation is a therapeutic tool to deal with the patient's feelings. The life story allows continuous assessment of psychological status and gives a patient the chance for life review and

identification of "unfinished business."
- **NEUROPSYCHIATRIC COMPLICATIONS OF HIV DISEASE** occur among 30% of patients and may range from myelopathy to AIDS dementia.

  AIDS dementia complex (ADC)
  - Caused by direct HIV infection of glial cells, targeting deep structures such as the thalamus, basal ganglia, and white matter. ADC may be the first clear symptom of AIDS.
  - ADC is a subcortical dementia that primarily affects mood and motor activity.
    - Cognitive symptoms: mental slowing, memory loss, poor concentration, and forgetfulness.
    - Motor symptoms: unsteady gait, leg weakness, tremor, spasticity, hyperreflexias, and loss of coordination.
    - Behavioral symptoms: apathy, withdrawal, agitated psychosis, social isolation, and personality changes such as irritability.
    - Organic denial: patient is unaware of cognitive deficits.
  - Symptoms may be confused with those of depression, anxiety, or psychotic disease.
  - Opportunistic infection of the central nervous system may be confused with ADC. A lumbar puncture is required for differential diagnosis.
  - Symptoms are progressive; the patient may be unable to walk, and in the terminal phase impairment is global with severe psychomotor retardation and mutism.
  - Family and friends may have to be decision makers due to the disabilities that result from neuropsychiatric and neurological impairment. Patients should inform family and friends of their wishes and get legal advice before ADC proceeds.

- **HIV-ASSOCIATED PSYCHOSIS IS UNCOMMON.**

  Etiology is undetermined, but may be related to substance abuse, antiretroviral treatment, central nervous system neoplasms, or HIV encephalopathy.

  Patients at risk are those with a history of stimulant, sedative, or hypnotic abuse.

Psychosis appears early in HIV disease; therefore, patients with first-time psychotic symptoms should be HIV tested.

- **AIDS ANXIETY SYNDROME** results from patient's ineffective coping. A range of destructive and debilitating symptoms are part of the syndrome.

  Symptoms range from panic attacks and morbid obsessions to persistent hypochondria and self-absorption.

  Symptoms are disruptive to normal routines. Patients tend to focus on their sexual orientation or their drug use.

  Approaches to caring for patients with AIDS anxiety are those that restore self-esteem and identify multiple aspects of the patient's personality. The patient is helped to understand that the origin of the anxiety involves more than the threat of AIDS. Health care providers need to show acceptance and endorsement.

- **DEPRESSION**

  A high incidence of depression has been shown in studies.

  Symptoms range from mild transient symptoms to mood disturbance or organic mood disorder.

  A lifetime history of depression may be assessed; one third of homosexual men have been reported to have this problem.

  Depression may be due to central nervous system impairment.

  Suicide may or may not be a risk; for HIV-positive individuals who abuse substances or for heterosexual partnerships involving intravenous drug users one needs to address the pessimistic attitude that comes with HIV infection. Addressing the pessimism is an important step toward providing the HIV-infected substance abuser with the rationale for drug or alcohol rehabilitation.

  Hospitalization may be helpful if the staff's attitude is empathetic.

- **PERSONALITY DISORDERS** are likely to occur when personality traits are inflexible, maladaptive, and cause significant functional impairment or subjective distress.

Disorders are common among the HIV-positive population. Inflexible traits that contribute to the risk of HIV infection include impulsiveness, overdramatization, poor recognition of future consequences of current behavior, and inability to tolerate discomfort or delay.

Denial and helplessness are used by patient as coping style, which may hinder patient's ability to accept and deal with HIV infection. Denial and helplessness also affect the relationship between patient and health care providers and the patient's compliance with treatment.

- More social conflict in patients with personality disorder.
- Need team approach to prevent splitting, identify target symptoms, and set firm limits with fixed consequences that are agreed upon in advance.

- **MEDICATING THE PATIENT INFECTED WITH HIV**

  Patients have a high rate of response to psychotropic drugs; however, dosage must coincide with the patient's potential reaction to the drug. "Start low and go slow." The tricyclical antidepressants can cause exaggerated anticholorenergic side effects.

  Psychotropic drugs increase the risk of seizure in neurologically compromised patients with HIV disease, as psychotropic drugs lower the seizure threshold.

  Zidovudine (AZT) is associated with mania and depression; **lithium and other antipsychotics** may be used for treatment.

  Drug overdose is the most common method of attempting suicide among patients infected with HIV.

- **PAIN MANAGEMENT OF PATIENTS WITH AIDS**

  Pain is second only to fever as the most frequently presenting complaint among people with AIDS.

  Pain has a profound impact on the level of emotional distress.

  Pain is intensified by psychological factors such as anxiety and depression.

  Barriers to pain control

  - Assessment of pain is difficult in patients with communication difficulties.

- Prescribing physician and staff may be afraid patients will become addicted.
- Respiratory depression may be a concern.

Nonpharmacological approaches to pain management including behavioral and cognitive techniques, such as relaxation, imagery, hypnosis, and biofeedback, have been effective when used alone or with medications.

Research indicates that patients with substance abuse histories do not complain of more pain nor do they require more analgesics for relief of pain than other patients.

Psychiatric disorders can complicate pain management. Opiates may worsen dementia.

Relief is best achieved on a fixed-time, fixed-dose schedule, rather than as needed. The schedule establishes a steady blood level and helps diminish memory and expectation of pain.

New noncyclic antidepressants, such as trazodone and fluoxetine, have potent analgesic properties and are widely used to treat chronic pain syndrome.

- **TEACHING PATIENTS WITH HIV DISEASE AND THEIR FAMILIES**

  Risky situations and strategies to avoid HIV need to be identified, which is accomplished by patient-staff collaboration. Barriers to learning include the perceived risk of infection, values, attitudes, beliefs, prejudices, and stigma.

  Safe-sex education is vital in dealing with patients who are in a psychiatric facility.

  Families and significant others, in order to support a patient with HIV disease, need help in accepting the patient and dealing with the patient's behavior and problems. They may need help relating to the patient when mental illness complicates HIV disease and during the grieving process.

TAKING ANOTHER LOOK

You are now ready to respond to the questions posed in Gaining a Perspective at the beginning of this chapter. After you have written or thought about your responses, you may wish to look at the Suggested Responses on page 334.

SECTION IV

PSYCHIATRIC NURSING PRACTICE

35 CONCEPTUAL MODELS AS GUIDES FOR PSYCHIATRIC NURSING PRACTICE

GAINING A PERSPECTIVE

Think about the following questions as you read the Key Concepts for this chapter. When you have finished reading, use the information to respond to the two questions.

1. Why is it important to have a conceptual model to guide your nursing practice?

2. What are some factors that Roy's, Neuman's and Johnson's models have in common?

KEY CONCEPTS

- **THE TERMS CONCEPTUAL MODEL, CONCEPTUAL FRAMEWORK, CONCEPTUAL SYSTEM, PARADIGM, AND DISCIPLINARY MATRIX ARE USED INTERCHANGEABLY.** They have the same definition: a set of abstract and general concepts and the statements that describe or link those concepts. Each conceptual framework presents a particular perspective about the phenomena of interest to a particular discipline, such as nursing. The works of several nurse scholars are currently recognized as conceptual models (see Study Guide Table 35-1).

  Each conceptual model has a different vo-

TABLE 35–1. OVERVIEW OF SEVEN CONCEPTUAL MODELS OF NURSING

Conceptual Model	Recipient of Nursing	Environment	Health	Nursing
Johnson's Behavioral System Model	A behavioral system with seven subsystems: attachment, dependency, ingestion, elimination, sexual, aggression, and achievement.	Internal External	Behavioral system balance and stability. Efficient and effective behavioral functioning. Purposeful, orderly, and predictable behavior.	*Definition:* A service that is complementary to that of medicine and other health professions, but which makes its own distinctive contribution to the health and well-being of people. *Goal:* Restore, maintain, or attain behavioral system balance and stability. *Actions:* Impose external regulatory or control mechanisms. Alter set or add choices for behavior. Provide protection, nurturance, or stimulation.
King's General Systems Framework	Personal system: Focus on perception, self, growth and development, body image, time, space, learning. Interpersonal system: Focus on interaction, communication, transaction, role, stress, coping. Social system: Focus on organization, authority, power, status, decision making, control.	Internal External	Dynamic life experiences of a human being. Ability to function in social roles.	*Definition:* Perceiving, thinking, relating, judging, and acting vís-a-vís the behavior of individuals who come to a nursing situation. *Goal:* Help individuals maintain their health so they can function in their roles. *Actions:* A process of action, reaction, interaction, and transaction directed toward establishment of goals and goal attainment.
Levine's Conservation Model	A holistic being, a system of systems. Organismic responses are fight or flight, stress, basic orienting system, visual system, auditory system, haptic system, taste-smell system.	Operational Perceptual Conceptual	Health and disease are patterns of adaptive change	*Definition:* A human interaction. *Goal:* Promotion of wholeness for people, sick or well. *Actions:* Conservation of energy, structural integrity, social integrity, and personal integrity.
Neuman's Systems Model	A patient system composed of five variables: physiological, psychological, sociocultural, developmental, and spiritual. Central core surrounded by flexible and normal lines of defense and lines of resistance	Internal External Created	Client system stability	*Definition:* A unique profession that is concerned with all the variables affecting an individual's response to stressors. *Goal:* To facilitate optimal wellness through retention, attainment, or maintenance of client system stability. *Actions:* Primary prevention, secondary prevention, and tertiary prevention.
Orem's Self-Care Framework	Self-care agent Therapeutic self-care demand made up of universal self-care requisites, developmental self-care requisites, and health deviation self-care requisites.	The person's external surroundings	Soundness or wholeness of developed human structures and of bodily and mental functioning	*Definition:* A helping service, a creative effort to help people. *Goal:* Help people to meet their own therapeutic self-care demands. *Actions:* Wholly compensatory, partly compensatory, and supportive-educative nursing systems. Assist by acting for or doing, guiding, providing physical and/or psychological support, providing a developmental environment, and teaching.
Rogers' Science of Unitary Human Beings	A unitary human being, a patterned, open, pandimensional energy field.	A patterned, open, pandi-mensional energy field	An expression of the life process	*Definition:* A learned profession that is both a science and an art. *Goal:* Help people achieve maximum well-being. *Actions:* Deliberative mutual patterning that involves environmental patterning to promote helicy, integrality, and resonancy.
Roy's Adaptation Model	An adaptive system with four response modes: physiological, self-concept, role function, and interdependence. Regulator and cognator coping mechanisms.	Focal stimuli Contextual stimuli Residual stimuli	Being and becoming an integrated and whole person	*Definition:* A theoretical system of knowledge that prescribes a process of analysis and action related to care of the ill or potentially ill person. *Goal:* Promotion of adaptation. *Actions:* Management of environmental stimuli, including increasing, decreasing, maintaining, removing, altering, or changing.

cabulary, which is the result of considerable thought about how to convey the meaning of that perspective. Each model also has a distinct frame of reference and a coherent, internally unified way to think about events and processes. Conceptual models also specify for nurses and society the mission and boundaries of the profession. The most tangible benefit of using a conceptual model of nursing is its delineation of goals of nursing practice. Another tangible benefit is the articulation of a nursing process format that encompasses parameters for assessment, labels for patient problems, a strategy for planning nursing care, a set of nursing interventions, and criteria for evaluating the outcomes of nursing practice. Three models are discussed here: Johnson's Behavioral System Model, Neuman's Systems Model, and Roy's Adaptation Model. Systems thinking is a comprehensive way of viewing clients and their environments.

- **WORK ON JOHNSON'S BEHAVIORAL SYSTEM MODEL** was begun by Dorothy Johnson in the early 1940s to clarify nursing's social mission from the perspective of a scientifically sound view of the person served by nursing and to identify the nature of the body of knowledge needed to attain the goal of nursing.

Philosophic Orientation

Johnson values a focus on the person's behavior and views it as a manifestation of the momentary condition of the whole behavioral system and the subsystems. She values nursing interventions before, during, and following illness, such as the use of contracts for intervention established between nurses and patients. Johnson also values patients' contributions to their own care. Johnson views patients as behavioral systems; medicine views patients as biological systems.

Pragmatic Orientation

Johnson's model focuses on the degree to which seven interrelated behavioral subsystems and the entire behavioral system function efficiently and effectively.

- The attachment, or affiliative, subsystem functions to attain security needed for survival, as well as for social inclusion and bonding and intimacy.
- Dependency subsystem succors behavior that encourages a response of nurturance and approval, attention, and physical assistance.
- Ingestive subsystem functions to satisfy appetite; is governed by social and psychological considerations, as well as biological requirements for food and fluids.
- Eliminative subsystem's function is the appropriate disposal of wastes, i.e., when, how, and under what conditions.
- Sexual subsystem functions to procreate and gratify; behaviors dependent on individual's biological sex and gender identity.
- Aggressive subsystem functions to protect and preserve self and society.
- Achievement subsystem functions for mastery or control of some aspect of self or environment with regard to intellectual, physical, creative, mechanical, social, or caretaking skills; measured against a standard of excellence.

The function of the behavioral subsystem reflects the drive or goal.

- Structural elements of each subsystem are:
-SET is a person's predisposition to act in a certain way.
-CHOICE refers to the person's total behavioral repertoire for fulfilling subsystem functions and achieving particular goals.
-ACTION is the actual organized and patterned behavior in a situation. Only structural element that can actually be observed, other elements must be inferred.
- For the subsystem to fulfill its function, three requirements must be met by the person or through outside assistance from a nurse:
-PROTECTION FROM NOXIOUS INFLUENCES with which the subsystem cannot cope.
-NURTURANCE through input of appropriate supplies from the environment.
-STIMULATION to enhance growth and prevent stagnation.
- Goal of nursing action is to restore, maintain, or attain behavioral system balance and dynamic stability at the highest possible lev-

TABLE 35–2.

THE NURSING PROCESS FOR JOHNSON'S BEHAVIORAL SYSTEM MODEL

I. Determination of the existence of a problem
  A. Obtain past and present family and individual behavioral system histories
  B. Specify condition of the subsystem structural components
    1. Determine drive strength, direction, and value
    2. Determine the solidity and specificity of the set
    3. Identify the range of behavior patterns available to the individual
    4. Identify the usual behavior in a given situation
    5. Assess and compare behavior with indices of behavioral system balance and stability
      a. Determine whether the behavior is succeeding or failing to achieve the consequences sought
      b. Determine whether more effective motor, expressive, or social skills are needed
      c. Determine whether or not the behavior is purposeful, that is, whether or not actions are goal-directed, reveal a plan, cease at an identifiable point, and are economical in sequence
      d. Determine whether or not the behavior is orderly, that is, whether or not actions are methodical, systematic, build sequentially toward a goal, and form a recognizable pattern
      e. Determine whether or not the behavior is predictable, that is, whether or not actions are repetitive under particular circumstances
      f. Determine whether or not the amount of energy expended to achieve desired goals is acceptable
      g. Determine whether or not behavior reflects appropriate choices
        (1) Determine whether or not actions are compatible with survival imperatives
        (2) Determine whether or not actions are congruent with the social situation
      h. Determine whether or not the individual is sufficiently satisfied with the behavior
    6. Determine the organization, interaction, and integration of the subsystems
II. Diagnostic classification of problems
  A. Internal subsystem problems
    1. Functional requirements not met
    2. Inconsistency or disharmony among structural components of subsystems
    3. Behavior inappropriate in the ambient culture
  B. Intersystem problems
    1. Domination of entire system by one or two subsystems
    2. Conflict between two or more subsystems

III. Management of nursing problems
  A. General goal of action
    1. Restore, maintain, or attain the patient's behavioral system balance and stability
    2. Help the patient achieve a more optimum level of balance and functioning when this is possible and desired
  B. Determine what nursing is to accomplish on behalf of the behavioral system
    1. Determine what level of behavioral system balance and stability is acceptable
    2. Determine who makes the judgment regarding acceptable level of behavioral system balance and stability
      a. Identify value system of nursing profession
      b. Identify own explicit value system
  C. Select a type of treatment
    1. Fulfill functional requirements of the subsystems
      a. Protect patient from overwhelming noxious influences
      b. Supply adequate nurturance through an appropriate input of essential supplies
      c. Provide stimulation to enhance growth and to inhibit stagnation
    2. Temporarily impose external regulatory or control measures
      a. Set limits for behavior by either permissive or inhibitory means
      b. Inhibit ineffective behavioral responses
      c. Assist patient to acquire new responses
      d. Reinforce appropriate behaviors
    3. Repair damaged structural elements in desirable direction
      a. Reduce drive strength by changing attitudes
      b. Redirect goal by changing attitudes
      c. Alter set by instruction or counseling
      d. Add choices by teaching new skills
  D. Negotiate treatment modality with patient
    1. Establish a contract with the patient
    2. Help patient understand meaning of nursing diagnosis and proposed treatment
    3. If diagnosis and/or proposed treatment are rejected, continue to negotiate with the patient until agreement is reached
IV. Compare behavior after treatment to indices of behavioral system balance and stability (c.f. I.B.5.a-h)

Reprinted from Fawcett J. *Analysis and Evaluation of Conceptual Models of Nursing.* 3rd ed. Philadelphia: Davis; 1995:82–83, with permission.

el for the person. The nursing process used is outlined in Study Guide Table 35-2.

Using Johnson's Model In Psychiatric Nursing. Example: Patient Classification Instrument (PCI) used at Neuropsychiatric Institute, University of California, Los Angeles (UCLA)

- PCI operationalizes each behavioral subsystem as a list of critical behaviors. Overall level of behavior for each patient is categorized as adaptive, in process of being learned, the minimally maladaptive, or maladaptive. Specific nursing interventions are designated for specific behaviors and categorized to the particular level of nursing care required.

  CATEGORY I. Patient behaviors are appropriate to patient's developmental stage and adaptive to the environment; linked to nursing interventions that provide general supervision, maintain and support appropriate patient behavior, and reinforce independent behavior.

  CATEGORY II. Patient behaviors are inconsistent, in the process of being learned, and maladaptive to the environment or inappropriate to the patient's developmental stage; linked to nursing interventions that provide moderate/periodic supervision, modify maladaptive behaviors and maintain adaptive ones, and structure the environment to provide limits. Interventions are carried out in the context of group settings and implement a medical treatment regimen.

  CATEGORY III. Patient behaviors are severely maladaptive to the environment and inappropriate to the patient's developmental stage; linked to nursing interventions that provide direct supervision, modify maladaptive behaviors, teach new behaviors, reinforce adaptive behaviors, and structure the environment to provide limits. Interventions implement the medical treatment regimen.

  CATEGORY IV. Patient behaviors are from Category III and of acute intensity, duration, and/or frequency, and represent self-destructive acts or aggression toward others; linked to nursing interventions that provide one-to-one supervision and that reduce intensity, frequency, and/or duration of maladaptive behaviors and protect the patient.

• NEUMAN'S SYSTEMS MODEL

Philosophic Orientation

Neuman's model values intervention before variances from wellness are manifested, as well as after they occur, and emphasizes the need to consider both the client's and the caregiver's perceptions of stressors. Nursing goals are effectively established when negotiated with the client. This model focuses on the extent of the client system's wellness rather than illness.

Pragmatic Orientation

The model regards the person as a client system that must defend its central core from the invasion of environmental stressors.

- The client system, which can be an individual, a family or other group, or a community, is a composite of five interrelated variables.

  - PHYSIOLOGICAL VARIABLES encompass bodily structures and functions.

  - PSYCHOLOGICAL VARIABLES include mental processes and relationships.

  - SOCIOCULTURAL VARIABLES encompass social and cultural functions.

  - DEVELOPMENTAL VARIABLES include the developmental processes of the life cycle.

  - SPIRITUAL VARIABLES include aspects of spirituality on a continuum.

- The client system is depicted as a central core, which is a basic structure of survival factors common to the species. Three types of concentric rings surround the core.

  - FLEXIBLE LINE OF DEFENSE is a protective buffer for the client's normal or stable state; prevents invasion by stressors, thus keeping the client system from stressor reactions or symptomatology.

  - NORMAL LINE OF DEFENSE represents the client system's normal or usual wellness state.

  - LINES OF RESISTANCE are involuntarily activated when a stressor invades. If the lines of resistance are effective, the system can reconstitute; if they are ineffective, death can occur.

- Environment

  - INTERNAL ENVIRONMENT consists of all forces or interactive influences internal to or con-

TABLE 35–3. THE NURSING PROCESS FOR NEUMAN'S SYSTEMS MODEL

I. Nursing diagnosis
  A. Establish database that includes the simultaneous consideration of the dynamic interactions of physiological, psychological, sociocultural, developmental, and spiritual variables
  1. Identify client/client system's perceptions
    a. Assess condition and strength of basic structure factors and energy resources
    b. Assess characteristics of the flexible and normal lines of defense, lines of resistance, degree of potential or actual reaction, and potential for reconstitution following a reaction
    c. Assess internal and external environmental stressors that threaten the stability of the client/client system
      (1) Identify, classify, and evaluate potential or actual intrapersonal, interpersonal, and extrapersonal stressors that threaten the stability of the client/client system through deprivation, excess, change, intolerance, etc.
      (2) Identify, classify, and evaluate potential and/or actual intrapersonal, interpersonal, and extrapersonal interactions between the client/client system and the environment, considering all five variables
    d. Assess and discover the nature of client/client system's created environment
      (1) Assess client/client system's perception of stressors
      (2) Determine degree of protection provided
      (3) Identify the cause and effect relationship between the created environment and client/client system in terms of bound versus available energy
    e. Evaluate influence of past, present, and possible future life processes and coping patterns on client/client system stability
    f. Identify and evaluate actual and potential internal and external resources for optimal state of wellness
  2. Identify caregiver's perceptions (repeat 1 a, b, c, d, e, and f from caregiver's perspective)
  3. Compare client/client system's and care giver's perceptions
    a. Identify similarities and differences in perceptions
    b. Facilitate client awareness of major perceptual distortions
    c. Resolve perceptual differences
  B. Variances from wellness
  1. Synthesize client database with relevant theories from nursing and adjunctive disciplines
  2. State a comprehensive nursing diagnosis
  3. Prioritize goals
    a. Consider client/client system wellness level
    b. Consider system stability needs
    c. Consider total available resources
  4. Postulate outcome goals and interventions that will facilitate the highest possible level of client/client system stability or wellness (i.e., maintain the normal line of defense and retain the flexible line of defense)

II. Nursing goals
  A. Negotiate desired prescriptive change or outcome goals to correct variances from wellness with the client/client system
  1. Consider needs identified in I.B.3.b.
  2. Consider resources identified in I.B.3.c.
  B. Negotiate prevention as intervention modalities and actions with client/client system
III. Nursing outcomes
  A. Implement nursing interventions through use of one or more of the three prevention as intervention modalities
  1. Primary prevention as intervention nursing actions to retain system stability
    a. Prevent stressor invasion
    b. Provide resources to retain or strengthen existing client/client system strengths
    c. Support positive coping and functioning
    d. Desensitize existing or possible noxious stressors
    e. Motivate toward wellness
    f. Coordinate and integrate interdisciplinary theories and epidemiologic input
    g. Educate or re-educate
    h. Use stress as a positive intervention strategy
  2. Secondary prevention as intervention nursing actions to attain system stability
    a. Protect basic structure
    b. Mobilize and optimize internal/external resources to attain stability and energy conservation
    c. Facilitate purposeful manipulation of stressors and reactions to stressors
    d. Motivate, educate, and involve client/client system in mutual establishment of health care goals
    e. Facilitate appropriate treatment and intervention measures
    f. Support positive factors toward wellness
    g. Promote advocacy by coordination and integration
    h. Provide primary preventive intervention as required
  3. Tertiary prevention as intervention nursing actions to maintain system stability
    a. Attain and maintain highest possible level of wellness and stability during reconstitution
    b. Educate, re-educate, and/or reorient as needed
    c. Support client/client system toward appropriate goals
    d. Coordinate and integrate client system health resources
    e. Provide primary and/or secondary preventive intervention as required
  B. Evaluate outcome goals
    1. Confirm attainment of outcome goals
    2. Reformulate goals
  C. Set intermediate and long-range goals for subsequent nursing action that are structured in relation to short-term goal outcomes

Reprinted from Fawcett J. *Analysis and Evaluation of Conceptual Models of Nursing.* 3rd ed. Philadelphia: Davis; 1995:234–235, with permission.

tained within the boundaries of the defined client system. It is the source of intrapersonal stressors.

- EXTERNAL ENVIRONMENT consists of all forces or influences external or existing outside the defined client system. It is the source of interpersonal and extrapersonal stressors.

- CREATED ENVIRONMENT is subconsciously developed by the client as a symbolic expression of system wholeness and encompasses the internal and the external environments. It functions as a subjective mechanism that may block the true reality of the environment and the health experience.

• Goal of nursing is to facilitate optimal wellness through retention, attainment, or maintenance of client system stability (see Study Guide Table 35-3).

Using Neuman's Systems Model (NSM) in Psychiatric Nursing. Example: Friend's Hospital, Philadelphia

As an outcome of the use of NSM, there was a fairly dramatic increase in the attention focused on the client's perceptions; the nurse's commitment to assessment of all five variables, even in the face of pressure to focus on most significant reason for hospitalization; and the scope of (client system) teaching and the creativity with which it was accomplished.

Example: A NSM-based continuing education program for psychiatric nurses

Project organized according to psychological, physiological, and sociological variables; the stressors and lines of defense relevant to each variable; and the nurse-client relationship in primary, secondary, and tertiary prevention.

NSM is equally effective with individual psychiatric clients and families.

• **ROY'S ADAPTATION MODEL** was developed in 1964 by Sister Callista Roy to articulate a body of scientific nursing knowledge that can be taught in a program of nursing education and used to guide practice.

Philosophic Orientation

Assumes that people are integrated wholes, capable of action. General principles are humanism and veritity.

• Humanism recognizes the person and subjective dimensions of the human experience as central to knowing and valuing.

• Veritivity asserts that there is an absolute truth and a common purposefulness of human existence.

Roy values the active participation of persons in their nursing care and believes that medicine focuses on biological systems and the person's disease, whereas nursing focuses on the person as a total being who responds to internal and external environmental stimuli.

Pragmatic Orientation

Roy's adaptive model focuses on the responses of the person, as a human adaptive system, to a constantly changing environment. Adaptation is the central feature. When the system is unable to cope with or respond to constantly changing stimuli from internal and external environments, problems arise in maintaining the integrity of the system.

• Three types of environmental stimuli:

- FOCAL STIMULUS: the one most immediately confronting the person.

- CONTEXTUAL STIMULI: all other stimuli that contribute directly to adaptation.

- RESIDUAL STIMULI: all unknown factors that may influence the situation.

• Adaptation occurs by means of two coping mechanisms:

- REGULATOR MECHANISM: receives input from internal and external environments and processes it through neural-chemical-endocrine channels to produce responses.

- COGNATOR MECHANISM: receives input from external and internal stimuli and process it through cognitive/emotive pathways including perceptual/information processing, learning, judgment, and emotion.

• Responses to environmental stimuli take place in four interrelated modes:

- PHYSIOLOGICAL MODE: concerned with basic needs requisite to maintaining the physical and physiological integrity of the human system.

- SELF-CONCEPT MODE: deals with person's con-

TABLE 35–4. THE NURSING PROCESS FOR ROY'S ADAPTATION MODEL

I. Assessment of behaviors
   A. Methods used to collect data
      1. Observation
         a. Sight
         b. Sound
         c. Touch
         d. Taste
         e. Smell
      2. Objective measurement
         a. Paper and pencil instruments
         b. Measures of physiological parameters
      3. Interviews
   B. Behaviors to assess
      1. Physiological mode
         a. Oxygenation
         b. Nutrition
         c. Elimination
         d. Activity and rest
         e. Protection
         f. Senses
         g. Fluid and electrolytes
         h. Neurological functions
         i. Endocrine functions
      2. Self-concept mode
         a. Physical self
            (1) Body image
            (2) Body sensation
         b. Personal self
            (1) Self-consistency
            (2) Self-ideal
            (3) Moral-ethical-spiritual self
      3. Role function
         a. Primary role
            (1) Instrumental component(s)
            (2) Expressive component(s)
         b. Secondary roles
            (1) Instrumental component(s)
            (2) Expressive component(s)
         c. Tertiary roles
            (1) Instrumental component(s)
            (2) Expressive component(s)
      4. Interdependence mode
         a. Significant others
            (1) Contributive behavior
            (2) Receptive behavior
         b. Social support
            (1) Contributive behavior
            (2) Receptive behavior
   C. Judgment of behaviors
      1. Adaptive or ineffective responses
         a. Nurse's judgment
         b. Person's perception
      2. Criteria for judgment
         a. Person's individualized goals
         b. Comparison of behavior with norms signifying adaptation
         c. Regulator mechanism activity
         d. Cognator mechanism effectiveness

II. Assessment of stimuli
   A. Criteria for priorities for further assessment of the person's behaviors
      1. Behaviors that threaten the survival of the individual, family, group, or community
      2. Behaviors that affect the growth of the individual, family, group, or community
      3. Behaviors that affect the continuation of the human race or of society
      4. Behaviors that affect the attainment of full potential for the individual or group
   B. Methods used to determine influence of stimuli
      1. Observation
      2. Objective measurement
      3. Interview
      4. Validate hunch about relevant stimuli with the person
   C. Stimuli
      1. Focal stimulus
      2. Contextual stimuli
         a. Culture
            (1) Socioeconomic status
            (2) Ethnicity
            (3) Belief system
         b. Family structure and tasks
         c. Developmental stage
            (1) Age
            (2) Sex
            (3) Tasks
            (4) Heredity
            (5) Genetic factors
         d. Integrity of response modes
            (1) Physiological mode and disease pathology
            (2) Self-concept
            (3) Role function
            (4) Interdependence
         e. Cognator effectiveness
            (1) Perception
            (2) Knowledge
            (3) Skill
         f. Environmental considerations
            (1) Change in internal or external environment
            (2) Medical management
            (3) Use of drugs, alcohol, and/or tobacco

      3. Residual stimuli
         a. Beliefs
         b. Attitudes
         c. Traits
         d. Cultural determinants
III. Nursing diagnosis
   A. Three approaches
      1. State behaviors within each response mode and with their most relevant influencing stimuli
      2. Provide a summary label for behaviors in each response mode with relevant stimuli
      3. Provide a label that summarizes a behavioral pattern across response modes that is affected by the same stimuli
   B. Arrange diagnoses in order of priority using criteria in II.A
IV. Goal setting
   A. Statement of behavioral outcomes of nursing intervention
   B. Determine that the person agrees with goal
V. Nursing intervention
   A. Management of stimuli
      1. Alter stimuli
      2. Increase stimuli
      3. Decrease stimuli
      4. Remove stimuli
      5. Maintain stimuli
   B. Priorities
      1. Manage focal stimulus first if possible
      2. Manage contextual stimuli next
   C. Selection of nursing intervention approach
      1. List possible approaches
      2. Outline consequences of management of each stimulus
      3. Determine probability for each consequence
      4. Judge value of outcomes of each approach
      5. Share options with the person
      6. Select approach with highest probability of reaching valued goal
VI. Evaluation
   A. Methods used
      1. Observation
      2. Objective measurement
      3. Interview
   B. Criteria for judgment of effectiveness of nursing intervention
      1. Goal attained or not attained
      2. Person does or does not manifest behavior stated in goal

Reprinted from Fawcett J. *Analysis and Evaluation of Conceptual Models of Nursing.* 3rd ed. Philadelphia: Davis; 1995: 462–464, with permission.

ceptions of the physical self, including moral, ethical, and spiritual self.

- ROLE FUNCTION MODE: concerned with the person's performance of roles, based on his or her position within society.

- INTERDEPENDENCE MODE: focuses primarily on relationships with significant others and social support system.

• Responses in each mode are judged as adaptive (promoting the integrity of the person in terms of the goals of the human adaptive system) or as ineffective (not contributing to these goals).

• The goal of nursing is to promote adaptation in each of the four adaptive modes, thereby contributing to the person's health, quality of life, and death with dignity (see Study Guide Table 35-4).

Using Roy's Adaptation Model (RAM) in Psychiatric Nursing

Example: RAM basis for organizing nursing history tool in a psychiatric hospital, Hull, Quebec, Canada

Patients said it was the first time they were fully evaluated; consequently, they realized that most problems interrelate. Nurses were satisfied because they came to know the patient better.

Example: Findings from a study that linked RAM to practice indicated that nursing interventions should be directed toward management of contextual stimuli to enhance the patient's adaptation.

Example: RAM has been used to guide nursing practice with patients who have various psychiatric symptoms and have been linked to particular types of therapy such as music therapy and group therapy.

• **SELECTING A CONCEPTUAL MODEL** for psychiatric nursing practice essentially has six steps.

State your philosophy of nursing in the form of beliefs and values about the nursing recipient, environment, health, and nursing goals.

• In what settings can psychiatric nurses practice?

• What is health? What is mental health?

• What are the appropriate goals of psychiatric nursing practice?

• What part do recipients of mental health nursing play in determining nursing goals and identifying interventions used to attain those goals.

Identify a particular patient population with which you wish to practice. Specify psychiatric diagnoses, age, and level of care (acute or chronic).

Analyze and evaluate several conceptual models of nursing, emphasizing philosophical claims and utility for psychiatric nursing practice.

Compare the philosophical claims upon which each conceptual model is based with your own philosophy of nursing.

Determine which conceptual models are appropriate for use with the patient population of interest.

Select the conceptual model that most nearly matches your philosophy of nursing and the population of interest.

Try using the model with several patients. If it is not successful, try another model.

• **THE CONSISTENT USE OF ANY MODEL TO INTERPRET OBSERVABLE PATIENT DATA IS NOT AN EASY TASK.** Much like the development of any habitual behavior, it requires thought, discipline, and the gradual development of a mind set of what is important to observe within the guidelines of the model.

TAKING ANOTHER LOOK

You are now ready to respond to the questions that were raised in Gaining a Perspective at the beginning of this chapter. After you have written or thought about your responses, you may wish to look at the Suggested Responses on page 334.

36 THE THERAPEUTIC NURSE-PATIENT RELATIONSHIP

GAINING A PERSPECTIVE

Think about the situations below, and after you have read the Key Concepts for this chapter describe your responses in more detail.

1. In practice as a psychiatric nurse, how will you use the idea that each individual is unique?

2. How would you, as a nurse, handle the situation described below?

   A patient that the nurse has developed a therapeutic relationship with is ready for discharge. The patient wants to buy the nurse a gift to show her gratitude.

KEY CONCEPTS

- **PSYCHIATRIC NURSING INVOLVES THE THERAPEUTIC USE OF SELF** in the care of individuals experiencing distress. The use of self therapeutically requires knowledge and a mastery of a therapeutic relationship. In the context of this relationship, the nurse provides information, empathy, nondirective listening, respect, and feedback as an actual treatment modality. The patient experiences the therapeutic relationship as an opportunity to address and redress sources of distress.

  Professional nursing embodies thoughtful, deliberate goals, as well as attitudes and actions of concern, to support the well-being of individuals and groups. In psychiatric nursing, care is based on accepting the patient as he or she is, focusing on the here and now, remaining nonjudgmental, and recognizing the person's uniqueness and potential for growth and self-actualization.

  Throughout a therapeutic relationship, the nurse has four interlocking roles: resource person, counselor, technical expert, and surrogate.

Resource Person
The nurse helps patients identify needs and the resources available to meet those needs.

- Patients must feel safe in the environment and be oriented to their role, including informed consent.

- Patients need to recognize and understand the crisis they are experiencing and the extent of help needed. The nurse acts as a resource by helping patients see how they are functioning and the relationship of their symptoms to illness. The nurse engages the patient as an active partner in identifying and assessing the present problems.

Counselor
Initially, patients are not completely ready to disclose difficult underlying issues related to their crisis. The nurse needs to respond unconditionally and assist the patient to focus on

the problem, allowing the patient to express feelings and develop increased awareness of what those feelings are. The initial focus for the nurse and the patient is to gain understanding of the situation as seen by the patient. The patient is encouraged to identify and express feelings. The nurse's advice, reassurance, suggestion, or persuasion is of little value when offered in response to feelings.

Technical Expert

The nurse has an understanding of the biological correlates of mental illness, diagnostic testing, and treatment options. In the role of technical expert, the nurse educates the patient about other aspects of treatment including medication, changes in diet related to medication, stress management techniques, and resuming activities of daily living.

Surrogate

This "substitute" role is often enacted through the unconscious dynamic process of transference and countertransference.

- Transference occurs when the patient projects onto the nurse feelings, thoughts, or wishes held by another person, such as a family member or other person in authority. Feelings can be intense, and negative or positive.

- Countertransference is the nurse's unconscious response to projected content. Countertransference also includes all feelings, negative and positive, that the nurse may hold in relation to the patient. These two processes occur naturally, but can impede the development of a therapeutic relationship, as psychiatric nursing requires a focus on the here and now.

- **THE NURSE-PATIENT THERAPEUTIC RELATIONSHIP (PEPLAU'S MODEL)** has four phases: orientation, identification, exploitation, and resolution. Each phase has overlapping purposes for the nurse and the patient.

Orientation Phase

Orientation is the beginning phase of the relationship when the patient and client first engage each other. The patient learns what to expect from the nurse, as well as what is expected of himself or herself. The goal of this phase is for the nurse and patient to become acquaint-

ed, and for the patient to identify the process of seeking help as a learning experience. The problem becomes one of a knowledge deficit rather than a personal or characterological deficit. The patient seeks assistance on the basis of a felt need in relation to a health crisis. The individual may be aware of changes in his or her mental health, or, with the support of a family member, friend, or the police, seeks assistance if experiencing a major mental health illness or psychiatric emergency. Expressed needs should be interpreted as "educative needs." What does the patient need to know about the present situation in order to resolve the crisis and develop adaptive, productive ways of coping with the present or future situations?

To the initial contact, the nurse brings all his or her prior knowledge, experiences, attitudes, and feelings. How the nurse feels about helping others makes a great deal of difference in patient outcome.

By the end of the orientation phase, a working understanding should be developed. The level of understanding will be reflected in the nursing diagnoses and interdisciplinary treatment plan that are developed and in the patient's knowledge of what the treatment situation can offer. The length of this first phase depends on whether the patient has the ability to trust and thereby establish a relationship.

Identification Phase

In this phase, patients may begin to indicate that they feel stronger and less helpless. In a close nurse-patient therapeutic relationship, the patient may begin to aspire to the strengths and healthy traits of the nurse. As the nurse models effective problem solving or expression of feelings, the patient begins to identify with those traits. The process of identification is natural and reasonable; however, it may evoke unsettling feelings for the nurse to know that his or her behavior is being so closely examined and incorporated into the action of another. It is necessary for the nurse to preserve self while caring for another and to define boundaries, i.e., where self leaves off and the other person begins. The nurse maintains defined boundaries through periodic review of the therapeutic relationship with the patient and the interdisciplinary team.

During the identification phase, a patient may express some powerful feelings, such as anger, helplessness, dependency, self-centeredness, or grief. The nurse's acceptance of these expressions will promote the patient's self-acceptance as he or she learns about those feelings and eventually how to manage them effectively.

- Difficulties with identification

  Sometimes due to symptoms of illness or earlier traumatic relationships, patients have difficulty moving into the identification phase. A patient may not feel worthy of care. Most resistance represents the patient's defense against feelings of discomfort. The nurse can creatively facilitate the therapeutic relationship with the resistant patient by engaging in routine care or participating in diversional activities with the patient.

Exploitation Phase

The true working phase of the relationship is the exploitation phase. Once the patient and nurse have learned enough about each other as unique individuals in a therapeutic relationship, the patient is ready to make full use of treatment resources; the patient takes advantage of all goods and services. The patient begins to demonstrate goal-oriented behavior. The more independent the patient (usually someone with greater interpersonal strengths), the more the patient may identify new and related issues and acknowledge progress toward goals. The nurse offers some clues. The dynamics of the interaction between the nurse and the patient should be a negotiated component of the treatment plan.

Exploitive behavior is characterized by an intermingling of needs and testing of new behaviors. The role of the nurse in this phase of the relationship is to facilitate exploitive learning whenever possible and to encourage the patient to develop insight into past behaviors through the application of newly learned skills. As in adolescent development, some dependence is needed; however, the patient must exercise new skills of independence.

The nurse may experience a variety of feelings during the exploitive phase: intense pride as the patient exercises increased independence; ambivalence as the patient's need for the nurse's support diminishes; or conflict as the nurse has a desire to protect the patient from anxiety and potential harm. The nurse should acknowledge these feelings as natural and identify their meaning both personally and in the therapeutic relationship.

Resolution Phase

In the final phase of resolution the hallmark is termination of the nurse-patient relationship. It is usually signaled by the patient's discharge or the meeting of patient goals.

- Resolution occurs on several levels for the patient.
  - ACUTE CRISIS OF ILLNESS IS RESOLVED and gradually integrated into the patient's life experience.
  - PATIENT PREPARES FOR LIFE AFTER TREATMENT, such as work, school, or outpatient follow-up.
  - GRADUAL FREEING FROM IDENTIFICATION WITH HELPING PERSONS and strengthening of ability to stand more or less alone.
- The focus for both the nurse and patient is often saying "good-bye." It is a time to review, synthesize, and consolidate what has been learned.
  - PATIENT SHOULD PARTICIPATE IN PLANS for discharge and follow-up.
  - ANXIETY MAY OCCUR and patient needs to exercise new coping skills to manage it.
  - PATIENT MAY WANT TO BUY A GIFT FOR THE NURSE; encourage patient to instead write or express feelings of gratitude.
  - MAINTAINING CONTACT WITH THE PATIENT AFTER TERMINATION conveys a subtle message of lack of confidence in the patient's independence.
- **THE NURSE'S ROLE IN THE THERAPEUTIC REALTIONSHIP REQUIRES A DYNAMIC BALANCE** between knowledge of the patient and knowledge of self. Skills are needed that specifically facilitate the relationship.

Empathy

Being able to accurately recognize the immediate emotional perspective of another person while maintaining one's own perspective is being empathetic; there is no loss of boundaries. On the other hand, when the therapeutic professional identifies with a patient, the professional not only recognizes the emotional state of the patient but feels the emotion of the patient as if it were his or her own; this leads to burnout and unrecognized countertransference. Empathy conveys the message to the patient that his or her feelings are understood and accepted by a helping professional.

Unconditional Positive Regard for the Patient

The nurse relates to and accepts the patient with deep and genuine caring, without attaching conditions such as moral judgment, relating from a position of power, or withholding care contingent on some behaviors of the patient. Regardless of the evocative issues that the patient brings to the relationship, such as violence, rape, or incest, it is essential for the nurse to relate to the patient as another person deserving care. To relate from the position of genuine caring, it is important for the nurse to periodically identify and assess potentially disturbing responses to the patient's feelings and issues. One's self-concept influences how the nurse and the patient relate to one another. Self-concept develops in interactions with the environment, society, and significant others. Actions and feelings on the part of the nurse can inhibit or enhance the formation of a therapeutic relationship. When the nurse identifies actions or feelings that can inhibit the progress of the therapeutic relationship, the nurse should consult peers or others for supervision in managing the feelings.

- **NURSING FACTORS AND THE TREATMENT DELIVERY SYSTEM MAY INHIBIT** the development of a therapeutic relationship.

Depersonalization

Depersonalization occurs when the patient is regarded as a diagnosis, bed number, or a quirk of the illness. This may also happen when the nurse refuses to "chat," does not make eye contact, or uses unnecessarily formal terms of address.

Maintaining an Efficient Attitude

Nurse needs a flexible style of interacting, which includes an honest presentation, a well-timed sense of humor, and a nondefensive attitude about questions the patient asks.

Failure to Trust the Patient

Not trusting the patient or being suspicious of ulterior motives can occur when the nurse feels he or she is being manipulated by the patient.

Ethnocentric Beliefs About Illness Behavior

When the nurse and patient do not share the same cultural beliefs or language, the nurse may fear the unknown and cling to his or her own beliefs. Instead, the nurse should spend time with the patient using nonverbal communication to help build a relationship. To facilitate a therapeutic relationship, the patient's belief system should be incorporated into the treatment plan.

Multiple Caregivers

Rotating shifts and days off may be perceived by the patient as lack of caring. The nurse needs to explain schedules and prepare the patient when the nurse is planning time off.

Charting Material Considered Confidential by the Patient

Realizing that some information is charted can inhibit the patient in further trust and disclosure. Patient needs to understand that sharing pertinent information with the treatment team is a safety measure.

Time Limits

Time is essential to building a therapeutic relationship, but the "system" may impose limits. Shorter therapeutic programs require that the nurse accurately prioritize patient needs and involve the patient in planning goals to be accomplished. The nurse may enhance therapeutic skills in a peer group that leads to development of self.

- **FOR STUDENT NURSES IN THERAPEUTIC RELATIONSHIPS** there are special considerations. Students worry they will say the wrong thing. Students must remember that for the patient the therapeutic relationship is to be a learning experience about the illness and self, and it may help the student to use the relationship in the same way. In addition, the student must be oriented to role responsibilities, boundaries, and available resources. The student needs to articulate his or her own learning needs and use available resources to expand professional knowledge.

By the end of the experience, the student should be able to recognize the skills that have been acquired. As in all learning experiences, the student is likely to experience some frustration. Research supports the use of journals to assist students in exploring and changing their attitude toward patients with mental illness. Clinical conferences with faculty and peers help to develop increased awareness about self in the therapeutic relationship.

- **A PATIENT MAY NEED HELP AND SUPPORT IN RECOGNIZING AND BEGINNING TO ADDRESS HIS OR HER NEEDS.**

Current Situation

The patient needs to recognize and understand the current situation and the extent of help that is needed.

- Nurses gently ask questions and probe the patient's understandings about the situation.

Plan of Care

The patient needs to collaborate in developing and implementing a plan of care.

- Patient must understand his or her situation and be aware of treatment options.
- Collaboration is dependent on patient's understanding and consent.

Focused Energy

Need to focus energy positively; define, understand, and meet problem at hand. Patient focus is on treatment. Focusing on problem is an opportunity for the patient to address and redress sources of distress and maximize situations for learning and growth.

- **PATIENT FACTORS MAY INHIBIT THE DEVELOPMENT OF A THERAPEUTIC RELATIONSHIP.**

Psychosis

Patient may not be able to focus on treatment goals because he or she is confused or overwhelmed. Symptoms need to be under control.

Lack of Trust

A lack of trust is evidenced by strategies to keep the nurse at a distance.

Behaviors

Specific behaviors signal inhibition in the relationship: withdrawing from contact, attempting to elope, and demanding, coercive and/or manipulative interactions.

Impaired Communication

A common language is needed.

Preconceptions

The nurse or patient having preconceptions about treatment can be an inhibiting factor in a relationship.

- **AN EXPLANATORY MODEL (MORSE, 1991) DESCRIBES FOUR OTHER TYPES OF MUTUAL NURSE-PATIENT RELATIONSHIPS:** clinical, therapeutic, connected, and overinvolved. The relationships are negotiated until a mutually satisfying relationship is reached. The type of relationship that is achieved depends on the contact between the nurse and patient, the needs and desires of the patient, the commitment of the patient, and the patient's inclination to trust the nurse.

Clinical

- Contact is relatively brief.
- Contact is sought by patient for a minor concern.
- Interaction between nurse and patient is courteous and superficial.

Therapeutic

- Contact is of short duration.
- Patient's needs are not great.
- Treatment interventions are not serious or life-threatening.

Connected

- Patient chooses to trust the nurse and nurse chooses to enter the relationship to meet the patient's needs; further trust evolves.
- The patient consults the nurse about the treatment plan, and the nurse serves as the patient's advocate.

Overinvolved

- This contact resembles a very close personal relationship; caring between nurse and patient exceeds professional boundaries.

TAKING ANOTHER LOOK

You are now ready to respond to the situations presented in Gaining a Perspective at the beginning of this chapter. After you have written or thought about your responses, you may wish to look at the Suggested Responses on page 335.

37 THERAPEUTIC MILIEU MANAGEMENT

TERMS TO DEFINE

containment

custodial model

involvement

managed care

milieu

milieu management

moral treatment

structure

support

therapeutic community

therapeutic milieu

validation

GAINING A PERSPECTIVE

Think about the meaning of the following statement, and after you have read the Key Concepts for this chapter present a detailed response.

What is meant by "The value of the milieu is the power of the group"?

KEY CONCEPTS

- **MILIEU IS THE GENERAL PSYCHOSOCIAL CONTEXT WITHIN WHICH CARE TAKES PLACE.** Health care reform and managed care incentives that mandate mental health services be provided in the least restrictive, or intensive, setting have created the need for a more dynamic formulation of milieu than the carefully planned environment previously provided in inpatient psychiatric settings. The term "milieu management" implies that the environmental factors in any setting can be assessed and managed on a continual basis. "Therapeutic milieu" refers to the efforts taken to release an environment's therapeutic potential.

- **THE EVOLUTION OF MILIEU IN PSYCHIATRY GENERALLY ENCOMPASSES FOUR MODELS:** moral treatment, custodial models, and two therapeutic community models — Maxwell Jones' model and therapeutic milieu. Each reflects the attitudes toward mentally ill people during various historical periods.

Moral Treatment

- In Europe and America at the end of the 18th century.

- A supportive, attractive environment emphasizing fresh air, rest, and recreation; retreats in aesthetically pleasing locations.

- Not a particular technique, but an approach based on Christianity, enlightenment, and reason.

- The rationale was that psychological stressors had robbed the "lunatics" of their reason and that physical setting and social influences were curative agents.

- Although this was an era of optimism for the mentally ill, leaders of the moral treatment movement failed to train successors; with the advent of the state mental institution, the moral treatment movement died.

Custodial Models

- By the end of the 19th century, Darwin's *The Origin of Species* was used as the rationale for inhuman treatment of the mentally unfit. Successful treatment was viewed as impossible, and institutions provided only shelter and safety. The mentally ill were socially isolated and institutionalized for many years.

- In the total institutional setting, all activities were organized to meet the institution's goals, not the goals of the resident or inmate. Residents were induced to conform through a complex organization of privileges and punishment.

Therapeutic Community Models

Factors that influenced the development of more therapeutic models were the many draftees who revealed mental illness when they were to be inducted into the U.S. armed forces, people's increasing sensitization to psychiatric disorders, and the combat neurosis that appeared in increasing numbers of soldiers, which resulted in the development of new methods for short-term treatment.

- Maxwell Jones' Therapeutic Community

Jones viewed the psychiatric hospital as a small society, a community, and believed in the patient's right to participation in treatment. The underlying premise is that all relationships and activities in the hospital can have therapeutic value.

The model focuses on social and group interactions, living-learning opportunities, and "shared responsibility," not only of the staff but of all community members. A democratic process is used to mediate problems; privileges are granted by the community as a whole.

The preconditions for establishing a therapeutic community are:
- a community sanctioned by administration
- a willingness to examine conflicts
- a stable patient population

Although this model was found to be impractical, many of its principles were used in the evolving therapeutic milieu models.

- Therapeutic Milieu Model

Any therapeutic milieu normally retains some of the elements of the therapeutic community, including the distribution of responsibility and decision-making power; the

clarity of treatment programs, roles, and leadership; and the high level of staff-patient interaction.

Elements that differ include the maintenance of a medical hierarchy and retention of staff control in decision making. During the 1980s, the advancement of somatic and medical treatments deemphasized the value of psychosocial treatments. Currently, however, the negative effects of some medications coupled with renewed interest in a psychosocial model has revitalized interest in milieu management principles.

Nursing's role in therapeutic milieus has evolved over the years.

- The milieu models have fostered collaboration among the disciplines of nursing, medicine, social work, and social sciences and helped to solidify psychiatric nursing as a specialty.
- The nurse's role as "sociotherapist" was defined.
- In inpatient settings, the nurse's 24-hour presence was fundamental to the nurse's centrality in the milieu.

Therapeutic processes in the milieu are containment, support, structure, involvement, and validation.

- Containment. Represents that which sustains the physical well-being of patients and prevents assaults, homicides and suicides, and physical deterioration in or accidents by those who lack judgment. In addition, the effect of containment reinforces the internal controls of the patient. Nursing interventions designed for medication-free psychotic patients include use of seclusion; cold, wet packs; time-outs; and suicidal observation. To establish safety, staff must create expectations for conduct and develop a hierarchy of interventions.
- Support. Assists patients to feel comfortable and secure. Support can be given by concrete provisions such as food and clothing, or as direction, advice, and education. Too much support may confirm a patient's sense of inadequacy and dependence. Sometimes withholding support is a pur-

TABLE 37–1.
ELEMENTS OF COMMUNITY MEETING

Preparation
Community members designated to prepare room.
Community leaders and staff meet to review agenda.

Meeting order
Chairperson calls meeting to order.
Roll is called and missing members are accounted for.
Minutes are read.
Agenda is followed.
Meeting is terminated on time with supportive ending (i.e., thought for the day).

Typical agenda
New members introduced and welcomed.
Members who are leaving say good-bye and where they are going.
Community jobs are filled if applicable.
Old business is discussed.
New business is discussed.
Committee and treasurer reports (if applicable) are given.
Daily schedule is read and reviewed.
Meeting ends on time.

Postmeeting process
Staff meet with community leaders to provide support and give feedback.

poseful way to prevent regression. Nursing interventions based on support include providing patient education on such topics as coping skills, medications, and stress and symptom management.

- Structure. All aspects of the milieu that provide a predictable organization of time, place, and person; involves all regulation, hierarchy, and role definitions. Support includes such nursing interventions as open reports, community meetings (see Study Guide Table 37-1), nursing rounds, and education groups.

- Involvement. Those processes that cause patients to attend actively to their social environment and interact with it — socialization. Involvement includes group therapy and informal and formal discussion groups. Provision is made for a consistent adult relationship in an atmosphere in which the patient can try new interpersonal skills which connect him or her to the environment.

- Validation. The unit processes that affirm a patient's individuality; characterized by respect and honor for the individual. The concept of norms relates to validation and helps build a climate of universality and shared experience. Norms are the values that underlie what is acceptable and tolerated behavior. The value of the milieu is the power of the group; however, the individual's needs are not subordinated to the group by coercion or a demand for behavior socially defined by the group.

- **THE CHANGING NATURE OF INPATIENT HOSPITALIZATION** renders some of the ideals of therapeutic milieu difficult to operationalize. These changes include:

Shorter hospital stays.

Higher acuity.

Heterogeneity of patients.

Increased physical complications/medical complexity.

Fewer or inconsistent staff.

Devaluation of psychosocial methods by biologically oriented psychiatrists.

The function of the inpatient unit has evolved from "storing the mentally ill" to "dispatching the mentally ill." Now, gathering diagnostic and assessment information and transferring patients to a suitable nonacute setting dominates the activities of staff on many inpatient units.

Impact of managed care

- Managed health care influences utilization, monitors costs, and measures performance.

- Managed care providers serve as gatekeepers for third-party reimbursement for services. Managed care companies have created incentives to develop several levels of care that decrease cost and intensity of services. A vertically integrated system results, offering crisis intervention, inpatient treatment, partial hospitalization, assisted living programs, outpatient services, and home care. Several of these settings are amenable to milieu interventions.

TABLE 37–2. THERAPEUTIC MILIEU PROCESSES APPLIED ACROSS SETTINGS

Milieu Function	Crisis Intervention Center	Inpatient Unit

Containment	Intensive care procedures:
	  Restraints
	  Sedatives
	  One-to-one staff
	  Quiet rooms
	  Staff trained in behavior management
		Intensive care procedures:
		  Restraints
		  Medication
		  One-to-one staff
		  Quiet rooms
		Level or privilege system
		Belongings restriction
		Access monitoring and restriction

Support	Nourishment if needed Clean clothes if needed Facilities for hygiene Medical screening Minimal bureaucracy for access to services	Clean attractive unit Availability of supplies Nutritious meals and snacks
Structure	Explanations of all procedures Introduction and role of all who contact patient	Clear hierarchy of staff Written expectations Opportunity to participate in a staff–patient forum Schedule of activities Predictable routines Patient handbook
Involvement	One-to-one contact with crisis worker	Opportunities to participate in unit planning Group activities and therapies Consistent therapist/RN Participation in treatment plan Family groups and meetings
Validation	Maintenance of privacy and confidentiality	Privacy Alternative track if needed Opportunities for growth and leadership

	Partial Hospital Program	Assisted Living
Containment	Plan for management of aggression and suicide Hot line for after hours Mechanism for admission to an inpatient unit, if necessary Clear behavioral expectations	Plan for management of aggression and suicide Hot line for after hours Therapist on call House rules Assistance with controlling drug and alcohol abuse
Support	Transportation to the center Assistance with budgeting Assistance with obtaining medication and prescriptions	Supervised ADLs if needed Assistance with meals Assistance with obtaining health care Medication self-administration program
Structure	Defined schedule Assistance with time management	Each member has a flexible schedule Assistance with time management Participation in the larger community through a job, school, or sheltered workshop
Involvement	Participation in program planning Community meetings Social as well as therapeutic activities Group excursions	Planned social activities Social skills education Celebration of important events, such as holidays and birthdays Facilitated family interventions
Validation	Opportunities for growth and leadership Education regarding the patient's specific illness Facilitation of completion of GED or college Opportunity for paid work	Access to patient advocate Ritualized acknowledgement of strengths and successes Focused education Tolerance of occasional regression

- Two programs listed above are described here: PARTIAL HOSPITALIZATION PROGRAMS. Day, evening, or weekend programs provide structured activities, medication monitoring, and living skills, as well as opportunities for socialization, positive reinforcement of strengths, and a connection with a consistent therapist. Programs include activities based on the patient's culture and community. Partial hospitalization is for subacute patients who are assessed for suicide and violence potential prior to admission.

  ASSISTED LIVING. Clients who are socially isolated from their families and who need continual supervision and monitoring may be placed in assisted living or personal care homes. These settings vary in quality, but most provide cooked meals, laundry services, safety screening, and medication monitoring. Resident supervisors manage the home, and patients participate in the upkeep and chores. Many patients attend day hospital programs for more structure.

- **THERAPEUTIC MILIEU PROCESSES MAY BE APPLIED ACROSS ALL SETTINGS** (Study Guide Table 37-2).

Containment

The most concrete examples of containment are crisis intervention centers, inpatient psychiatric hospitals, and maximum security units. Involuntary commitment, and locked doors and windows, as well as restraints and staff observations, are forms of constraint. Less restriction can be facilitated through a level or privilege system.

A minimal degree of containment is experienced in partial programs, residential programs, and intensive outpatient settings. A plan is in place for emergency management if patients lose impulse control.

Nurses assess the degree of restriction that is necessary by evaluating patients and their need for safety. If patients perceive that an environment is too restrictive, they may act out or elope (leave hospital without permission).

Support

In inpatient settings, patients depend on staff for assistance with basic needs until they are able to reintegrate and attain stability. Staff will encourage patients to develop coping skills and recognize and draw upon their inner strengths. Too much support creates dependency on the institution and staff and can retard patient growth and promote further dysfunction.

In partial-setting and assisted-living programs nurses provide support to patients by facilitating negotiation with social agencies, assisting with job placement, and improving life skills so that patients can maintain independence.

Structure

In inpatient settings, staff provide boundaries and limits, and they schedule patient activities.

In other settings, patients learn to structure their time and to choose among alternatives. Patient schedules need to be individualized and realistic, and staff can assist with them.

Involvement

In all communal settings participation and socialization play important roles in treatment. Any member of the community can have an opportunity to develop leadership skills.

Community meetings generally focus on community living issues. During the meetings, there is also the potential of assessing the patient's level of functioning. Emergency meetings may be held during or following a crisis such as a suicide attempt, death, or violence.

Validation

Validation acknowledges and affirms patients as individuals and as deserving of treatment that maintains their dignity and uniqueness. Patients are not labeled or dehumanized, and activities are appropriate to the patient's age, culture, and developmental level. Regressed behavior, while not encouraged, is acceptable.

TAKING ANOTHER LOOK

You are now ready to respond to the statement in Gaining A Perspective at the beginning of this chapter. After you have written or thought about your response, you may wish to look at the Suggested Responses on page 335.

38 CLINICAL ASSESSMENT AND NURSING DIAGNOSIS

GAINING A PERSPECTIVE

Think about the questions listed below, and after you have read the Key Concepts for this chapter respond to the queries in greater detail.

1. What would your initial thoughts be when you, as a nurse, are asked to conduct an assessment interview with a patient who is attending a mental health clinic for the first time?

2. What do you think is the purpose of making a nursing diagnosis?

KEY CONCEPTS

- **THE PSYCHIATRIC NURSING ASSESSMENT GUIDES THE ENTIRE NURSING PROCESS AND IS THE BASIS FOR INTERACTIONS** between the nurse and the person receiving psychiatric nursing services. Assessment is also basic to the interactions the nurse has in the health care system as a coordinator and care manager. It is the critical step that leads to developing nursing diagnoses that direct the planning of patient care.

  In looking beyond the medical model of disease and cure, symptoms and psychosis, a holistic approach to assessment connects mind-body-spirit and environment to determine their impact on the person's well-being, self-advocacy, rehabilitation, and recovery. A holistic approach to nursing process promotes mental, emotional, motivational, environmental, spiritual, systems, and biological outcomes. The approach is particularly useful for behavioral health because medical cure is elusive and pharmacological interventions do not address all the issues, concerns, and desired outcomes involved in providing care and assisting recovery.

- **NURSING ASSESSMENT AND EMPOWERMENT**

  Empowerment

  Through the process of empowerment, people are supported and valued as they learn about themselves, make decisions, mobilize resources, and accept power, control, and direction for their lives. The empowerment process begins with assessment.

  Self-Awareness as a First Step in Assessment

  Is the nurse prepared to advocate for the diversity of people who may seek services? Stigmatizing attitudes could inhibit assessment and contribute to the failure of obtaining adequate data for the nursing care plan.

  Nonlabeling Assessment

  Patients with mental illness are people, not

symptoms or psychiatric labels. Labeling and pathologizing are two mechanisms of professional distancing that usually relate to the practitioner's fear, sense of superiority or inadequacy, and powerlessness.

Therapeutic Use of Self

Self-awareness develops into a higher level of knowledge and skill in identifying transference, countertransference, and defense mechanisms that affect assessment and interaction.

- **THE ELEMENTS IN PSYCHIATRIC NURSING SITUATIONS ARE THE NURSE, THE PATIENT, AND WHATEVER GOES ON BETWEEN THEM** that can be characterized as a nursing problem, a patient problem, or a theme of the relationship. To recognize and validate themes in nursing situations is difficult.

- **THE FIRST STEP OF NURSING PROCESS, ASSESSMENT,** is described in the Statement on Psychiatric Mental Health Nursing Practices, along with the other steps of the nursing process. The statement includes standards of care, which relate to the direct clinical care a patient receives as demonstrated through the nursing process.

Assessment begins the nursing process. The standards cite two important guidelines: first, the nurse has the responsibility to inform the patient of their mutual roles, while getting feedback from the patient about his or her intent; and second, the nurse uses clinical judgment to determine what information is needed.

Data Collection

During an initial interview, data are collected on functional areas and the behavioral and mental status of the patient (see Study Guide Figure 38-1). The nurse observes, encourages the patient to talk, listens, and keeps the interview focused.

To formulate a nursing diagnosis, the nurse needs to know the patient's patterns of interaction, methods of coping, emotional status, and general lifestyle. While gathering data, the nurse must remain in touch with the patient's feelings.

Beginning the Assessment Interview

The nurse introduces self and orients patient.

In explaining the purpose of the interview, the nurse asks why the patient is there and what the patient's understanding is of how past experiences have influenced his or her being there now. Appropriate questions include:

- What problem brings you here?
- When did you first notice the problem?
- What do you believe is causing or contributing to it?
- What, if anything, alters or relieves the problem?
- What do you believe has to be done? By whom?
- How will you know if the problem has been solved?
- What resources are available?

In writing narrative comments, it is critical that nurses use the patient's own words rather than relying on the nurse's interpretation of the language.

Coordinating Care

The nurse also coordinates care. In so doing, the nurse assesses the resources available as each person moves through the system. What functions can be integrated in the patient's care? What areas of the system or process need improvement?

Processing Data

Integral to assessment is eliciting accurate information and transmitting it correctly and efficiently to the persons receiving services, their support networks, professional peers and colleagues, as well as to individuals and groups who are responsible for system processes. In assessing if a person receiving services is satisfied with them, the nurse might ask:

- Do you feel you received value for the money, time, and effort spent?
- Do you perceive that the services have improved your quality of life?

- **EMPOWERMENT IN ASSESSMENT** is achieved as the nurse and patient enter into an interactive role with the health care system, other providers, and significant others to collect and present information and formulate interventions. During the admission interview and subsequent interactions, the psychiatric nurse and the patient assess the problem that resulted in admis-

(continued on page 259)

Study Guide Figure 38–1.

Middletown Psychiatric Center		Form 444 MED (MPC 5/93)

NURSING ASSESSMENT

INSTRUCTIONS: (this form must be completed by a Registered Nurse)
- Part I must be completed within 24 hours of admission to the extent possible
- Part II must be completed within 11 days of admission.
- Update annually thereafter.

Patient	Last Name	First Name	M.I.
C#		DOB / / 70	
Unit/Ward		Sex ☐ Male ☒ Female	

Part I - Initial Assessment

1. IDENTIFYING DATA

A. Physical Characteristics:

Height _5'0"_   Eye Color _brown_

Weight _150 lbs_   Hair Color _brown_

Race/Ethnicity _Caucasian_

Physical Disability _none noted_

Scars/Birthmarks/Tatoos _see skin integrity_

B. Vital Signs:

Blood Pressure _130/78_

Temperature _98_

Pulse _100_

Respirations _22_

C. Language:

Primary _English_   Secondary _--_

D. Religion:

Religion _Catholic - states no_

Practice _longer believes in God_

E. Cultural Issues:

Cultural Identification _Caucasian_

Practice _____

F. For Women:

Pregnant	Menopause	Last Menstrual Period	Last Pap Smear	Last Breast Exam	Last Mammogram
☐ Yes ☒ No	☐ Yes ☒ No	1992	1995	1995	n/a

2. ALERTS *List risk factors including danger to self/others, elopement risk, fire setting risk, allergies, compromised gag reflex, h/o violence or suicide, h/o drug/etoh use, etc.* Ms. _____ reports that she has been

hospitalized since age 10. She describes several suicide attempts and
multiple episodes of self-inflicted violence. Denies allergies. Denies
drug and alcohol use.
States suicide attempts were by "drinking bleach" and O.D. Self-inflicted
violence includes cutting and self-induced vomiting (using "little girl
voice" here).

3. PATTERNS *The following classification represents an arrangement of human responses into categories or patterns based on their relationships. Note 'P' = Past, 'C' = Current, 'NA' = Information Not Available.*

A. Exchanging: *(Human responses involving mutual giving and receiving between systems)*

• **Circulation** *(Include edema, chest pain, hypo/hypertension, tachycardia, bradycardia, cyanosis, pacemaker)*
States past and current "low blood pressure" and "palpitations"

• **Elimination** *(Include incontinence, fluid intoxication/hyponatremia/DWB, constipation, diarrhea, urination problems, ostomy device)*
Past and current constipation - "from meds" and from not eating.

• **Nutrition** *(Include food allergies, dentures, special diet, altered appetite, abnormal weight gain/loss, eating disorder, underweight, obesity)*
Vegetarian; states she has had periods in past where she has refused to eat
and was fed through a "tube in my nose"; current - self-induced vomiting.
Reports she takes "Tagamint" (Tagamet) for "an ulcer in the stomach."
Reports weight gain in last year. Overweight.

Page 2	Patient	Last Name	First Name	M.I.	C#	NURSING ASSESSMENT Part I - Initial Assessment

A. Exchanging: *(Continued)*

• **Oxygenation** *(Include cough, difficulty breathing, respiratory problems, pattern of smoking)* Smokes two packs per day. Sometimes at night feels like being "smothered."

• **Skin Integrity** *(Include bruises, lacerations, rashes, pale/flushed skin)* Multiple scars on both arms - mid-biceps to wrist; all perpendicular to veins and arteries. About 50 1/2" x 1/4" scars on each arm. Superficial scars "on top of" scars described above.

• **Potential for Infection** *(Include HIV, TB, Hepatitis B, sexually transmitted disease; note HIV testing)* States no risk "can't have sex when you're locked up." "They can't get in" - "don't want to have sex with anybody." (Marked change in appearance from pleasant to defiant/angry)

B. Communicating: *(Human responses related to sending and receiving messages)*
Listens and responds to questions; marked changes in body language and affect during interview.

C. Relating: *(Human responses relating to establishing bonds with others)*

• **Support Systems** *(Include whether family is involved, visitors are expected, socially isolated, comfortable with groups* Father, foster mother, and paternal grandmother in area. States does not want visits - does not want family to know she is "still in hospital."

• **Sexuality** *(Indicate whether sexually active outside the hospital, sexual orientation, sexual acting out, knowledge of safe sex practices, use of contraceptives)* States she is celibate, heterosexual, "innocent but not a virgin." Has a Norplant, placed 2 years ago, was sexually active with men "by choice" since 15.

• **Trauma** *(Include history of child abuse/neglect as victim/abuser, rape, spouse abuse, sexual abuse)* "I don't remember anything about my childhood. I was in foster care." (head down, face averted, eyes closed)

D. Valuing: *(Human responses related to selecting and implementing alternatives)*

• **Spiritual Concerns** States she used to believe in God, but God doesn't help her. "Hates" God now.

E: Choosing: *(Human responses related to selecting and implementing alternatives)*

• **Adjustment to Hospitalization** Would like to get help but "no one can help me." "You should just let me die." "I desire to die."

CLINICAL ASSESSMENT AND NURSING DIAGNOSIS

Page 3	Patient	Last Name	First Name	M.I.	C#	NURSING ASSESSMENT Part I - Initial Assessment

F. Moving: *(Human responses related to activity)*

• **Mobility** *(Indicate whether ambulatory, needs ambulatory aides, needs safety devices, needs staff assistance)* _____
Ambulatory

• **ADL** *(Indicate whether well-groomed, dresses appropriately, bathes independently, toilets self)* Well-groomed, clean,
light makeup, slightly provocatively dressed. Can bathe and toilet self.
Demands privacy in showering/bathroom.

• **Sleep Patterns** *(Describe and note any changes)* States she has nightmares and difficulty
falling and staying asleep nightly. States she has had this for years
(at least 10 years that she can remember)

G. Perceiving: *(Human responses relating to sending and receiving/integrating information)*

• **Hallucinations** *(Describe)* States she hears voices - always male, always say the
same things - "you're bad," "it's your fault," "don't tell anybody," "drink
the bleach/cut yourself - you should die." Describes feelings of being
touched at night, but nobody there.

• **Self-esteem** *(Include coping/dysfunctional coping, problems expressing anger, self-destructive behavior, h/o or current drug/etoh
use, psychological response to physical/mental illness)* _____
Multiple episodes of self-destructive behavior

H. Knowing: *(Human responses related to cognitive functioning)*

• **Thought Content** *(Include delusions, obsessions, preoccupations; describe)* _____
Reports many rituals around bathing and eating, induced vomiting and cutting
and blood.

• **Altered Thought Processes** *(Describe)* Limited insight into behaviors, large memory
gaps

• **Orientation** *(Person, place, time)* Oriented x 3

• **Educational Needs** *(Consider medication, symptom management, coping skills, safe sex, health, HIV counselling, discharge planning)*
Psychoeducation to decrease self-harm; individual therapy; symptoms management

I: Feeling: *(Human responses related to subjective awareness)*

• **Mood** Showed euphoria to depression during interview

• **Affect** Marked changes

• **Physical Pain** Stomach ache

Page 4	Patient	Last Name	First Name	M.I.	C#	NURSING ASSESSMENT Part I - Initial Assessment

SUMMARY AND TREATMENT RECOMMENDATIONS *Identify and prioritize nursing diagnoses/patient needs. Include strengths/assets relevant to nursing interventions and recommended interventions.*

Assessment of Strengths/Needs *(Psychiatric)* Intelligent, would like help, young. Needs to reduce harm to self behaviors and explore effect of past events in present situation

Nursing Diagnosis *(Psychiatric)* Unresolved post-traumatic response related to altered memory, altered perceptions, spiritual distress, altered sleep and altered self-concept as evidenced by self-mutilation, reports "voices," nightmares, insomnia, no early memories, "I deserve to die," suicide attempts, rituals.

Nursing Interventions (1) Assessment of lifetime history of traumatic events. (2) "No harm" contract to maintain her safety. (3) Psychoeducational interventions to manage distress during flashbacks/memory recovery - keeping log, create a safe space, ice for hands for orientation. (4) Careful evaluation of any psychotropic medications for effectiveness and side-effects. (5) Individual counselling or psychotherapy.

Assessment of Strengths/Needs *(Medical/Other ie: MICA, DWB, functional, etc.)* _____

Nursing Diagnosis *(Medical/Other ie: MICA, DWB, functional, etc.)* Altered nutritional processes related to altered eating, reported gastric ulcer, and obesity as evidenced by self-induced vomiting, taking Tagamet, many rituals with mood, obesity, vegetarian.

Nursing Interventions (1) Ask for dietary consult/monitor labs/weight. (2) Supervise meals to prevent vomiting. (3) Administer Tagamet. (4) Observe rituals around food and document.

RN Signature	Title	Date

sion, attend to and analyze responses, assess expectations and capacity. The patient's experiences are the bedrock that creates his or her behavior. It is essential for the nurse to be attentive to the patient's experiences, as the patient's understanding of them forms the basis for recovery. Assessment, when viewed as a partnership, is a tool to engage the patient in the treatment process and so empower him or her.

- **FUNCTIONAL BEHAVIOR STATUS** is assessed by gathering information using an organized set of questions and dialogue or a self-assessment form. Some questions that might be asked to assess the patient's functional behavior status are: Are you able to communicate with others in a socially acceptable manner? (assertiveness); Are you able to identify your future goals? (rehabilitation); Do you budget your money for rent, food, bills, etc.? (daily living skills); Do you take your medication on time as prescribed (medication management).

- **MENTAL STATUS ASSESSMENT** is an objective determination of observable aspects of the patient's psychological functioning. Findings are recorded objectively.

  Performing and recording a mental status assessment has several major functions.
  - It is a method of organizing clinical observations.
  - It provides a clinical baseline for a patient's psychological state.
  - It provides specific information to help establish certain diagnoses.

  Four major categories of mental status are assessed: presentation and appearance; motor activity and behavior; cognition/intellect; and mood and affect.
  - Presentation and Appearance: general appearance, dress, grooming, facial expression, posture, gait, and hygiene.
  - Motor Activity and Behavior: gait, posture, tics, tremors, posturing, grimaces, and other abnormal body movement. The speed of movement is important: slowed, tense, or rapid. Is there nail biting, wringing of hands, tapping feet, or chewing movement? Do any behaviors increase or decrease as interview progresses and deals with emotionally charged materials? Are there any abnormal motor behaviors such as:

ECHOPRAXIA: pathological repetition (imitation) of the movements of another person
CEREAFLEXIBILITAS: waxy flexibility
CATALEPSY: a general condition of diminished responsiveness.
  - Cognition/Intellect: generally assessed by listening to history and considering level of functioning, family and cultural background, and vocabulary. Is patient able to abstract?

  Content of Thought
  Assessed by listening to patient's preoccupations, ambitions, and dreams and by assessing major themes and issues discussed by patient. Is there suicidal or homicidal ideation?

  Thought Process
  - Forms: Does patient think and communicate in a clearly understandable manner? If not, consider it a thought disorder/abnormality.
  - Disorders of perception
    ILLUSION: the misinterpretation of some real external sensory experience.
    HALLUCINATION: may be visual, auditory, olfactory, tactile, gustatory, or visceral.
    DEPERSONALIZATION: a feeling that one is outside of one's body.
  - Delusions
    PERSECUTORY: thinks there is conspiracy to harm him or her.
    SOMATIC: thinks that his or her body is deteriorating or someone is in the brain.
    GRANDEUR: believes self to be a famous person.
    GUILT: thinks his or her bad thoughts can affect others.
    INFLUENCE: thoughts are being controlled by objects.
  - Phobias
    ACROPHOBIA: fear of heights
    AGORAPHOBIA: fear of open places
    CLAUSTROPHOBIA: fear of closed spaces
    PANPHOBIA: fear of everything
    SPEECH is assessed.

- Volume
- Rate
- Tone
- Productivity
- Goal direction

SENSORIUM is assessed.

-Level of attention
- Does the patient know who he or she is?
- Time, place?

MEMORY, past and present

CONCENTRATION

Is patient easily distracted? Can patient perform simple mathematic additions and subtractions?

ABILITY TO ABSTRACT

Can patient interpret a proverb in a less literal and personal manner? Can the patient find similarities between objects?

INSIGHT. Does the patient recognize emotional or mental problems?

JUDGMENT. Is patient able to make and carry out plans or to discriminate accurately? Are patient's thoughts inconsistent with reality?

ATTITUDE. Is patient cooperative, evasive, arrogant, ingratiating, spontaneous, assertive, or withdrawn? What is patient's attitude about treatment, interview? Attitudes may be clues to defense mechanisms.

• Mood and affect

Affect is what the individual is feeling at the moment—the emotional state and outward appearance. Affect can be noted by measuring a variety of factors.

RANGE. Are only a few emotions expressed? Is the range wide or labile, meaning are there frequent shifts between different emotions?

INTENSITY. Is the quality of emotion expressed flat or exaggerated?

TYPES, or categories, of emotion, for example, fear, happiness, or anger. Is what is expressed an appropriate emotion?

Mood is the individual's subjective description of his or her feelings. Does a patient's mood change?

• **TO CONCLUDE THE ASSESSMENT INTERVIEW**, a series of questions may be asked followed by discussion. For example, Are there any questions you wish to ask? Of the ideas we have discussed, what are some that you think are important in relation to what is presently concerning you? Such questions can help the nurse formulate patient care. The final interaction may be recorded in narrative form.

• **CASE FORMULATION** evolves with the assessment of data collected during assessment. Data are studied and summarized, and the nurse and patient together prioritize areas that will require work. The nurse and patient will recognize behaviors that are manifested, determine which need improvement or change, what strengths are available, and what resources are needed. Nursing diagnoses are formulated, and a plan of care begins to take shape.

Nursing Diagnosis

Formulating relevant nursing diagnoses is expressing the needs and goals of the patient. Diagnoses conform to accepted classification systems, such as North American Nursing Diagnosis Classification (NANDA). Diagnoses can be organized into nine "human response patterns."

Pattern 1. Exchanging: mutual giving and receiving

Pattern 2. Communicating: sending and receiving messages

Pattern 3. Relating: establishing bonds with others

Pattern 4. Valuing: assigning relative worth

Pattern 5. Choosing: selecting alternatives

Pattern 6. Moving: activity

Pattern 7. Perceiving: receiving information

Pattern 8. Knowing: meaning of information

Pattern 9. Feeling: subjective awareness of information

A nursing diagnosis is the conceptualization of the patient's health problems identified from the assessment process. In establishing diagnoses, whatever need there is to interface with other care providers becomes evident.

Based on the hypotheses (diagnoses), implementing an intervention plan is proposed. Thought is given to what treatment services, combined with what patient strengths, will promote the desired outcome cost effectively and in a satisfying way.

Outcome Identification

Outcomes are individualized for the patient; the ultimate goal is to influence health and improve the patient's health status.

Planning Care

Care is planned that prescribes interventions to attain expected outcomes. The plan is used to guide interventions systematically and to achieve the expected patient outcomes. In planning care, nursing diagnoses are identified and prioritized in terms of patient's needs. Discharge plans are included in any plan of care.

Implementing Care

Nurses implement a range of interventions designed to prevent mental and physical illness and to promote, maintain, and restore mental and physical health. Interventions are usually selected according to the nurse's level of practice.

Evaluation

As with any hypothesis or intervention, it is essential to continue evaluation and assessment in order to determine whether the desired effects are being achieved.

TAKING ANOTHER LOOK

You are now ready to respond to the questions raised in Gaining a Perspective at the beginning of this chapter. After you have written or thought about your responses, you may wish to look at the Suggested Responses on page 335.

39 CRISIS INTERVENTION

affect

crisis

crisis reaction

crisis theory

hazardous event

homeostasis

maladaptive coping responses

precipitating event

therapeutic alliance

transition states

GAINING A PERSPECTIVE

Think about the crisis situations described below, and after you have read the Key Concepts for this chapter respond to the questions in greater depth.

1. What would you think has the highest priority when a nurse assists a patient who is in crisis?

2. What do you think would happen if a patient in crisis is not helped to deal with the situation?

KEY CONCEPTS

- **A CRISIS SITUATION DEVELOPS WHEN** stress or stressors overwhelm an individual. Crisis is a period of psychological disequilibrium, experienced as a result of a hazardous event or situation; it constitutes a significant problem that cannot be remedied using familiar coping strategies or patterns. A crisis occurs when a person faces a seemingly insurmountable obstacle to important life goals.

- **THE GOAL OF CRISIS INTERVENTION** is to resolve the most pressing problem within 1 to 12 weeks through focused, directed intervention aimed at helping the patient develop new adaptive coping methods.

- **CRISIS REACTION REFERS TO THE ACUTE STAGE**, which usually occurs soon after the hazardous event. The reaction may take various forms including helplessness, confusion, anger, anxiety, shock, or disbelief. Low self-esteem and serious depression are often produced by the crisis state. The person in crisis may appear incoherent, disorganized, agitated, and volatile or calm, subdued, withdrawn, and apathetic. It is during this crisis reaction period that the individual often is most willing to seek help, and crisis intervention is usually more effective at this time.

- **DEVELOPMENT OF CONTEMPORARY CRISIS INTERVENTION THEORY AND PRACTICE** was not formally elaborated until 1940. Erich Lindemann and Gerald Caplan were primarily responsible.
  Erich Lindemann
  Lindemann's work focused on the psychological symptoms of survivors and on preventing unresolved grief among relatives of persons who die. Many individuals experiencing acute grief have five related reactions:
  - Somatic distress

- Preoccupation with the deceased's image
- Guilt
- Hostile reactions
- Loss of patterns of conduct

Duration of grief appears dependent on the success with which the bereaved person mourns (grief work). Grief work involves:

- Achieving emancipation from the deceased
- Readjusting to changes in the environment from which the loved one is missing
- Developing new relationships

People need to be encouraged to have a period of mourning, and eventually accept the loss and adjust to life without the deceased. By delaying grieving, negative outcomes of the crisis develop.

Gerald Caplan

Caplan's work described four stages of crisis reaction:

- The initial rise of tension that comes from the emotionally hazardous the crisis-precipitating event.
- An increased level of tension and disruption in daily living because the individual is not able to resolve crisis quickly.
- As the individual attempts and fails to resolve the crisis by emergency problem-solving mechanisms, tension increases to such an intense level that the individual may go into depression.
- The person may experience a mental collapse or breakdown or may partially resolve the crisis with new coping methods.

Contemporary Crisis Theory

Contemporary theory from a biopsychosocial perspective is based on the concept of homeostatic balance and the relationship of coping processes to stable psychological functioning. For each individual a reasonably consistent balance exists between affective and cognitive experience. The primary characteristic of this balance is its stability for that individual. A healthy homeostatic balance requires stable psychological functioning with a minimum of dysphoric affect, the maintenance of a reasonable cognitive perspective on the experience, and

the retention of problem-solving skills.

Coping mechanisms, which individuals have a repertoire of, are designed to reduce, control, or avoid unpleasant emotions in order to reestablish homeostatic balance and thereby facilitate the person's return to normal functioning. Maladaptive coping responses are typically used in situations where the individual feels vulnerable. Coping behaviors, however, should be view as a continuum, with behaviors manifesting various levels of adaptiveness depending on the person and the situation.

Four distinct phases in the life cycle of an emotional crisis were identified by B.A. Baldwin:

- Phase 1. Emotionally hazardous situation occurs
- Phase 2. An emotional crisis occurs
- Phase 3. Crisis is resolved; either adaptive or maladaptive resolution
- Phase 4. Postcrisis adaptation: either adaptive or maladaptive resolution

Transitional Situations

Migration and retirement are among the transitional situations that can cause crisis. Generally three phases overlap:

- Impact
- Recoil
- Post-traumatic recovery.

Each phase has specific interventions. Basically, persons in a transitional crisis should not be removed from their life situations; interventions should focus on bolstering the network of relationships.

Linda Rapoport

Rapoport's work, built on Lindemann's and Caplan's, defines a crisis as an upset state that places an individual in a hazardous condition. Three interrelated factors create a state of crisis:

- Hazardous event
- Threat to life goals
- Inability to respond with adequate coping mechanisms

Rapoport conceptualized the content of crisis intervention practice. She found that rapid access to the crisis worker was essential for the patient, as initially the patient is more emotionally available. During the first interview, the task is to develop a preliminary diagnosis of the presenting problem. A sense of hope and optimism must be conveyed by focusing on mutual exploration, problem solving, and delineated goals and tasks.

- **THE PRESSURE TO ACT, TO SEEK HELP, COMES FROM A SUFFICIENT AMOUNT OF BOTH DISCOMFORT AND HOPE** for the individual in crisis. The person must have a conscious purpose to live and grow, but needs to ventilate and be accepted, and to receive support, assistance, and encouragement to discover the path to crisis resolution.

  That the individual is helped to understand the meaning of the event and how it conflicts with expectations, life goals, and belief system is important. The nurse needs to listen carefully for cognitive errors or distortions (overgeneralizing, catastrophizing) or irrational beliefs and help the patient to recognize them. Carefully worded questions may be helpful.
  - How do you view yourself now that you realize everyone with less than five years seniority got laid off?
  - Have you ever asked your doctor whether he thinks you will die from cancer at a young age or what the actual risk is of your having cancer?

  Persons in highly stressful events may use denial and express anger and fear, grief and loss; however, crisis intervention can help individuals see that they can survive.

- **CRISIS INTERVENTION MODELS**
  Golan's Model
  This model provides the crisis nurse with examples of empathetic statements for each phase of treatment: beginning phase, first interview; middle phase, first to fourth interviews; and ending phase, last one or two interviews. At first, the focus is on the here and now of the precipitating event, including its scope, persons involved, outcome severity of effect, and

the time the event occurred. Then the patient is allowed to verbalize, while the nurse elicits subjective reactions from the patient, trying to obtain affective responses and the part that the patient played in them. Golan's prompting statements include:

You must have felt terrible about it.

No wonder you sound so upset.

Can you put your finger on what started this?

Things really began to change after you....

I suppose in the beginning you were in a state of shock.

You're in a real dilemma. I guess the most important thing is to come to a decision as to whether to....

Roberts and Burgess Model
Roberts and Burgess developed a seven-stage crisis intervention model that can be applied to specific patients (see Study Guide Table 39-1).

The order of stages 1 and 2 can be reversed, depending on the type of crisis and the level of lethality of the situation.

- Stage 1: Assess Lethality and Safety Needs. Determine the person's degree of risk for serious injury or death from self-destructive acts or from the violent acts of another person. On the telephone, it is necessary to assess the level of seriousness of threats to the caller's safety. Examples of questions that crisis workers might ask battered women include:

  Are you or your children in danger?

  Is the abuser there now?

  Do you want me to call the police?

  Do you want to leave and can you safely?

- Stage 2: Establish a Therapeutic Alliance. Initial rapport is set up when the nurse lets the patient know that he or she did the right thing by coming to a crisis unit and conveys a willingness to help. The patient, who feels vulnerable and frightened, must be made to feel safe and secure. The nurse directly supports patient or helps mobilize support. The personal resources of the patient are assessed and identified as essential to developing adaptive responses to the crisis.

TABLE 39–1.

ROBERTS AND BURGESS SEVEN-STAGE CRISIS INTERVENTION MODEL

Stage	Intervention
1	Assess danger and safety Are patient and family in danger or safe from others? Is patient safe from himself or herself?
2	Establish therapeutic alliance Contract for meeting Active listening Provide support
3	Identify the precipitating event Time and place of precipitating event Interpersonal dimensions of the event Physical and emotional response to event Psychodynamic issue of the crisis Processing the precipitating event
4	Meaning of the crisis Effect of crisis on present and future Changes to life plan or goals
5	Explore coping alternatives Past and present coping Adaptive and maladaptive coping
6	Develop action plan Short-term approach for the crisis Long-term approach for mastery
7	Follow-up Evaluation of crisis resolution Referral

- Stage 3. Identify the Precipitating Event. Explore with the patient the immediate past, that is, the "last straw" that precipitated the crisis. The nurse may want to know how the patient was functioning just prior to the crisis, as many patients have multiple problems. Prioritize problems and attend to the immediate major one. It cannot be assumed that the patient is aware of or understands the relationship of the precipitating event to the emotional crisis; in creating an understanding, the patient is helped to organize the experience.

  The nurse often needs to scrutinize several aspects of the crisis to identify the pre-

cipitating event. The information is primarily gotten from discussions with the patient. Topics to explore include: time and place of the event; the interpersonal dimensions of the problem situation; the patient's affective response to the precipitating event (the dysphoria experienced with disruption of homeostatic balance); psychodynamic issues in the crisis (unresolved conflicts from the past that are brought to the surface by the current crisis), and the actual detection and working through of the event that precipitated the crisis.

The precipitant may be activated in two basic ways:
- The individual has an experience that is somehow directly analogous to a past conflict or trauma.
- An event activates anticipatory fear of experiencing a past trauma.

Some questions the nurse may ask the individual to help define the crisis precipitant are:
- When have you felt this way before?
- When has this type of experience happened before?
- Who are you reminded of in this situation?
- Is this time of the year reminiscent of a painful stressful experience?
- What would be the worst outcome now and has such an outcome happened before?
- How is your current response helping you and has that helped in the past?
- Have you had prior difficulty dealing with stress?
- Who have you known that reacts like this to stress and are you like that person?
- What have you been dreaming about at night?
- What types of thoughts have popped into your mind recently?

- Stage 4: Process the Meaning of the Crisis. The nurse focuses on the individual's current feelings (affect) and the effects of the crisis. The nurse's active listening and communicating through empathetic statements will help the patient express intense feelings. Cognitive distortions should be noted.

- Stage 5: Explore Coping Alternatives. To identify coping alternatives, past adaptive and maladaptive coping methods are explored. Patterns at the preconscious and conscious levels are identified and, if appropriate, modified. To counteract a patient's feelings of helplessness or despair, the nurse may encourage alternative ideas, coping methods, and solutions.

- Stage 6: Develop Plan of Action. In resolving a crisis, the individual in crisis is prevented from using maladaptive coping responses; the person is helped to learn new more adaptive coping responses, resulting in a more mature, stable reintegration postcrisis; the individual is helped to become aware of and resolve underlying conflicts that were manifest during the crisis; and the individual is helped to integrate changes resulting from adaptive crisis resolution at both the cognitive and affective levels.

- Stage 7: Follow Up. In terminating the crisis intervention process, the patient's attainment of goals is evaluated. Anticipating possible difficulties will help prepare the individual to meet future similar situations more adequately. Information is shared about community resources. A direct referral is made to continue therapy if appropriate.

TAKING ANOTHER LOOK

You are now ready to respond to the questions that were raised about crisis situations in Gaining a Perspective at the beginning of this chapter. After you have written or thought about your responses, you may wish to look at the Suggested Responses on page 335.

40 TREATMENT MODALITIES: CRISIS, BEHAVIORAL, RELATIONSHIP, AND INSIGHT

GAINING A PERSPECTIVE

Think about the situations presented below, and after you have read the Key Concepts for this chapter answer the questions in greater detail.

1. What factors would you, as a nurse, consider before deciding what kind of treatment modality to use with a patient?

2. Describe why insight therapy might be an appropriate treatment modality for your nurse colleague who seems to be functioning well, but complains about not being satisfied with life.

KEY CONCEPTS

- **DIRECTION FOR SELECTING THE THERAPEUTIC FOCUS** comes from patient assessment and diagnosis. The context (community or inpatient facility) also defines what resources are available.

- **THERAPEUTIC MODALITIES**

Crisis Management

THE TASK is to provide support.

THE STRATEGIES are to modify and stabilize acute symptoms, control impulsive behaviors, and foster rational problem solving.

THE TECHNIQUES are active guidance, stress reduction, medication, environmental manipulation, self-control procedures, and focused problem solving.

THE GOAL is to reduce the patient's sense of being overwhelmed and strengthen coping ability through the use of community and social support resources.

Behavioral Change

Behavior is targeted that is excessive, lacking, or inappropriate.

THE TASK is to provide a setting where the patient will be motivated to participate and learn new behavior; first, internal and external triggers for a behavior are identified, as are the consequential factors that support continuation of the behavior pattern.

THE STRATEGIES for learning include classic conditioning, operant techniques, modeling, and self-regulating procedures, such as biofeedback.

THE GOAL is to change behaviors that are related to symptoms, that have unwanted consequences, or that are antisocial.

Relationship Therapy

THE TASK is to provide a corrective emotional experience.

THE STRATEGY is therapy relationship, which employs attachment, cognitive, psychodynamic, and humanistic theories.

THE GOAL is to change interpersonal expectations, reduce debilitating social behaviors, foster affectionate and trusting relationships, and enhance a positive self-image.

Insight Therapy

For patients who experience few or no dysfunctional patterns.

THE TASK is to help build self-awareness and insight.

STRATEGIES are to increase verbalization and insight (self-exploration), and focus and direct emotional experiences, behavioral-emotional change, and analysis of the therapeutic relationship.

THE GOAL is to reduce defensive behaviors and increase self-awareness and self-control without defensive patterns.

- **THERAPEUTIC TECHNIQUES** assist with the therapeutic tasks and the outcomes. The techniques are the basic tools organized by a theoretic orientation to the therapy task.

Linking Technique to Task

- Communication is the common denominator of therapeutic modalities.

- Therapeutic techniques seek to accomplish one or more of the following: separating, combining, changing, or sorting patterns for positive and negative effects, changing criteria to alter priorities, and rehearsing new behaviors.

- A basic strategy in therapies is asking questions. Questions must be posed carefully so that they elicit the type of information sought. The theoretic orientation often becomes the framework for interpreting feedback.

Crisis Management (Chapter 39)

This therapeutic modality can be viewed as a series of steps: evaluation, stabilization, and protection.

EVALUATION: How severe is the crisis? What are the personal resources of the individual? What are the risk factors?

- Ask what is overwhelming the patient. Is it in events external or internal to the patient?

- Assess the patient's answers in terms of how much anxiety is increased or decreased

and the regaining of personal control. From the patient's information, an assessment of personal resources is made as well as the degree of hope or hopelessness.

- Evaluate the patient's intellectual resources to better understand the appropriate number and level of questions, explanations, and directives the patient can absorb. A patient's capacity to respond interpersonally gives an indication of the patient's capacity to attach or relate, and whether the engagement is dependent, hostile, rejecting, or simply absent with no connecting.

STABILIZATION: derived from assessment.

- Does contact with the nurse have a calming effect? Does talking help the patient calm down?

- Directing patient to note what he or she is thinking, feeling, and experiencing supports the capacity for self-observation.

- Focusing on reality and concrete events helps divert patient from unsettling fantasies of what might have been or should have been.

- A patient, in gaining mastery, will build upon resources and move toward a more problem-solving approach to distress.

PROTECTION:

Restrictive and less reactive strategies are incorporated to protect patient.

- Assessment indicates how restrictive the strategies should be.

- If hospitalization is required, have patient participate as much as possible in decision making; patient will experience less loss of control and fantasy about others being in control.

- Patient may be removed from the stressful circumstances or stressors, or stressors may be manipulated.

- Following assessment, supportive efforts can be directed at restoring logical thinking and inner controls by improving and developing coping behaviors.

- Problem-solving strategies are the focus, and new ways of coping are fostered by direct advice, suggestion, modeling, encouraging independent discovery through such sources as books and other people. New behaviors are implemented through rehearsal and by manipulating the environment to reduce stress.

- Preparation for termination and follow-up are accomplished through a gradual decrease in therapeutic content, refinement of coping skills, and anticipation and preparation for future stress (positive and negative).

Behavioral Change

- Assessment in behavioral change therapy emphasizes measurement; symptom or problem is the focus. The procedure for assessment is outlined below.

IDENTIFY THE FREQUENCY AND INTENSITY of symptoms and problem behaviors.

EVALUATE THE CONDITIONS (INTERNAL AND EXTERNAL) under which symptoms or problematic behaviors occur. Conditions refer to environmental stimuli, such as thoughts and emotional reactions.

DEVELOP HYPOTHESES about the functional relationship between the symptoms and problems and the conditions that elicit them.

TEST HYPOTHESES by using specific treatment methods derived from the functional analysis of the interaction, and measure the effect on problem behaviors.

REVISE TREATMENT APPROACHES depending on the basis of the measured effect.

- Examples of treatment approaches: drinking is the problem.

-Antibuse might be one treatment.

- If drinking is perceived as a loss of self-control, operant conditioning may be used. (Monitoring self involves recording self or bringing into awareness the frequency and intensity of the unwanted behavior.)

- Covert conditioning, in this situation the imagining and ideation processes generated in the drinking, will be used to reduce drinking behavior.

- Cognitive learning strategies focus on detailing thoughts and the underlying promises that are associated with reasons for

drinking, and on problem solving to overcome obstacles.

- Observation learning and rehearsal may be used. The patient's attention is captured and retention downloaded. The information, practice, and correct feedback assist the drinker to rehearse and correct behavior, i.e., interpersonal relations with groups or individuals.

- For individuals with severe mental illness, efforts to design a community that rewards the patient for nonpsychotic behavior have been useful. A process of arranging reinforcers, strengthening the capacities and skills basic for coping, and refraining from self-defeating thought patterns can aid not only in change but in solidifying the retention of therapeutic effects.

Relationship Therapy

- The central task is providing a corrective emotional experience. The object is to adapt more positive behaviors and insights that reduce inner distress.

- Stages in the therapy process include:

-Dealing with issues of motivation and resistance and suspiciousness

-Preventing premature closure with the therapist

-Maintaining commitment to patient

-Managing testing and heightened anxiety

-Providing verbal emotional support

-Responding to patient's attachment and dependency

-Assisting patient in self-observation, self-discovery, and self- evaluation

-Pursuing active efforts to change patient's perceptions, expectations, and behaviors

-Encouraging and monitoring new relationships

-Decreasing therapeutic intensity and therapeutic relationship

- The initial stage of therapy is making contact with the patient. At that time, the patient is educated about the therapeutic process and how the relationship is used for therapy. Emergencies and premature ruptures in the relationship are anticipated, and procedures for dealing with these events are detailed.

- A testing period, not always on the conscious level, ensues once the patient begins therapy. The patient tries to get the nurse to agree to patterns of participating that cannot be fulfilled (no medication, no reporting of self-injurious behavior). Efforts are made by the nurse to contain anxiety, by increasing the patient's awareness through reframing and reflection.

- A stage of increased closeness evolves in the context of a supportive relationship. There is increased self-awareness on the patient's part. With closeness, however, comes increased potential for crises, as anxiety is stimulated by the depth of emotion and sensations. Strategies, such as focusing and questioning, are shifted to either contain or heighten the anxiety. Irrational thinking is challenged, and the patient prompted to seek alternatives.

- The patient's emotional commitment and attachment to the nurse emerge in the next stage, with a deep drop in anxious, hostile responses. The patient is assisted in self-discovery and self-evaluation.

- A working stage emerges, in which the patient actively engages in changing his or her behavior with others, revaluates goals and sets new ones. Therapeutic work involves strategies that help the patient enhance self-monitoring, set priorities, expose self to anxiety-provoking situations, and learn how to control and express anger. Gradually the patient moves to the stage of implementing the goals in interpersonal situations. Attachment shifts from the therapist to outside relationships.

- The close of therapy is marked by decreased contact with the therapist.

Insight Therapy

The two broad areas of work in insight therapy are self-exploration and insight, and becoming commited to behavior changes while enacting them.

- The process of insight therapy includes:
  - Learning to identify and analyze repetitive patterns of behavior.
  - Becoming oriented to internal patterns of thinking.
  - Evaluating internal patterns of thinking.
  - Identifying defensive behavior and emotional presentations.
  - Analyzing origins of emotional conflicts and defensive mechanisms.
  - Developing areas of behavioral change, moving to make changes, and extinguishing old behaviors and developing new ones.
  - Solidifying changes.
  - Preparing for termination, enhancing independence from therapy and commitment to change.

TAKING ANOTHER LOOK

You are now ready to address the situations that were raised in Gaining A Perspective at the beginning of this chapter. After you have written or thought about your responses, you may wish to look at the Suggested Responses on page 336.

41 THERAPEUTIC GROUPS

GAINING A PERSPECTIVE

Think about the questions listed below, and after you have read the Key Concepts for this chapter respond to each.

1. How would you, as a nurse, prepare a patient for therapy in a group that uses the interpersonal model?

2. When dealing with an adolescent, why may it be appropriate to place him or her in group therapy?

3. What might lead to problems in a multiethnic therapy group that is led by a nurse?

KEY CONCEPTS

- **GROUP THERAPY IS A PROFESSIONALLY GUIDED PLANNED ENTERPRISE TO TREAT PSYCHOLOGICAL DISTRESS.** An American invention of the 20th century, the concept has been greatly expanded in the last decade. Pioneering efforts in group psychotherapy represented a psychoeducational approach. Group leaders incorporated a holistic body-mind concept that was coined "collective counseling."

Joseph Pratt introduced therapy with a group in a medical setting (1905). He met with 20 to 30 patients to discuss their disease; the group was generally supportive and encouraging. Patients responded well, and the positive therapeutic results were transferred to other groups of patients.

I. Cody Marsh, a minister and psychiatrist, used group methods with mentally ill institutionalized patients. He lectured them about their diseases, and arranged discussion groups with all who came into contact with the patients. In a sense, Cody Marsh was a pioneer of the hospital as a therapeutic community.

E.W. Lazell lectured schizophrenic patients about their diseases. Patients improved, in part, because education reduced their fears. The socialization process — patients getting to know one another — accounted for the positive changes observed.

Joseph Moreno (1925) introduced psychodrama, in which patients act out problem situations in a group setting to achieve a heightened awareness of the patients' actual conflicts.

Sigmund Freud, although he never ran therapeutic groups, recognized the curative value of group participation. Freud differentiated the leaderless group (a mob capable of great excesses) from the leader-centered group (a vehicle with the potential to diminish anxiety). The leader was seen as a parental surrogate, and members reacted to each other as siblings in a family.

Kurt Lewin focused on group dynamics (1939) with the premise that the acts of the individual can be explained on the basis of the nature of the social force—the field to which the person is exposed.

Post-World War II

In 1950, the psychodynamic group model was the characteristic approach, and theoreticians, such as Freud, Sullivan, Horney, and Rogers, explored applications of their conceptual frameworks to group therapy, theory, and practice.

During the 1960s, new types of groups, such as encounter and transcendental meditation, functioned and shed light on the need for short-term models. Three types of group work have been described: traditional interpersonal group therapy, psychoeducational groups, and self-help groups that are therapeutic and responsive to the sociocultural needs of people.

- **GROUP THERAPY IS DEFINED AS A FORM OF INTERVENTION IN WHICH** carefully selected persons are placed in a group and guided by a trained therapist for the purpose of changing the maladaptive behavior of the individual members.

Traditional group therapy is based on the assumption that people are consistent in their stylistic manner of behavior and that the formal group gathering is one mechanism by which people can be helped to become more aware of their interactions and coping patterns. One role of the nurse in group therapy is to help patients understand their characteristic manner of relating by examining their interaction with the leader and other group members.

- **INTERPERSONAL MODEL OF GROUP THERAPY** (based on Sullivan and Yalom) is used widely in both inpatient and outpatient settings. Members must be both affectively and cognitively engaged in the process of interpersonal learning. The central focus in applying the model is use of the here and now. The therapy is a two-stage process:

FIRST STAGE: Members are plunged into a richly affective expression of their immediate reaction to one another.

SECOND STAGE: The affective expressions are analyzed.

Goal of Treatment

The goal is to foster group members' development of effective social interactions that will enable them to achieve more intimate, gratifying interpersonal relationships.

In inpatient settings, the goal is to assist patients to overcome feelings of isolation.

Therapist Style

The therapist's interactive style must be strong, authoritative, and yet egalitarian. An egalitarian approach is important to promote self-disclosure. Self-disclosure on the part of leader must be constant with the group and should concern the therapist's reaction to some aspect of the group process. Conflict, including exploration of anger, must not be fully evoked or totally squelched.

Two Types of Groups

- The agenda group is for higher functioning patients.
    - Fosters a positive attitude toward therapy.
    - Enables members to appreciate that talking is helpful.
    - Helps isolate problems to be addressed in long-term therapy.
    - Relieves iatrogenic anxiety.
- Focus group is suited to lower functioning patients; has the same goals as agenda group.
    - Stresses the need to socialize in a non-threatening manner.
    - Increases reality orientation.

Patient Preparation

- Leader explains the processes to which the patient will be exposed and emphasizes the need to be open and honest. The patient is alerted to the possibility that he or she may not like all group's members or that the others might not like the patient; however, the leader explains that by examining interactions, self-knowledge and more adaptive ways of feeling, thinking, or behaving will develop.
- More positive feelings are developed in the patient by being prepared for the process; group members who are prepared have a lower dropout rate, and are more communicative, and the group has a greater cohesiveness.

Patient Selection

Careful selection and group organization are essential clinical responsibilities. Group psychotherapy is not appropriate for all types of emotional disorders. The dynamics of a potential group member are assessed and discussed — the dynamics of that individual in current and past relationships with peers and authority figures, including commonly used defensive mechanisms.

Individuals with authority anxiety often do well in group therapy; individuals with peer anxiety present another situation.

- Authority Anxiety. Patients whose primary difficulties center on their relationship to authority and who are anxious in the presence of authority often do better in group than in didactic one-on-one settings. The patients gain support from peer groups and are helped to deal more realistically with the therapist. Adolescents often have authority anxiety and may be good candidates for the group.
- Peer Anxiety. Patients who have destructive relationships, particularly within the nuclear family or with peers or who have been extremely isolated from peer group contact, generally react negatively or with increased anxiety when placed in the group setting. The group leader needs to evaluate patients' ability to tolerate the anxiety produced. If patients can interact in a group, these individuals often have greater insight into their problems than if they were to verbally reconstruct situations in individual therapy. For individuals raised without siblings, the group setting rather quickly causes their dynamics to unfold; they are either unwilling to share or long to share. Their dynamics are subject to examination and ultimate resolution.

- **THE THERAPEUTIC PROCESS IN GROUP WORK INVOLVES THREE FACTORS THAT ASSIST THERAPEUTIC CHANGE:** actional, emotional, and cognitive.

Actional Factors

The action in a group is the expression of thoughts and feelings and related discussion.

- Reality Testing. The group setting is a forum for objective evaluation of oneself and the world. Through the process of consensual validation, the group defines the beliefs and actualities for its participants. Honest and open communication, which is encouraged by the therapist, helps the group maintain an accurate assessment of reality. The group leader, depending on the theoretical framework, may or may not choose to share much about himself or herself. The group creates a family setting for many patients, which may revive previous familial tensions and conflicts. In successful reality testing, the patient is able to separate his or her reactions that are appropriate to current stimuli from those that carry over from past conflicts.
- Ventilation and Catharsis. Ventilation is the open expression of one's innermost thoughts and secrets. Catharsis is the evocation of feeling tones and affect that may be attached to the ventilated thought or secret. Ventilation ameliorates guilt feelings and anxiety and provides the group with important information about the person's thoughts, feelings, and problems. It also stimulates in other members associations that may bring to awareness their repressed feelings.
- Abreaction. Although similar to catharsis, abreaction is a more heightened process in that the discharge of affect is greater when reliving past events. It is associated with increased insight, as it usually deals with emotions previously blocked from consciousness. As emotions unfold during highly therapeutic events, they may produce distress in all concerned. Motor abreaction may take the form of hysterical paralysis, psychosomatic illness, and anxiety states.

Emotional Factors

The emotion of the therapeutic group is "togetherness."

- Cohesion. Working groups are marked by their sense of cohesion, a willingness to maintain the group's integrity. A cohesive group is one in which members are accepting and supportive and have meaningful relationships with one another. Individual evaluation of group members is often done using the measure of cohesion. A cohesive member takes responsibility for effective group function by participating actively, even when goals are difficult.

- Transference. In group therapy, when transference happens between an individual member and the leader, other group members will often help the individual recall earlier treatment by a parent or significant other which was similar to the experience in the group. The patient is assisted in seeing the distortion and experiencing reality.

Cognitive Factors

Cognitive factors are universalization, intellectualization, interpretation, and identification.

- Universalization. Group members recognize that they are not alone in having emotional problems and that others may be struggling with the same or similar problems. Sharing experience fills an important human need; group members sense that they are important in the lives of one another, and they seek to help each other. The process is called altruism, or support. The mechanics of universality — altruism, advice giving, and reassurance — are processes that continue throughout the life of the group.

- Intellectualization. The process of intellectualization implies a cognitive awareness of oneself, others, and various life experiences and how they relate to the present. Receiving feedback is a learning experience.

- Interpretation. A derivative of intellectualization, interpretation is a cognitive framework for group members that can help them understand themselves better; interpretation may come from the therapist or another group member.

- Identification. Many psychiatric patients have modelled themselves using faulty models. In groups, a variety of models are available, and patients identify with certain qualities of the other models. Other group mechanisms can also be understood within the framework of the identifications that take place between members. For example, the sense of alienation is lost as patients develop feelings toward one another and the group as a whole;

acceptance is therapeutic, as members realize that there is a place for differences of opinion; and arguments or negativity do not disrupt the positive forces linking members of the group.

- **CO-THERAPY** is when two or more professionals treat one individual or group. The process can use an individual, couple, family, or group approach.

Benefits of Co-Therapy

- Professionals have an opportunity to discuss and learn through a collaborative process.
- A wider or different perspective of a situation permits different interventions.
- A broader transference between the patient and therapists is possible, if that is the goal.
- Patients have a greater opportunity to expand their learning.
- Therapists have an opportunity to check their behavior.

Criteria in Choosing a Co-Therapist

- Ability to communicate.
- A co-therapist of the opposite sex allows for parental transference and modeling of male-female communication.

Success of a Co-Therapy Team

It is beneficial for the therapists' abilities to be balanced. Theoretical compatibility needs to be present, as well as openness in communication. Participating equally, sharing the leadership and responsibility of decision making, and having mutual respect are important.

Dysfunction of the Co-Therapy Team

When therapists do not function as a treatment team, do not communicate as peers, or both, the team is often oblivious to mistakes that occur, and thereby fails to correct errors. Co-therapist teams should somehow be supervised. Five factors contribute to dysfunction:

- Competition
- Countertransference, when not identified or addressed
- Confusion and lack of communication
- Incongruence
- Co-dependency

TABLE 41–1. THE LEADER'S ROLE IN EDUCATIONAL AND INTERPERSONAL PSYCHOTHERAPY

Educational	Interpersonal
Uses contract to set limits	Encourages discussion of contract violations
Contract renegotiable	Contract renegotiable
Focuses on external reality outside the therapeutic hour	Focuses on interpersonal issues within the group
Encourages dependence on the leader as an authority	Encourages self-reliance
Actively directs sessions	Actively directs sessions
May use formal agenda	Follows patients' agenda
Explains symptoms, feelings, behavior	Explores symptoms, feelings, behavior
Teaches	Provides interpersonal feedback
Stimulates positive transference	Allows negative transference
Explains away negative feelings	Explores negative feelings
Stimulates use of secondary process	Stimulates use of secondary process
Helps patients explain what they mean	Helps patients say what they mean
Helps patients use words, instead of behavior	Helps patients use words, instead of behavior
Provides structure to sessions	Less structured than educational therapy
Focuses on real-life issues	Focuses on relationships in group
Urges asking questions, instead of making assumptions	Urges asking questions, instead of making assumptions
Urges thinking before acting	May promote spontaneity
Accepts members' inability to tolerate emotional tension	Challenges members' attempts to avoid emotional tension
Avoids or explains intense feelings	Explores subjects that stimulate intense feelings
Emphasizes finding means to control symptoms	Relates symptoms to interpersonal events
Accepts members' defects in self-observation	Uses interpersonal feedback to promote self-awareness
Observations concern effective coping strategies	Leader has members observe and reflect back to each other
Maladaptive behaviors that occur in the group are redirected or reshaped	Maladaptive behaviors that occur in group members are considered in terms of their effects on others
Accepts defensive operations	Challenges maladaptive interpersonal defenses
Members' use of projection, denial, etc., is not confronted	Members' use of projection, denial, etc., is noted openly
Defensive operations used to gauge progress	Defensive operations used to gauge progress
Encourages accurate perception of reality	Encourages accurate perception of reality
Distracts from distorted ideation	Confronts distorted view of group members
Accepts real external problems	Examines members' roles in creating real problems
Encourages members to see themselves as ill	Encourages members to see themselves as having interpersonal problems
Develops ego by teaching and modeling coping skills	Develops ego by interpersonal learning
Fosters identification with healthier group members	Fosters identification with healthier group members
Helps patients see that they can function despite illness	Emphasizes use of will to overcome symptoms

Weiner MF. Role of the leader in group therapy. In Kaplan HI and Sadoch BJ (eds) Comprehensive Group Psychotherapy Baltimore, Williams & Wilkins, 1993, p. 89. Used by permission.

- **A GROWING NEED HAS EMERGED FOR NURSES TO DEVELOP SKILLS IN GROUP APPROACHES TO THERAPY.** That need has grown along with the importance of group process for coping and adapting in our society. The group method is effective, appeals to patients and practitioners, and can be combined with individual therapy, and therapists can treat more people. With the waning of natural social groups, small group networks have emerged to counter social isolation. There is also an increasing need to educate patients about medications and their illness. Nurses are designing psychoeducation groups to provide a more comprehensive interventions framework. Study Guide Table 41-1 compares the leader's role in working with educational and interpersonal groups.
- **MULTIETHNIC GROUPS HAVE UNIQUE DYNAMICS** and require interventions that are culturally appropriate. Multiethnic groups offer an opportunity for members to address their reactions to cultural diversity, to recognize their internalized biases and prejudices through exploration of cross-cultural issues, as well as to develop problem-solving skills to handle their individual life concerns.

Definition of Ethnicity

From a clinical point of view, ethnicity is more than distinctiveness defined by national origin, race, language, or religion; it involves unconscious processes that fulfill a deep psychological need for an individual's secure identity in a group.

Ethnicity-Bound Values

- Language. May be a subgroup issue. Language is used to form alliances. Even when only one is used, slang expressions may be interpreted differently.
- Physical Appearance. May see subgrouping according to race.
- Race-linked Conversational Differences. May result in misperceived verbal messages and nonverbal clues. Examples include eye contact, physical contact, use of titles.

Specific Group Dynamics Within Multiethnic Groups

- Power struggle within the group. Groups become microcosms of the struggles and prejudices played out in the larger, social context. Stereotyping, scapegoating, and polarization can easily occur.
- Understanding the culture of family of origin. Awareness and openness toward cultural patterns may help the leader and group understand individual group members' behaviors within the context of their ethnic heritage.
- Cohesion. Group issues are frequently framed in terms of race in a multiracial group. It is not uncommon, however, for the same concerns to connect different groups.
- Group attendance. If, as therapy sessions progress, ethnic group representation drops, the group should quickly inquire as to the reason. It may be that support systems are needed for minority ethnic group members.
- Silence. Some ethnic group members remain quiet and withdrawn although language proficiency is not the issue.
- Racial balance in group work. The degree of intimacy in a group-proposed activity is influenced by the size of the group. The goal of biracial groups should be to sustain intergroup contact until both parties are able to readjust themselves to what may be for them an atypical racial configuration.
- Stereotype of the ethnic group. The focus should be the individual in order to avoid stereotyping. A norm must be established in which diversity is valued rather than shunned.
- Cultural awareness of the group leader. Leaders need to examine their own biases toward certain racial or ethnic groups before beginning to work with a new group. Leaders need to anticipate their own biased reactions, which might contaminate responses.
- Modeling. Group leaders act as role models and must be willing to work through cross-ethnic issues with group members. Leaders must create a safe, accepting environment.

CLINICAL CONSIDERATIONS

- Preparing the group. The nurse must know patient's expectations and perceptions of group therapy and use culturally appropriate methods to address them.

- Elicit biases and prejudices of the group to facilitate a positive multicultural environment. In a society that devalues differences, ethnic and minority group members often internalize a negative sense of self. Building a positive cultural identity is an important part of transcultural therapeutic work.

- Be neutral. Group leaders should become neither overprotective of other ethnic group members nor overly confrontational.

STRATEGIES AND INTERVENTIONS

- Confront the issue. When issues of color, race, and/or ethnicity are discussed openly, the group becomes a safer place where multicultural interaction and learning can occur more easily.

- Deal with problematic behavior.

- Use group rules.

- Discuss stereotypes at all levels. Move from the individual to the family and peers to societal means of indoctrination, such as media images.

- Point out group commonalities.

- Be sensitive to language shifts and choices.

TAKING ANOTHER LOOK

You are now ready to respond to the questions that were raised in Gaining a Perspective at the beginning of this chapter. After you have written or thought about your responses you may wish to look at the Suggested Responses on page 336.

42 PHARMACOTHERAPY

TERMS TO DEFINE

akathisia

anticholingeric agents

anticholingeric syndrome

anticonvulsant

antiparkinsonian agents

antipsychotic drugs

anxiolytics

benzodiazepine

bioavailability

biotransformation

buspirone

choreoathetoid movements

discontinuance syndrome

dyskinesia

dystonia

extrapyramidal symptoms (EPS)

idiosyncratic effect

lithium

medication effects

parkinsonian syndrome

pharmacodynamics

pharmacokinetics

steady state

tardive dyskinesia

GAINING A PERSPECTIVE

Think about the pharmacotherapy issues described below, and after you have read the Key Concepts for this chapter respond in greater depth to the questions.

1. What do you think is the purpose of the nurse's assessment of a patient prior to starting drug therapy?

2. Why might you, as a nurse, empathize with some patients who become noncompliant with drug therapy?

KEY CONCEPTS

- **SOMATIC, OR BIOLOGIC, INTERVENTION** is an important aspect of the nurse's work with patients. Although the physician has traditionally been responsible for prescribing drugs, the role of the advanced practice nurse has expanded to include prescriptive authority in many states. The nurse's role in pharmacotherapy, at both the specialist and generalist levels, goes beyond the dispensing of drugs. In the mental health field, nurses are the primary evaluators of behavior and have great influence over patients who receive drugs.

    During the past 40 years, the development of psychopharmacology has expanded to include widespread use of antipsychotic, antidepressant, antianxiety, and mood stabilizing medications. The development of such techniques as magnetic resonance imaging (MRI) and positron emission tomography (PET) has made possible the evaluation of medication effects on brain structure and function.

    Serious issues accompany the use of drugs. Informed consent is imperative. Nurses must know the risks of drug therapy and convey that information to patients and families in an appropriate manner. Key to the patient's overall treatment plan are preliminary observations to distinguish between the side effects emerging

TABLE 42–1. BRIEF PSYCHIATRIC RATING SCALE

	Not Present	Very Mild	Mild	Moderate	Mod. Severe	Severe	Extremely Severe
Somatic concern: Preoccupation with physical health, fear of physical illness, hypochondriasis.	☐	☐	☐	☐	☐	☐	☐
Anxiety: Worry, fear, overconcern for present or future, uneasiness.	☐	☐	☐	☐	☐	☐	☐
Emotional withdrawal: Lack of spontaneous interaction, isolation deficiency in relating to others.	☐	☐	☐	☐	☐	☐	☐
Conceptual disorganization: Thought processes confused, disconnected, disorganized, disrupted.	☐	☐	☐	☐	☐	☐	☐
Guilt feelings: Self-blame, shame, remorse for past behavior.	☐	☐	☐	☐	☐	☐	☐
Tension: Physical and motor manifestations of nervousness, overactivation.	☐	☐	☐	☐	☐	☐	☐
Mannerisms and posturing: Peculiar, bizarre unnatural motor behavior (not including tic).	☐	☐	☐	☐	☐	☐	☐
Grandiosity: Exaggerated self-opinion, arrogance, conviction of unusual power or abilities.	☐	☐	☐	☐	☐	☐	☐
Depressive mood: Sorrow, sadness, despondency, pessimism.	☐	☐	☐	☐	☐	☐	☐
Hostility: Animosity, contempt, belligerence, disdain for others.	☐	☐	☐	☐	☐	☐	☐
Suspiciousness: Mistrust, belief others harbor malicious or discriminatory intent.	☐	☐	☐	☐	☐	☐	☐
Hallucinatory behavior: Perceptions without normal external stimulus correspondence.	☐	☐	☐	☐	☐	☐	☐
Motor retardation: Slowed weakened movements or speech, reduced body tone.	☐	☐	☐	☐	☐	☐	☐
Uncooperativeness: Resistance, guardedness, rejection of authority.	☐	☐	☐	☐	☐	☐	☐
Unusual thought content: Unusual, odd, strange, bizarre thought content.	☐	☐	☐	☐	☐	☐	☐
Blunted affect: Reduced emotional tone, reduction in formal intensity of feelings, flatness.	☐	☐	☐	☐	☐	☐	☐
Excitement: Heightened emotional tone, agitation, increased reactivity.	☐	☐	☐	☐	☐	☐	☐
Disorientation: Confusion or lack of proper association for person, place, or time.	☐	☐	☐	☐	☐	☐	☐

Adapted from Overall and Gorham (1962) The brief psychiatric rating scale. *Psychol Rep.* and Overall (1988). The brief psychiatric rating scale. *Psychol Bull.*

from treatment and the worsening symptoms of the psychiatric condition. Assessment and reassessment of patient behaviors are key tasks.

- **THE NURSE'S ROLE IN PHARMACOTHERAPY DEMANDS CRITICAL ASSESSMENT OF THE PATIENT,** including the sociocultural, psychological, as well as physiological contexts in which the behavior is manifest.

Baseline Assessment and Monitoring of Behavior

- Functional status assessment protocols and mental status examinations assist the nurse to assess, with the help of the patient, past response to drug therapy and the patient's total drug history.
  - Functional health history includes the patient's beliefs and expectations regarding the drugs, the patient's willingness to use the drugs, and understandings about potential side effects and risks.
  - Behavior and thought patterns that interfere or limit the patient's understandings must be fully noted by the nurse.
  - Assessment can strengthen the therapeu-

TABLE 42–2.
GLOBAL ASSESSMENT SCALE

Rate the subject's lowest level of functioning in the last week by selecting the lowest range that describes his or her functioning on a hypothetical continuum of mental health–illness. For example, a subject whose "behavior is considerably influenced by delusions" (range 21 to 30) should be given a rating in that range even though he or she has "major impairment in several areas" (range 31 to 40). Use intermediary levels when appropriate (e.g., 35, 58, 63). Rate actual functioning independent of whether or not the subject is receiving and may be helped by medication or some other form of treatment.

Points	Functioning
100	No symptoms, superior functioning in a wide range of activities, life's problems never seem to get out of hand, is sought out by others because of his or her warmth.
90 to 81	Transient symptoms may occur, but good functioning in all areas, interested and involved in a wide range of activities, socially effective, generally satisfied with life. "Everyday" worries that occasionally get out of hand.
80 to 71	Minimal symptoms may be present but no more than slight impairment in functioning. Varying degrees of "everyday" worries and problems that sometimes get out of hand.
70 to 61	Some mild symptoms (e.g., depressive mood and mild insomnia) OR some difficulties in several areas of functioning, but generally functions pretty well, has some meaningful interpersonal relationships and most untrained people would not consider him sick.
60 to 51	Moderate symptoms OR generally functioning with some difficulty (e.g., few friends and flat affect, depressed mood and pathological self-doubt, euphoric mood and pressured speech, moderately severe antisocial behavior).
50 to 41	Any serious symptomology or impairment in functioning that most clinicians would think requires treatment or attention (e.g., suicidal preoccupation or gesture, severe obsessional rituals, frequent anxiety attacks, serious antisocial behavior, compulsive drinking).
40 to 31	Major impairment in several areas, such as work, family relations, judgment, thinking or mood (e.g., depressed woman avoids friends, neglects family, unable to do housework) OR some impairment in reality testing or communication (e.g., speech is at times obscure, illogical, or irrelevant) OR single serious suicide attempt.
30 to 21	Unable to function in almost all areas (e.g., stays in bed all day) OR behavior is considerably influenced by either delusions or hallucinations, OR serious impairment in communication (e.g., sometimes incoherent or unresponsive) or judgment (e.g., acts grossly inappropriately).
20 to 11	Needs some supervision to prevent hurting self or others or to maintain minimal personal hygiene (e.g., repeated suicide attempts, frequently violent, manic excitement, smears feces) OR gross impairment in communication (e.g., largely incoherent or mute).
10 to 1	Needs constant supervision for several days to prevent hurting self or others, or makes no attempt to maintain minimal personal hygiene.

Adapted from Endicott et al., The global assessment scale. *Arch Gen Psych.* 1976.

tic alliance because of the shared thought patterns and the decisions that the patient must make. This empowerment of the patient can prevent regression.

- Mental status examination provides information about behavioral movement patterns (e.g., spasms, flexibility, and tremors) and psychological processes (e.g., perception, hallucinations, illusions).
- Several valid and reliable rating scales are available for clinical practice (see Study Guide Tables 42-1 and 42-2). These scales can be used when a drug is initiated and to monitor progress at specific points along the course of therapy.

- Assessment for the presence of side effects requires careful monitoring.
  - Nursing observations and the patient's self-appraisal are part of continued assessment and monitoring.

- Data derived from monitoring are recorded on a patient status sheet, which also includes physiological indicators, such as weight and blood pressure.

Drug Education

- Nurses must be knowledgeable about drugs and must share the information with the patient. If patients are knowledgeable, it enhances their independence and self-reliance.

- An educational paradigm should emphasize that a chemical imbalance left uncorrected will influence thoughts, perceptions, and interpretation of information. This approach is likely to counteract negative assumptions by patients.

- Patients need to know that drugs do not solve problems, but rather aid thinking processes, which allows for problem-solving.

- It is important to teach patients self-monitoring procedures and how to communicate their need for increased or decreased medication.

- **KEY BIOLOGICAL ASSUMPTIONS IN PSYCHOPHARMACOTHERAPY** concern drug actions and interactions within the human being. Research into drug action, interaction, dosage, etc., is focused on identifying and understanding signal molecules (neurotransmitters, receptors, signal transducing proteins, and second messengers) as they relate to psychopharmacological mechanisms. The mechanisms are the molecular means by which exogenous and endogenous chemicals travel biochemical pathways. The primary functions of the pathways are to alter cellular activity, information flow, and, ultimately, behavior. Drug therapy seeks to maintain functional pathways.

The Brain and Neuronal Functioning

- Neurochemical dysfunctions related to mental illness appear to involve various subcortical structures of the brain, limbic system, basal ganglia, reticular system, and brain stem. Irregularities in chemical transmission of information by neurotransmitters/hormones, as well as structural lesions and abnormalities, can upset the relationship of these areas; the disruption is manifest as a mental disorder. Mental illness is not associated with any one dysfunction or pathology in a brain structure or neurotransmitter. Certain neuroanatomical areas, however, have been implicated in the distribution of neurotransmitters and associated with containment disorders. Examples of such neurotransmitters are norepinephrine in depression and anxiety; dopamine in schizophrenia and certain depressions; and serotonin in depression, particularly associated with post-traumatic stress disorder, and in obsessive compulsive disorder.

Every region of the brain is both activated and controlled by millions of neurons. Of particular concern in psychopharmacology is neurotransmission, the influence of drugs, and sites of malfunction.

- Neuronal processing is described by the two-compartment (central and peripheral) model.

  - Central compartment. Intravenous drugs enter directly into this compartment, for example the blood. Irreversible drug elimination occurs by hepatic biotransformation, or renal excretion.

  - Peripheral compartment. Intracellular processes, and synaptic processes are examples. The compartment usually is not accessible to direct measurement or study nor are the sites of drug elimination.

  - Reversible distribution of drugs occurs between the peripheral and central compartments and usually requires a finite time for distribution and equilibrium to return (30 to 60 minutes after intravenous injection).

Pharmacokinetics

- Absorption. Drugs taken orally are usually absorbed in the stomach or small intestine. Many factors influence absorption. What is central is knowing the bioavailability of a drug; some drugs are metabolized before reaching the bloodstream. Whether a drug is able to penetrate the blood/brain barrier of the central nervous system is also a factor in bioavailability.

- Distribution. A drug enters the bloodstream and is distributed to various organs or sites of action. Some drugs are stored in tissues; at times, more drug is stored in tissues than in the bloodstream. Blood levels of a drug, therefore, are not always an accurate estimate of the amount of drug in an individual's body.

Individual physiologic patterns of drug distribution vary greatly; thus there is great variability in how quickly a person reaches a therapeutic dose and how much is in reserve. When patients do not take the drug correctly, or stop taking it, or a planned reduction is implemented, there is great variability in how rapidly the drug will be eliminated from the system.

- Biotransformation, or Metabolism. Biotransformation is one way the body rids itself of a drug. Metabolism occurs mainly in the liver. When metabolism is impaired, toxicity is a danger. Or, with increased enzymatic function of the liver, a drug can be metabolized too quickly, resulting in a decreased drug level.

- Excretion. Elimination occurs primarily via the kidneys, although some other routes are the GI tract, sweat, saliva, and breast milk. Clinically and pharmacologically, a balance is needed between the ingestion of the drug and its elimination. Has a steady state been achieved?

Drug Effect

To understand the time required for a drug to reach a steady state, the drug's half-life is measured. Half-life is used to determine dose and the intervals between doses.

Pharmacodynamics

- The pharmacological effect is the therapeutic effect.

- Side effects, such as dry mouth, are extensions of the pharmacologic properties of drugs. Some side effects, such as assisting patients to sleep, can be useful.

- Idiosyncratic effects are extremely rare, adverse effects.

- Allergic reactions are drug effects resulting from the response of an individual's immune system to therapy.

- Discontinuance syndrome results from the effects of stopping or interrupting a medication regimen.

- Pharmacodynamics—drug action and interaction—may occur immediately or over time. When a drug is administered with a primary psychotherapeutic medication, the potential effect of the combination of drugs on the kinetic properties of absorption, distribution, biotransfortion, and excretion must be recognized.

The Neurobiologic Basis of Psychopharmacology

- Neurotransmitters. Most neurons are selective and release only one neurotransmitter. Neurotransmitters either activate or inhibit. Identified neurotransmitters (Study Guide Table 42-3) within the brain associated with mental illness and drug therapy are dopamine, serotonin (5HT), acetylcholine, norepinephrine, glycine, and gamma-aminobutyric acid (GABA).

- Receptor Binding. Receptors are coiled proteins that have on their exterior surface areas that bind to specific neurotransmitters. In early efforts to understand neurotransmission, receptors were classified by their ability to interact with specific drugs. Now, we can also determine the amino acid sequence of a receptor. This has lead to an understanding of their signal molecules, which can excite or inhibit neural activity.

- Signal Transduction. Information via signal molecules (neurotransmitters, receptors, signal transducing proteins, and second messengers) is transmitted through structures of the neuron and continues across the space (synapse) between the terminal bouton of the neuron to the dendrite of the next neuron.

- Second Messengers. The messengers are identified by the production of enzymes, which ultimately lead to regulation of cellular enzymatic function and gene expression within the DNA of certain genes within the cell. They also regulate transmitter responsiveness.

Neural Malfunction

Neural malfunction that leads to neural misfiring is the basis for understanding what underlies major mental illnesses.

- Insufficient neurotransmitters, which may be due to a failure in synthesis or production.

- Diminished or excess neurotransmitters at the presynaptic bouton can be caused by certain disorders and drugs.
- The process of recycling neurotransmitters (by re-uptake) can be overstimulated or retarded by physiological malfunctions and/or medications.
- Receptors on the membrane of cells that break the firing of neurotransmitters can, under certain conditions, increase (up-regulation) and result in overinhibition and decreased neuronal excitability, or receptors with a down-regulation can decrease, resulting in increased neuronal sensitivity.
- Excessive enzymatic activity may deplete neurotransmitters.
- **PSYCHOTROPIC DRUGS ARE GENERALLY BROADLY CLASSIFIED ACCORDING TO THE SYMPTOMS THEY ARE USED TO TREAT.** Antipsychotic drugs are used to treat disorders of thought and perception. Antianxiety drugs reduce anxiety, and are therefore often used in crisis situations, major problems of adjustment, as well as short-term adjunctive treatment for many major mental disorders. Antidepressant agents are primarily utilized to treat major depression, although they have been successful in the management of eating and obsessive compulsive disorders. Mood stabilizing drugs, such as lithium carbonate and certain anticonvulsive drugs, have proven effective in the treatment of affective disorders.
- **ANTIPSYCHOTIC DRUGS** (Study Guide Table 42-4) may be used after psychosis has been identified. A clear history of the onset of the illness is critical, as well as an accurate assessment of patients' symptoms.

     Target symptoms most affected by antipsychotic drugs are delusions, hallucinations, changes in the flow of ideas, changes in the structure and rate of association, ideas of reference, suspicious behavior, incoherence, and marked illogical thinking. Agitation accompanying psychiatric symptoms responds well to antipsychotic drugs, and symptoms, such as withdrawal, anorexia, and self-neglect, improve. Personality structure and communication styles remain unchanged.

Antipsychotic Drug Action
- Antipsychotics are extremely effective and safe, but are often referred to as neuroleptics because they have many neurological side effects.
- Antipsychotics alter the kinds and amounts of amines at the synapse. The drugs block postsynaptic (D2) dopamine receptors, which is believed to be critical in selectively changing the transmission of information along the dopamine pathways.
- Many neuroleptics have alpha-androgenic blocking effects, which result in lowered blood pressure, decreased pulse rate, and sedation. Sedation often contributes to the patient's overall improvement and is useful for manic and agitated states.
- Antipsychotic drugs are extremely useful in treating acute psychotic states and managing individuals with chronic psychotic symptoms.
- A major serious consequence of prolonged use of antipsychotic drugs is tardive dyskinesia. That it will occur is unpredictable, and no corrective treatment is known. New antipsychotics, such as clozapine and risperidone, have not been associated with tardive dyskinesia.

TABLE 42–3.
KNOWN AND POSTULATED NEUROTRANSMITTERS

Name	Group	Distribution in CNS
Adrenaline	Catecholamine/Monoamine	Subcortical
Noradrenaline	Catecholamine/Monoamine	Everywhere
Dopamine	Catecholamine/Monoamine	Everywhere
GABA	Amino acid	Supraspinal interneurons
Glycine	Amino acid	Spinal interneurons
Glutamic acid	Amino acid	Interneurons generally
Enkephalines	Neuropeptide	In numerous CNS regions
Substance P	Neuropeptide	In numerous CNS regions
Vasopressin	Neuropeptide	Sometimes together with
Angiotensin	Neuropeptide	other neurotransmitters
Somatostatin	Neuropeptide	
Serotonin	no specific group	Everywhere
Acetylcholine	no specific group	Everywhere

Adapted from Spiegle R. An Introduction to Pharmacology. 2nd ed. New York: Wiley; 1990.

Dosage Considerations

- Dosage schedules vary according to potency of the drug and individual differences. Drugs are available to minimize the unwanted pharmacologic effects of sedation, androgenic blocking activity, and extrapyramidal effects.
- Antipsychotic drugs are long-acting. Once a dose level to control symptoms is achieved, a single dose can be given at bedtime, diminishing the problem of daytime sedation.
- In acute psychotic episodes, treatment may be brief; however, for newly treated chronic patients, 3 to 6 months of treatment may be required before a change in medication is warranted. For patients with schizophrenia, maintenance doses should be as low as possible.

Pharmacokinetics of Antipsychotic Drugs

- Antipsychotic drugs are metabolized in the liver and may cause hepatic toxicity. They are excreted via the kidney.
- Most fatalities occur among children or when the drug is mixed with other drugs.

Side Effects

Side effects and toxicity are not infrequent (see Study Guide Table 42-5). In general, the high-

TABLE 42–4.
SEVERITY OF ADVERSE EFFECTS OF ANTIPSYCHOTIC DRUGS

Drugs	EPS	NMS	Anticholinergic	Hypotension	Sedation
Thorazine	++	++	+++	++	+++
Mellaril	+	+	+++	+++	+++
Stelazine	++	++	++	+	+++
Trilafon	++	+	++	++	++
Prolixin	+++	+++	+	——	+
Haldol	+++	+++	——	——	+
Moban	++	++	++	+	+
Loxitane	+++	+++	++	++	++
Clozaril	——	——	+++	+++	+++
Risperdal	+	——	+	+	+

EPS, extra pyramidal symptoms; NMS, neuroleptic malignant syndrome; mild, +; moderate, ++; severe, +++; no information, ——.

TABLE 42–5.
ANTIPSYCHOTIC DRUGS AND ANTI-PARKINSONIAN DRUGS

Brand Name	Generic Name	Daily Dose Range (mg)
I. Antipsychotic agents		
A. Phenothiazine derivatives		
1. Aliphatics		
a. Thorazine	Chlorpromazine	100 to 1,000
b. Vesprin	Triflupromazine	20 to 150
2. Piperidines		
a. Mellaril	Thioridazine	30 to 800
b. Serentil	Mesoridazine	50 to 400
3. Piperazines		
a. Stelazine	Trifluoperazine	2 to 30
b. Trilafon	Perphenazine	2 to 64
c. Prolixin, Permitil	Fluphenazine	0.5 to 20
d. Prolixin enanthate or decanoate	(long-acting injectable)	4 cc (½ to 4 cc every 2 or 3 weeks)
B. Thioxanthene derivatives		
1. Navane (piperazine)	Thiothixene	6 to 60
C. Butyrophenone derivative		
1. Haldol	Haloperidol	1 to 100
2. Haldol decanoate	Haloperidol	
D. Dihydroindolone derivative		
1. Moban	Molindone	20 to 225
E. Dibenzoxazepine derivative		
1. Loxitane	Loxapine	20 to 250
F. Diphenylbutylpiperidines		
1. Orap	Pimozide	0.3 to 0.5
II. Atypical antipsychotic agents		
A. Dibenzodiazepines		
1. Clozaril	Clozapine	200 to 450
B. Benzioxazols		
1. Risperdal	Risperidone	4 to 10
III. Antipsychotics under study		
A. Amperozide		
IV. Antiparkinsonian agents (drugs used in the control of side effects. They also have anticholinergic properties that can lead to toxic reactions.)		
A. Artane	Trihexyphenidyl	1 to 10
B. Benadryl	Diphenhydramine	25 to 200
C. Cogentin	Benztropine mesylate	1 to 6
D. Symmetrel	Amantadine	100 to 300

er the dose, the greater the risk of side effects. Low-potency antipsychotics produce a different side effect profile than high-potency drugs. With the exception of clozapine, most antipsychotic drugs cause or have the potential to cause extrapyramidal symptoms (EPS) such as dystonia, dyskinesia, akathisia, parkinsonian syndrome, tardive dyskinesia, and choreoathetoid movements. With the exception of tardive dyskinesia, symptoms occur and disappear within the first several weeks of treatment.

- Tardive dyskinesia is a syndrome that occurs later in the use of antipsychotic drugs.
  - Repetitive, involuntary movements, involving the mouth, lips, tongue, trunk, and extremities, occur. Chewing, smacking and licking of lips, sucking, tongue protrusions, tongue tremor with open mouth, wormlike movements on the surface of the tongue, blinking, and facial distortion are also common. Choreic movements (involuntary twitching) of the limbs and rhythmic dystonic contractions of the axilla muscle (giving rise to torticollis) and pelvic thrusting may also occur. Movement is constant, although it may increase with emotional arousal and decrease with relaxation or volitional effort. Movements are absent during sleep.
  - Tardive dyskinesia is usually preceded by parkinsonism syndrome.
  - Early detection of disorder will reduce the seriousness of the condition. Subtle signs including wormlike movements of the tongue surface and subtle spasmodic signs must be evaluated immediately.
  - The only known treatment at this time is to discontinue the drug.
  - Clozapine, and perhaps risperidone, can be used as alternatives for individuals who have developed tardive dyskinesia.
- Dystonia is involuntary, irregular clonic contortions of the muscles of the trunk and extremities. Initially, patients complain of a thick tongue and inability to hold their neck straight. Other early symptoms include cogwheeling respirations and difficulty speaking and swallowing.

  - Dystonia requires immediate treatment.
  - Treatment, as for all extrapyramidal side effects except tardive dyskinesia, is with antiparkinsonian drugs such as benzotropine mesylate (Cogentin) or diphenhydramine (Benadryl).
- Dyskinesia is impaired power of voluntary movement, resulting in fragmentary or incomplete movements.
- Akathisia is an extreme inability to sit or remain still. The body is in constant movement. It is frequently mislabeled agitation or severe anxiety.
- Parkinsonian syndrome is marked by muscular rigidity, immobile face, involuntary movement of the head, tremors and pillrolling movements of the forefingers, and excessive salivation and drooling. Patient appears rigid (not free to move), yet agitated.
- Agranulocytosis is a life-threatening blood dyscrasia associated mainly with clozapine. Although agranulocytosis is rarely associated with other neuroleptics, it can occur. It is initially recognized by a sore throat, fever, and general malaise. White blood cell counts must be monitored.
- Neuroleptic malignant syndrome (NMS) is a rare side effect, which has been referred to as an extrapyramidal crisis. Symptoms include labile blood pressure, elevated pulse rate and temperature, anxiety, dyspnea, profuse perspiration, cyanosis, and seizures. Treatment is to discontinue the antipsychotic drug and treat the patient's symptoms.
- Progressive obstructive jaundice is, most notably, an increased yellowing of the skin and the sclera of the eyes. Antipsychotic drug must be stopped and another drug administered.
- Seizures may result from a lowered convulsion threshold; they may occur with clozapine use.
- Hematologic system symptoms are rare, with the exception of agranulocytosis caused by clozapine. When symptoms do occur, they are generally in the form of leukopenia and thrombocytopenia. Drug must be stopped. Periodic blood counts may help detect abnormalities.

- Psychiatric symptoms, which include drowsiness and akathisia, are often perceived as depression and anxiety; therefore, the reported symptoms need to be carefully assessed. A decrease in drug dosage corrects the problem.
- Anticholinergic effects include blurred vision, flushing, pallor, and dry mouth. Reassuring the patient usually helps. Urinary retention may occur with thioridazine (Mellaril).
- Cardiovascular symptoms (mild form) include syncope and ECG changes, which need to be evaluated before decisions about stopping the drug are made.
- Hypersalivation is associated with clozapine.
- Dermatologic symptoms include photosensitivity which usually occurs with the use of chlorpromazine (Thorazine) and thioridazine (Mellaril). Staying out of the sun and wearing protective clothing are suggested. Less common effects are skin rashes with edema of the face, feet, or hands. Diphenhydramine chloride (Benadryl) may be used for treatment.
- Endocrine system symptoms include obesity, menstrual irregularity, edema, abnormal lactation, and decreased sex drive among men, and increased sex drive among women. Reassuring the patient or trying another class of drugs is a method of handling these side effects.
- Ophthalmologic symptoms include a mild disturbance in accommodation in which the eye is not able to focus images and the pupil is small. Other rare side effects include glaucoma and ulceration of the cornea. An ophthalmologist is contacted to treat these problems.
- Gastrointestinal symptoms are uncommon, but may include fecal impaction, constipation, or diarrhea. Symptoms can be managed by diet supplements or mild medications, as needed.

Nursing Management of Patients with Extrapyramidal Side Effects

- Management of Paitients with Neuroleptic Malignant Syndrome (NMS)
  - Exhaustion and dehydration place individuals at risk. NMS affects all ages, both sexes, but predominately young males. NMS is underdiagnosed and a potentially dangerous condition.
  - Assessment is critical. The four cardinal signs are:
  Muscular lead-pipe rigidity
  Hyperthermia
  Disturbance of consciousness
  Autonomic dysfunction
  - Elevated serum phosphokinase levels generally confirm diagnosis.
  - When symptoms are reported, medication is withheld.
  - Close observation and comfort measures are essential: cool blankets to reduce temperature and intravenous fluids to prevent dehydration and renal complications. Education and support of family and significant others are vital to help decrease anxiety and fear throughout this medical psychiatric emergency.
- Management of Patients with Parkinsonian-Syndrome
  - Syndrome usually occurs after the first week of administering drug, but before the second month of treatment. Symptoms are akinesia, lack of interest or ambition, fatigue, slowness, heaviness, vague bodily discomfort, muscular rigidity, masklike facies, shuffling gait, hypersalivation, drooling, alterations in posture, tremor, and pillrolling.
  - The akinesia associated with parkinsonian syndrome is often interpreted as depression or negativism. Lack of facial expression is often mistaken for a sign of chronic schizophrenia or depression.
  - Symptoms usually improve slowly with the reduction of drug dosage and addition of an anticholinergic drug. Switching to a different antipsychotic drug may remove symptoms. After 2 to 3 months, the symptoms usually disappear.
- Management of Patients with Dyskinesia and Dystonias
  - Dystonic reactions, acute dyskinesias, and oculogyric crisis typically occur during the early hours or the day following an increase

in the dose of antipsychotic drugs. These symptoms are episodic and recurrent and last from minutes to hours.

- It is important to recognize dyskinesia and dystonias, as they can be misdiagnosed as an emergency situation.
- Symptoms are painful and frightening and may be acute or mild. Once they occur, dosages of medications are lowered to avoid further episodes.

• Management of Patients with Akathisia

- Feeling restless and agitated may be mistaken for anxiety. To test if symptoms are caused by the drug, increase the dose and watch to see if symptoms persist. Also, walking makes patients with akathisia feel better.
- Incidence of symptoms peaks in 6 to 10 weeks, with a decline in 12 to 16 weeks. Symptoms can also be treated with antiparkinsonian drugs or short-acting benzodiazapines.

• Management of Patients with Tardive Dyskinesia

- Patients, especially those on long-term therapy, must be screened every 3 months.
- Earliest signs of tardive dyskinesia are excessive blinking, fine vermiform movements of the tongue, and subtle spasmodic movements, particularly of the arms. Then, symptoms progress until they interfere with activities of daily living.
- Change antipsychotic drug or lower dose; taking "holidays" from drug is another option when symptoms appear. Do not administer drugs used to treat extrapyramidal reactions as therapy.

• Management of Patients with Other Side Effects

- Postural hypotension is evaluated by taking patient's blood pressure sitting and lying down before and after drug is administered. Advise patient to rise slowly in the morning and be careful when stooping in order to avoid fainting.
- Drowsiness is usually controlled by taking drug at night.

- Nasal stuffiness, should it occur, is another side effect.
- Among men, impotence and inhibition of ejaculation or retrograde ejaculation may occur, as well as urinary retention. For the latter, documentation in intake and output records may be necessary.
- Several anticholinergic side effects may occur.

DRY MOUTH: Suggest sugarless gum or gum drops or salvia substitutes.

CONSTIPATION: Stool softeners may be given.

CARDIAC CHANGES: Periodically check pulse and have ECGs done.

BLURRED VISION: If blurred vision is a severe problem, treat with physostigmine.

- Atropinelike psychosis is marked by confusion, incoherence, visual hallucinations, disorientation, and impaired concentration. Symptoms are reduced by using physostigmine and withdrawing antipsychotic medications.
- Hypothalamic side effects include disturbances in menstruation, temperature deregulation, fever, and appetite change. A daily program of evaluation and reporting is established.
- Lowered seizure threshold is monitored.
- Photosensitivity necessitates staying out of sun and wearing protective clothing.

• Management of Patients Who Overdose with Antipsychotic Drugs

- Hypotension is the most serious symptom, and it responds to volume expansion. Because of beta-adrenergic blockade, ephedrine or norepinephrine (Levophed) is used.
- Other serious complications of overdose are hypertension and hyperthermia, urinary tract infection with oliguria and renal failure, cardiac arrhythmias, skin lesions, and clinical relapse. Treatment is best approached symptomatically. Use of stimulants is avoided because of convulsions.

Drug Interactions with Antipsychotic Drugs

The most critical antipsychotic drug interactions are with other central nervous system depressants because of the synergistic and cumulative effects.

- Antacids. Concurrent administration of chlorpromazine and alum or magnesium gel-type antacids lowers serum levels.
- Haloperidol. When given with anticoagulants, haloperidol produces prothrombin, enhancing the anticoagulant effect.
- Dibenzodiazepines, phenothiazines, and thioxanthenes. These drugs lower the seizure threshold of some patients, making it necessary to increase seizure-controlling medication.
- Antipsychotic agents and central nervous system depressants. Addictive central nervous system depression may develop when these drugs are taken together.
- Monoamine oxidase inhibitors. Antipsychotic agents and monoamine oxidase inhibitors used concomitantly may cause an additive hypotensive effect.
- Tricyclic antidepressants and phenothiazines. Taken together, these drugs increase anticholinergic effects and may lead to toxic psychosis.
- Epinephrine. When used with antipsychotics, epinephrine has a paradoxical effect on blood pressure: it lowers blood pressure.
- Propranolol. Chlorpromazine inhibits propranolol's metabolism, resulting in hypotension.

Nursing Principles Regarding Antipsychotic Drugs

- The nurse must understand the major objective of drug treatment.
- Side effects must be distinguished from targeted symptoms.
- Severely and chronically disturbed patients are among the medically underserved; therefore nurses must take initiative, when necessary, to establish adequate protocols for the health surveillance of patients taking drugs.
- The nurse must initiate drug education for patient, family, and auxiliary health personnel.
- Dosage ranges are wide and relate to the high therapeutic index of this drug class. Patient

reactions must be monitored. Usually start with low dose and observe patient for side effects. Within five to ten days symptoms are usually controlled. Positive drug responses occur within three to six weeks.

RAPID NEUROLEPTIZATION, used by some physicians, is the administration of extremely large doses of antipsychotic drugs in the acute treatment phase of patients who are very excited or dangerous. There are increased untoward reactions. The nurse must be prepared to monitor the administration of the drugs and the patient's response. Following the acute phase, in 4 to 12 weeks the dose is slowly lowered.

DURATION OF TREATMENT

- A patient who has had an acute psychotic episode perhaps can be slowly removed from the drug.
- Patients with recurrent psychotic episodes usually receive long-term intermittent maintenance drug therapy.
- Patients must be removed from the drug slowly. Because antipsychotic drugs tend to be stored in the body, time must elapse before beginning any new drug.
- Nurses must make it clear to patients who have decided independently to discontinue medications that they have that right; however, they need to work closely with the nursing and medical team when the drug is discontinued.
- During withdrawal of the drug, for whatever reason, the nurse, patient, and physician must work together, as symptoms may exacerbate. The increase in symptoms demoralizes patients.
- Drug information must be written down for patients and families. The nurse should also consider making group presentations for families and patients to teach the objectives of drug intervention and how patients can monitor themselves.

- **ANTIPARKINSONIAN AGENTS** are administered to correct a neurotransmitter imbalance (dopamine deficiency and acetylcholine excess in the corpus striatae). Levodopa or amantadine enhances dopaminergic action. Centrally active anticholinergic agents help inhibit acetyl-choline (see Study Guide Table 42-4). Antiparkinsonian agents reduce the incidence and severity of akinesia, rigidity, and tremor that are often seen in patients taking antipsychotic drugs.

Anticholinergic Syndrome

The syndrome is a consequence of excessive antiparkinsonian and antipsychotic drugs.

- Neuropsychiatric signs of toxicity include anxiety, agitation, restlessness, purposeless-ness, overactivity, delirium, disorientation, immediate and recent memory impairment, dysarthria, hallucinations, and myoclonic seizures.
- Systemic signs of toxicity include tachycardia and arrhythmias; large, sluggish pupils; flushed, warm, dry skin; increased temperature; decreased mucosal secretions; urinary retention; and reduced bowel motility.
- Treatment includes physostigmine salicylate (e.g., neostigmine, pyridostigmine).

Physostigmine-Induced Cholinergic Excess

- Neuropsychiatric signs include confusion, seizures, nausea, vomiting, myoclonus, and hallucinations. They often occur after treatment with physostigmine for anticholinergic syndrome.
- Systemic signs are bradycardia, miosis, increased mucosal secretions, copious bronchial secretions, dyspnea, tears, sweating, diarrhea, abdominal and/or biliary colic, and urinary frequency or urgency.
- Treatment and prevention involve the use of atropine sulfate, physostigmine, meth-scopolamine bromide (Pamine), and gly-copyrrolate (Robinul).

The Effect of Antiparkinsonian Agents on Disease

- Incipient glaucoma may be precipitated.
- When used to treat extrapyramidal syndrome (EPS), antiparkinsonian agent can exacerbate psychotic symptoms and precipitate a toxic psychosis; they may mask development of persistent EPS.

Symptoms of Overdose and Their Management

- Symptoms of overdose of an antiparkinsonian agent are similar in extent to those of an antihistamine overdose. Severe central nervous system depression is followed by, or preceded by, stimulation. (See description of anticholinergic syndrome in previous coumn.)
- Overdose management includes gastric lavage or emesis. Treatment is symptomatic.

• MOOD STABILIZERS

Identifying Mood Disorders

- Affective disorders are characterized by disturbances in mood (Chapter 20). Mood disorders include mania and depression, as well as cyclothymic and dysthymic disorders. A diagnosis of bipolar affective disorder is made when an individual who has experienced depression has had at least one manic attack. Unipolar affective disorder is diagnosed when an individual has had depressive episodes but no manic episode. Two types of medications are currently being used to treat mood disorders: lithium and anticonvulsants.

Lithium As a Treatment for Mood Instability

The best response with lithium occurs in manic individuals; however, it is also used to treat depression and cyclothymic and dysthymic disorders. In major depression lithium may be used with an antidepressant drug. Lithium has been used to treat many problems where mood is a prominent feature, including impulse and personality disorders.

When lithium is used to treat mania, the patient may be aware of a slowing of thought processes and acts. Lithium is used for maintenance therapy to prevent recurrence of an affective disorder. Lithium has also been used to augment the antidepressant effect of tricyclics in the treatment of many kinds of depression.

- Lithium Absorption and Action
  - Readily absorbed through the gastrointestinal system; peak blood levels occur within a few hours.
  - Eliminated almost entirely by renal excretion; sodium diuresis and sodium deficiency tend to increase the retention of lithium, potentially leading to toxicity.
  - Mechanism of action is not clear.
- Dosage
  - Unlike most drugs, the dosage range for

TABLE 42–6.
LITHIUM DOSAGE

Preparation	Adult Dosage	Lethal Dose
Lithium carbonate (Eskalith, Lithonate, Lithotabs)	Initial: 300 to 600 mg (1,200 to 1,800 mg/day) until lithium blood level is reached (0.8 to 1.2 for therapeutic effect).	Toxicity results in blood levels >2.0 mEq/L. Lethality generally occurs at levels greater than 3.0.
Lithium citrate Syrup (Cibalith)	Same as above.	
Lithium carbonate– Slow release (Lithobid, Eskalith CR).	Initial: 450 mg. Increase dosage to reach serum levels 0.8 to 1.2 mEq/L for therapeutic effect.	

lithium is not indicative of its clinical effects (see Study Guide Table 42-6).

- Dosage adjustment is slow and blood levels should be checked with any change in dose. Once blood level has stabilized, monthly checks suffice. Significant changes in patient's activity level should be followed by monitoring lithium blood level.

• Lithium Toxicity

Therapeutic levels of lithium closely approximate toxic levels; the margin of safety is quite low (see Study Guide Table 42-7).

- Prolonged blood levels greater than 1.5 mEq/L usually result in toxicity; greater than 2.0 mEq/L can result in a lethal situation.

- Early symptoms of toxicity include nausea and vomiting, diarrhea, abdominal pain, and general malaise.

- Severe symptoms associated with serious toxicity include somnolence, confusion, motor restlessness, disturbed behavior, ataxia, incoordination, dysarthria, stupor, and coma. Incontinence of urine and feces and seizures may also occur, as well as irregular pulse, decreased blood pressure, ECG changes, and peripheral circulatory failure.

- Management of early symptoms of toxicity includes the essential withdrawal of lithi-

um and replacement of fluids. Serum levels fall rapidly once drug is discontinued.

Serious symptoms indicate a life-threatening event requiring immediate medical intervention. Dialysis and intravenous fluid replacement may be indicated.

• Side Effects

- Chronic ingestion of lithium may lead to a diabetes insipidus-like syndrome, in which urine does not become concentrated. Polyuria may occur, which seems to be controlled with a lower maintenance single dose of the drug. Problems associated with polyuria are inconvenience and excessive liquid calories to replace lost fluids.

- Lithium interferes with the production of thyroid hormones. Goiter may occur; however, the drug does not need to be discontinued. Replacement therapy with synthetic form of T4 (Synthroid) may be used.

- A fine motor tremor exacerbated by anxiety may occur that may become worse about 1 to 2 hours after the dose is taken, due to rising blood levels.

- Other Side Effects

FEELING UNEXCITABLE OR DISCONNECTED from affect.

WEIGHT GAIN, making nutrition education important.

DERMATOLOGICAL PROBLEMS include dry skin, progressing to psoriasis and severe acne.

• Drug Interactions

- Drugs, such as thiazide diuretics, furosemide, and ethacrynic acid, decrease renal clearance and may lead to lithium toxicity.

- Indomethacin and other nonsteroid anti-inflammatory agents can increase the plasma level of lithium by 30% to 60%, which may lead to toxicity.

- Drugs, e.g., mazindol, phenytoin, methyldopa, thioridazine, and carbamazepine, may increase the central nervous system toxicity of lithium.

- Lithium and haloperidol in combination can cause an encephalopathic syndrome with irreversible brain damage.

- Nursing Responsibilities
  - Lithium blood levels are monitored frequently until stability is reached. Patients exhibit great individuality as to when side effects or toxicity may occur. When antipsychotic drugs are used in conjunction with lithium, they may mask side effects and toxicity because of their antinausea property.
  - Prevention is the best intervention. Patient education and frequent assessment, including blood level monitoring, are necessary.
  - Most side effects are reversible if doses are decreased and as time increases from the onset of treatment.
  - Patients must be reminded to keep well hydrated, as dehydration (caused by excessive heat, fever, or exercise) can cause toxicity.
  - Renal disease may cause toxicity.
  - Nurses must gain patient's cooperation for blood level assessment. Blood must be drawn 10 to 14 hours after the last dose of lithium or false readings will occur. Careful planning, therefore, is necessary, as well as patient education about toxicity.

Anticonvulsants As Treatment for Mood Instability

Carbamazepine (Tegretol) and valproic acid (Depakene) have shown significant results in treating mood instability. They are used singly or in conjunction with lithium. Depakene is used primarily for mania.

- Action

  The neurophysiologic action of these drugs is not known; they may cause alterations in the limbic system, which is responsible for thought and perception.

- Dosage

  Based on blood level. Therapeutic range of Tegretol is 4 to 12 ug/mL and Depakene is 50 to 100 ug/mL. When Tegretol is given with antipsychotic drugs, a resurgence of psychotic symptoms may occur.

- Side Effects
  - Nausea, vomiting, dizziness, ataxia, clum-

TABLE 42–7
LITHIUM TOXICITY AND SIDE EFFECTS

Lithium Concentrate (mEq/L)	Signs of Lithium Toxicity at Different Serum Levels
< 1.5	Nausea, vomiting, diarrhea, thirst, polyuria, lethargy, slurred speech, muscle weakness, fine hand tremor.
< 2.0	Persistent GI upset, coarse hand tremor, mental confusion, hyperirritability of muscles, ECG changes (moderate), drowsiness, incoordination.
> 2	Ataxia, giddiness, large output of dilute urine, serious ECG changes, tinnitus, blurred vision, clonic movements, seizures, stupor, severe hypotension, coma. (At this concentration, fatalities are secondary to pulmonary complications.)
> 3.0	Beginning of breakdown of many organ systems in the body.

Note: Treatment of toxicity: gastric lavage, hemodialysis (rapidly effective).

siness, drowsiness, slurred speech, and diplopia are frequently seen in early treatment. As the dose is lowered, symptoms subside.
  - Serious side effects include heart block, decreased white blood cell counts, and liver toxicity.

- Nursing Management of Patients Taking Anticonvulsant Drugs
  - Drug interactions may occur and should be watched for.
  - A baseline complete blood count and differential and an ECG are done; and a careful history regarding renal and hepatic function also is done.
  - Patients are carefully observed for colds, fevers, and flu-like symptoms, because of the hematologic effects of these drugs.
  - Anticonvulsant drugs should not be administered within 2 weeks of receiving MAO inhibitors.

- **ANTIDEPRESSANT DRUGS**

  Identifying Depression (Chapter 20)

  Depressive states have been classified as: bipolar disorder, depressed; major depressive disorders; dysthymic disorders; bereavement and adjustment disorders with depressed mood; and mood disorder due to a general medical condition or secondary to substance abuse.

- Bipolar disorder depressions are depressed states associated with a history of mania or hypomania. Bipolar depression is treated with antidepressants and lithium. While treatment of bipolar affective disorders with antidepressants is often effective, the potential exists for development of mania secondary to pharmacotherapy.

- Major depressive disorders, both a single episode and chronic depressions, are treated effectively with antidepressants. Major depressive episodes frequently coexist with other psychiatric or medical disorders, such as personality disorder, and may be treated with antidepressants. Persons with anxiety disorders or schizophrenia often benefit from antidepressants if depression is part of their symptomatology.

- Mood disorders secondary to medical conditions

  - If the depressed mood is thought to be a direct consequence of a major medical problem, then the appropriate diagnosis is mood disorder due to a medical problem; antidepressants may not be used. If, however, the depression is thought to be a psychological sequela from the medical condition, then the diagnosis is major depression and antidepressants can be used.

  - In persons who abuse drugs, if the history and evaluation clearly reveal present and past depressive symptoms, a major depressive episode is diagnosed and may be treated with antidepressants.

- Dysthymia usually requires a two-year history of depressive syndrome. The ongoing quality of the person's life and the ability to live it to its full potential are impaired. Antidepressants are being used to treat these mild depressive symptoms, to prevent worsening of the condition and to help people improve their overall social and occupational functioning and level of happiness.

- Situation depressive states are marked by a clear precipitant. Symptoms may include tearfulness, brooding, feelings of tension, preoccupation with a loss, loss of appetite, and insomnia. These states are usually self-limiting, but occasionally become symptomatic of a major depression, requiring more intensive treatment with antidepressants.

Antidepressive Drug Action (Study Guide Table 42-8)

The main predictor of what will be an effective therapy for a patient is a history of positive or negative responses to psychiatric drugs in the patient or in the patient's immediate blood-related family.

- Antidepressant medication is used primarily to treat depression, but may also be used for anxiety, eating and personality disorders, and other previously mentioned conditions.

- Antidepressants increase the concentration of certain neurotransmitters, e.g., norepinephrine and serotonin, within hours to days.

TABLE 42–8.
ANTIDEPRESSANT DRUGS

Class	Generic (Trade) Names	Daily Dosage
Tricyclic antidepressants (TCAs)	Amitriptyline (Elavil)	75 to 300 mg
	Clomipramine (Anafranil)	100 to 250 mg[a]
	Desipramine (Norpramin)	75 to 300 mg
	Doxepin (Sinequan)	50 to 300 mg
	Imipramine (Tofranil)	75 to 300 mg
	Nortriptyline (Pamelor)	75 to 150 mg
	Protriptyline (Vivactil)	15 to 60 mg
	Trimipramine (Surmontil)	75 to 300 mg
Monoamine oxidase inhibitors (MAOIs)	Isocarboxazid (Marplan)	20 to 40 mg
	Phenelzine (Nardil)	30 to 90 mg
	Tranylcypromine (Parnate)	10 to 60 mg
Serotonin re-uptake inhibitors (SSRIs)	Fluvoxamine (Luvox)	50 to 200 mg[a]
	Fluoxetine (Prozac)	10 to 80 mg
	Sertraline (Zoloft)	50 to 200 mg
	Paroxetine (Paxil)	10 to 50 mg
Miscellaneous antidepressants	Trazodone (Desyrel)	50 to 450 mg
	Bupropion (Wellbutrin)	150 to 450 mg[b]
	Venlafaxine (Effexor)	75 to 375 mg
	Nefazodone (Serzone)	200 to 600 mg
	Lithium carbonate (Lithane, Eskalith)	750 to 2,500 mg

[a] Currently approved only for obsessive compulsive disorder.
[b] No single dose may exceed 150 mg.
Reproduced from Schatzberg and Nemeroff, 1995.

The monoamine oxidase inhibitors are one exception.

MONOAMINE OXIDASE INHIBITORS (MAOIs)

- Monoamine oxidase inhibitors have both peripheral and central neuronal action. MAO is responsibile for destroying many substances within the body; inhibition of this action within the cell reduces the metabolism of endogenous amines and exogenous monoamines, thereby increasing their concentration.
- When MAOIs are used in conjunction with foods containing tyramine (closely related structurally to epinephrine and norepinephrine, with similar but weaker action), MAOIs can cause severe hypertension and stroke.
- Hypertensive crisis is characterized by marked increase in blood pressure and accompanied by one or more of the following: severe occipital headache, neck pain, sweating, nausea, and vomiting. Consequences may include stroke, coma, or death. Because MAOIs have significant adrenergic effects, a patient's food intake becomes most important when MAOIs are being taken. Hypertensive crisis may be caused by the ingestion of foods that contain tyramine as well as by sympathomimetic drugs. Foods containing tyramine include aged cheese, red wine, sherry, beer, fermented foods.
- MAOIs may cause hypotension and relief from angina pectoris.
- MAOIs can antagonize some of the pharmacologic and biochemical effects of reserpine, which is used to treat hypertension.

SELECTIVE SEROTONIN REUPTAKE INHIBITORS (SSRIs)

- SSRIs are among the newer antidepressants. They target one specific neurotransmitter: serotonin. Act acutely primarily at the nerve synapse to block the processes that allow endogenous amine to be absorbed into the presynaptic neurons.
- SSRIs have fewer of the uncomfortable side effects of some of the other antidepressants, e.g., the anticholinergic, sedative, and cardiac effects.

OTHER NEW ANTIDEPRESSANTS: TRAZODONE, BUPRO-
PION, VENLAFAXINE, AND NEFAZODONE

- Have varied effects on the pre- and postsynaptic norepinephrine and serotonin receptors and little effect on cholinergic, histaminergic, and alpha-adrenergic receptors.

Catecholamine Theory of Depression

It is hypothesized that certain depressive states are caused by a depletion of catecholamines at receptor sites and that mania is caused by excesses of catecholamines at receptor sites.

Theory has been expanded to include indolamine and other biogenic amines, hormones, and ionic changes.

Current thinking underscores that a cogent theory of depression must integrate observations at the chemical, anatomical, and behavioral levels.

Dosage Considerations and Clinical Treatment of Depression

• Trends show that SSRIs and new agents are the most widely prescribed antidepressants, primarily due to the different side effect profiles that these drugs have. They are relatively safe from overdose when compared with the tricyclic antidepressants and the MAOIs.

• When initiating the dosage of most antidepressants, the objective is to move slowly to a dose that can be tolerated by the patient.

• Usually morning doses are given of drugs that lead to insomnia, and afternoon or evening doses of drugs that have sedative effects.

• Administering a single-dose drug is preferable; however some drugs require multiple doses (bupropion, venlafaxine, and nefazodone).

• Preventing suicide is important. Taking a drug must begin in a cooperative, safe, interpersonal context. Overdose can be fatal.

• The drug effect of tricyclics is achieved 2 to 3 weeks after the maximum dose has been reached. This time lag is dangerous for suicidal patients.

• Safety has not been established for any antidepressant medications for pregnant or lactating women.

Nursing Management of Patients Taking Antidepressant Drugs

TABLE 42–9
MAJOR SIDE EFFECTS OF SELECTED ANTIDEPRESSANT DRUGS

| Antidepressant | Relative Side Effects | | | |
	Anticholinergic	Anxiety	Insomnia	Sedation
Tricyclic antidepressants (TCAs)				
Desipramine	Mild	Mild	Rare	Mild
Nortriptyline	Mild	Mild	Rare	Mild
Amitriptyline	Moderate	Rare	Mild	Moderate–severe
Imipramine	Mild	Mild	Mild	Moderate–severe
Clomipramine	Moderate	Moderate	Mild	Severe
Serotonin reuptake inhibitors (SSRIs)				
Huoxetine	Rare	Moderate	Moderate	Mild*
Fluvoxamine	Rare	Moderate	Moderate	Mild*
Sertraline	Rare	Moderate	Moderate	Mild*
Paroxetine	Rare	Moderate	Moderate	Mild*
Atypical antidepressants				
Trazodone	Rare	Mild	Rare	Moderate–severe
Bupropion	Rare	Moderate	Moderate	Mild
Venlafaxine	Rare	Moderate	Moderate	Mild
Nefazodone	Rare	Mild	Rare	Moderate
MAO inhibitors				
Phenelyzine	Mild	Mild	Moderate–severe	Moderate–severe
Tranylcypromine	Mild	Mild	Moderate	Moderate–severe

*Increased levels of sedation have been reported with higher doses.
Adapted from Teicher et al., 1993.

- Assessment of Side Effects

    MAOIs AND HETEROCYCLICS have a higher incidence of anticholinergic and adrenergic effects on body systems.

    STUDY GUIDE TABLE 42-9 lists major side effects of antidepressant drugs.

- Beginning Treatment

    CARDIOVASCULAR SYMPTOMS, such as postural hypotension, dizziness, tachycardia, and palpitations, are common at the beginning of tricyclics and MAOI use. Before starting the drug, check patient's blood pressure while he or she is lying and sitting; then check it weekly, with the patient in both positions, after the drug is started. Advise the patient to arise slowly in the morning.

    GASTROINTESTINAL SYMPTOMS may include nausea and vomiting. Advise patients to take drug with food. There may be weight gain and increased appetite. Teach patients about exercise and diet. For constipation, a stool softener is appropriate.

    INTERNAL ANXIETY AND AKATHISIA are difficult to tolerate. The nurse should try to assist patients to identify and distinguish between the two states.

    SEXUAL DYSFUNCTION may occur and needs to be addressed.

    INSOMNIA AND DAYTIME SEDATION may be addressed by timing medication administration.

    HEADACHES should be assessed to determine whether they are part of the depression symptomatology; if they are not, treat them with an analgesic.

    SYMPTOMS OF MANIA may develop. Patients and families should be instructed about what symptoms to watch for.

    OVERDOSE is a serious problem with the tricyclics, MAOIs, and bupropion; a patient should not be given large amounts of these

medications. One week's supply is sufficient.
- Determining Blood Levels
  Antidepressant drug blood levels are generally obtained only for those drugs that show a relationship between response to the drug and the therapeutic level. Determining plasma levels of antidepressant drugs will assist the clinician to:
  - Identify those patients who develop very high plasma levels with low doses.
  - Document the therapeutic plasma level in an individual patient at the time of clinical response as a guide to treating future episodes.
  - If patient responds and then relapses with a given dose, document compliance or possible short-term metabolic changes.
  - Explore why a patient fails to respond to a standard dose of an antidepressant drug.
  - Investigate possible causes for pronounced side effects using small drug doses.
- **ANXIETY, LIKE DEPRESSION, IS A HUMAN EXPERIENCE THAT TOUCHES EVERYONE** (see Chapter 14). Anxiety that is severe (panic) and that may be associated with physical problems must be reduced. Antianxiety drugs are beneficial, and their effectiveness is often immediate. The drugs may reduce immediate symptoms of anxiety, such as narrowed perception, disrupted thinking, and the distracting muscular and autonomic symptoms of tension that interfere with the person's taking charge of his or her life. In the case of anxiety associated with physical illness, reducing anxiety is essential to facilitate more specific interventions.

  In assessing anxiety, the following principles will be useful guidelines:
  - Anxiety is an essential dimension of the human condition.
  - Symptoms associated with anxiety can be understood as emanating from social (psychological), somatic, or biological events.
  - Intense anxiety is usually one symptom of a major psychiatric disorder. It must be effectively reduced, as it disrupts rational thinking and problem solving.
  - Treating anxiety disorders with medication

may require long-term measures. Other interventions, such as cognitive restructuring and behavior therapy, are often combined with pharmacotherapy. Frequently, both strategies are used and they enhance each other's effectiveness. Psychotherapy often helps persons suffering major trauma. Understanding the nature and severity of anxiety can offer a framework for more enduring intervention.
- Continued use of drugs to manage anxiety presents many health professionals with ethical considerations; the drugs can be abused and, in some instances, lead to addiction.

Anxiolytics (Antianxiety Drugs)

Anxiolytics, also called antianxiety drugs, are used to treat anxiety (see Study Guide Table 42-10). Antidepressants may also be administered.

Antianxiety drugs are beneficial in treating acute or chronic distress; however, their true usefulness depends on the patient's attitude concerning the drug.

Choice of the Antianxiety Drug

Diagnosis of the patient is usually the deciding factor regarding the drug used. Benzodiazepines have hypnotic and muscle relaxant qualities, and clonazepam has anticonvulsive properties. The benzodiazepines and SRRIs are safer for the potentially suicidal patient because they have a wider margin of safety (toxic versus therapeutic dose). Toxic effects are rare. Antidepressants are preferred for patients with panic disorders and for those with a history of substance abuse, as benzodiazepine has an addictive potential. Benzodiazepines are effective in treating symptoms of panic disorder and generalized anxiety disorder.

Antianxiety Drug Action

- Acts at all levels of the central nervous system, particularly the limbic system and reticular formation.
- Benzodiazepines increase the effects of the inhibitory neurotransmitter GABA in the brain, and thereby produce a calming effect. GABA is the major neurotransmitter involved in the etiology of anxiety.

General Precautions and Contraindications

TABLE 42–10
ANTIANXIETY DRUGS AND ANTIDEPPESSANTS USED TO TREAT ANXIETY DISORDERS

Chemical Group	Generic (Trade) Names	Average Daily Dosage
Benzodiazepines	Alprazolam (Xanax)	0.75 to 6 mg
	Adnazolam	
	Chlordiazepoxide (Librium)	15 to 100 mg
	Clonazepam (Klonopin)	1 to 4 mg
	Diazepam (Valium)	5 to 40 mg
	Halazepam (Paxipam)	60 to 160 mg
	Lorazepam (Ativan)	2 to 6 mg
	Oxazepam (Serax)	30 to 120 mg
	Prazepam (Centrax)	10 to 60 mg
Nonbenzodiazepine anxiolytic	Buspirone (Buspar)	15 to 60 mg
Antidepressants	Fluoxetine (Prozac)	5 to 80 mg
	Sertraline (Zoloft)	25 to 200 mg
	Paroxetine (Paxil)	10 to 50 mg
	Fluvoxamine (Luvox)	50 to 200 mg
	Imipramine	50 to 300 mg
	Clomipramine	25 to 250 mg
	Phenelzine (Nardil)	30 to 90 mg

Adapted from Schatzberg and Nemeroff, American Psychiatric Press Textbook of Psychopharmacology. Washington, DC: American Psychiatric Press, 1995.

- Any patient with a hypersensitivity to drugs within the anxiolytics classification should not use these drugs.
- Antianxiety drugs should not be taken in combination with other central nervous system depressants.
- Contraindications include pregnancy and lactation, narrow-angle glaucoma, shock, and coma.
- Be cautious with patients, especially the elderly, who have hepatic or renal dysfunction.
- No alcoholic beverages should be consumed with these drugs.
- Certain people with diagnoses such as borderline personality disorder may respond paradoxically.

Side effects
- Drowsiness, confusion, lethargy (most common side effects)
- Tolerance: physical and psychological dependence (does not apply to buspirone)
- Potentiates the effects of other central nervous system depressants
- Paradoxical excitement and disinhibition
- Dry mouth
- Alteration in sleep, particularly the stages of sleep

Physical Dependence
Physical dependence can occur. Abrupt discontinuation may be life-threatening or lead to serious effects that persist for 2 to 3 weeks. Patient has withdrawal symptoms, such as increased anxiety, palpitations, sweating, and insomnia.

Advantages of the Benzodiazepines
These drugs relieve anxiety rapidly; there is high tolerability, and serious side effects are few. The drugs break down in the liver and tend to have a long half-life. They are not excreted rapidly from the body; in the elderly, the benzodiazepines can become toxic. Whether the benzodiazepine is long- or short-acting determines how often it is given.

Buspirone
This anxiolytic is thought to be as effective as a benzodiazepine without the potential for addiction. It does not interact with alcohol. Anxiety is not effectively relieved, however, for 4 weeks. A patient taking buspirone should not drive or operate other dangerous equipment because sedation is a potential side effect. If headache does not subside with time, analgesics may be ordered. To minimize gastrointestinal distress, instruct the patient to ingest the drug with food.

TAKING ANOTHER LOOK

You are now ready to respond to questions that were raised in Gaining a Perspective at the beginning of this chapter. After you have written or thought about your responses, you may wish to look at the Suggested Responses on page 337.

43 CRITICAL PATHWAYS FOR MENTAL HEALTH AND PLANNING CARE

GAINING A PERSPECTIVE

Think about the issues suggested in the questions below, and after you have read the Key Concepts for this chapter discuss your answers in more depth.

1. What benefits do critical pathways have for mental health care planning?

2. What problems do you foresee in using critical pathways in nursing practice?

KEY CONCEPTS

- **A PLAN OF CARE IS FORMULATED AFTER A NURSING ASSESSMENT AND DIAGNOSIS ARE COMPLETED.** Together, the patient and nurse will recognize behaviors that are manifested and determine which need improvement or change, what strengths are available to bring to bear on the process, and what resources are needed. Critical pathways will provide the framework for implementation of Standards of Care III, IV, V, and VI.

- **PATHWAYS FOR MENTAL HEALTH**

  What Is a Pathway or Map?

  A pathway is the basis for a treatment plan for clinical care of patients with a given psychiatric diagnosis. A pathway can also be used to describe the care processes used for patients admitted to a level of care within a continuum. The pathway is a multidisciplinary care plan, replacing single disciplinary plans. Other pathway functions relate to cost and quality improvement and provider process improvement.

    An example of a pathway is the CareMap® (see Study Guide Table 43-1).

    Elements of a pathway include a problem list, outcomes and suboutcomes, a time line, task categories, and a variance coding system. When a map is used as the care plan, it describes the typical approach for the average patient in a case type, such as major depression or psychosis. Interventions, process tasks, and expected outcomes are described in relation to each other across time. Study Guide Table 43-2 shows the pathway concept.

  Why Might Mental Health Systems Use Pathway and Map Systems?

  - Trends in mental health care delivery demand that systems have coordinated case management and outcome measurement systems.
  - All patients deserve to be managed efficiently and effectively.
  - Pathway tools and systems are strategies for

TABLE 43–1
PARTIAL COPY OF A CAREMAP® FOR ADOLESCENTS WITH DEPRESSION

Problems/Focus or Outcomes	Day 1	Day 2
1. Axis I Concerns: Diagnostic assessment: clarification, neurological, major MI or other developmental disorder. Safety: SI/HI, impulse dyscontrol Mood: depression, anxiety, veg.s/s. Behaviors: rejection of authority, limit testing, regression, non-compliance, poor socialization, poor adaptation, impulse dyscontrol.	Meets team, discusses safety plans, states understanding of rights and responsibilities, no behavioral incidents or injury.	Participates in treatment planning, groups, individual counseling. Completes assignments with assistance, as necessary. No behavioral incidents or injury.
2. Axis II: Character or personality traits effecting depression.	Begins MMPI.	Identifies staff to whom they are able to talk.
3. Axis III: Co-existing medical conditions; medical management.	Patient/family share medical history. Completes health activities or medical testing as prescribed.	Completes health activities or medical testing as prescribed.
4. Axis IV: Psychosocial stressors: Family, school, or community service provider (CSP) issues.	Discusses recent stressors and supports or lack of supports.	Discusses emotional response to stressors in group/individual meetings.
5. Axis V: GAF, other scores.	GAF:_____	Other scores:_____
Assessments/consults.	Physical examination, psycho-social–behavioral assessment, vital signs (VS), weight, mental status exam (MSE), safety/suicide risk assessments, pediatrician, OT/RT, education, neurological, psychological.	Assess: MSE, VS, adjustment to milieu, safety behaviors, degree of participation in care, family/significant other (SO) involvement, visits, OT/RT, psychology.
Specimens/tests.	Adolescent screens, U/A, toxic screen, drug levels.	GAF: 1 to 50, Hamilton, BPRS, BSI, ASI, or other.
Safety, containment, milieu management and treatment.	Unit restriction until first team meeting, precaution checks as necessary, discuss safety contracts, counseling within groups and individually.	Form activity schedule; Develop coping plans: anger, depression, behaviors, increase privileges as appropriate. Identify motivators; encourage strengths.
Medications.	Obtain medical history; meds as ordered.	Evaluate for prn or standing doses.
Nutrition/diet.	Diet as tolerated	Monitor intake.
Teaching.	Orientation to unit layout and routines, staff, team, rights, responsibilities.	Teaching re: coping skills, anger management, substance use, meds, school.
Discharge planning.	Family/SO identified, agrees to be involved; CSP or other agencies contacted.	Team meeting, family meeting scheduled.

Day 3	Day 4	Day 5
Participates in treatment planning, groups, individual counseling. Completes assignments with assistance, as necessary. States +/– gains. No behavioral incidents or injury.	Participates in treatment planning, groups, individual counseling. Completes assignments with assistance as necessary. States +/– gains. No behavioral incidents or injury.	Participates in treatment planning, individual counseling. Completes assignments with assistance, as necessary. States +/– gains. No behavioral incidents or injury.
Continues to form working relationships with staff.	Continues to form working relationships with staff.	Continues to form working relationships with staff.
Completes health activities or medical testing as prescribed.	Completes health activities or medical testing as prescribed.	Completes health activities or medical testing as prescribed.
Identifies steps to take to cope with stressors.	Uses coping plans as able.	Uses coping plans as able.
Other scores:_____	Other scores:_____	Other scores:_____
Assess: MSE, VS, adjustment to milieu, safety behaviors, degree of participation in care, family/SO involvement and patient's response to the involvement, school functioning.	Assess: MSE, VS, adjustment to milieu, safety behaviors, degree of participation in care, family/SO involvement and patient's response to the involvement, school functioning.	Assess: MSE, VS, adjustment to milieu, safety behaviors, degree of participation in care, family/SO involvement and patient's response to the involvement, school functioning.
As ordered :	As ordered.:	As ordered.:
Encourage activities per plan, strengths, use of coping plans: anger, depression, behaviors, increase privileges as appropriate. Identify and use appropriate motivators.	Encourage activities, strengths, use of coping plans: anger, depression, behaviors, increase privileges as appropriate. Identify and use appropriate motivators.	Encourage activities, strengths, use of coping plans: anger, depression, behaviors, increase privileges as appropriate. Identify and use appropriate motivators.
Prn or standing doses.	Prn or standing doses.	Prn or standing doses. Best med plan determined.
Monitor intake.	Monitor intake.	Monitor intake.
Teaching re: coping skills, anger management, substance use, meds, school.	Reinforce teaching as necessary. Continue school/ tutoring schedule.	Reinforce teaching as necessary. Continue school/ tutoring schedule.
Team meeting, include CSP in DCP discussions.	Case conference (include CSP, patient if possible).	Team meeting.

From Andolina K. The Center for Case Managemet, 1996. *The CareMap® Tool and System.* Copyright The Center for Case Management, South Natick, Mass.

TABLE 43–2.
PATHWAY CONCEPT

Outcomes/ Problems/Focus	Time
1.	Patient/family outcomes, goals written progressively across time.
2.	Outcomes: patient/family participation, knowledge, behaviors, skills, agreements, etc.
	Example Staff Tasks and Processes for Care
1. Assessments	Vital signs, OT assessment, nursing assessment, mental status assessments.
2. Specimens/tests	Toxic screens, blood tests, psychiatric testing.
3. Treatments	Milieu therapy, one-to-one counseling, therapeutic approach, group programs.
4. Medications	Medical protocols, MD medication preferences, standing orders, medical consents.
5. Nutrition/diet	Diet orders, monitor intake.
6. Safety/activity	Privileges, precautions.
7. Teaching	Coping, anxiety management.
8. Discharge planning	Contact community providers, refer to home care, family meetings, team meetings, etc.

achieving care coordination in mental health systems.

What Are Some of the Benefits of Using Pathways?

- Lengths of stay are stabilized within the proper level of care.
- Consistent care approaches and processes for care management are facilitated.
- A path is a method for implementing quality changes.
- Paths provide a process for improvement, such as improved consistency in assessments, discharge planning, patient education, and team communication.

Are Pathways Developed by Psychiatric Diagnosis?

- Pathways often use "case types"; case typing is describing characteristics common to a population.
- Psychiatric population characteristics include the psychiatric diagnosis, age/gender groupings, medical needs, complexities, and other information that details the patient who will fit the case type.

How Is the Pathway a "System"?

- A pathway must have policies and procedures for development, implementation, and evaluation.
- The pathway provides for continuity of the plan among all disciplines and departments concerned with the case type/patient.
- Pathway system designs are unique in many ways to each organization, but they accomplish the same goal of provider-controlled managed care for patients.
- A variance is the difference between what has been planned as stated on the map and what actually occurs. Variance data are neither good or bad; they are simply pieces of information. Variances can be related to the patient or family, provider, system, or community; however, in mental health they tend to be more patient related. Variance data, which can be numerically coded for computer analysis, are used by care givers to improve organizaitonal performance, design plans of action, provide evidence of aggregate clinical outcomes, and problem-solve for quality concerns.

How Are Pathways Used to Manage Quality?

Revisions of pathways provide a track record of improvement. For example, when variance data indicate that the outcome "patient involvement in care planning" is below expectation, the path design group details what specific actions to take to improve outcome. This is an example of "retrospective continuous quality improvement" (CQI). In concurrent CQI, caregivers implement corrective actions to manage variances detected day by day.

What Is the Relationship of Clinical Case Management to Pathways?

- Clinical case management is a clinical system that focuses on the accountability of an identified individual or group for coordinating a patient's care across a continuum.
- Clinical case managers may or may not use pathways to help manage complex cases. Often case managers are called to assist in

the management of a patient on a pathway whose care has become complex. Clinical case managers may facilitate writing the map, collect data from or for a path development, or rely on paths to document outcomes.

How Would A Pathway Be Helpful If a Good System of Care Management Is in Place?

- The pathway helps provide evidence of care.
- Communicating expected results across all disciplines is becoming more important to caregivers across shifts/departments/settings, to payors, cost managers, and administrators.

How Does the Patient/Family Benefit From the Care Plan?

- When patients and their families see the path, they view it as a contract.
- It controls expectations, allowing caregivers to negotiate the context and results of care in the absence of an emotionally charged environment.
- A path describes a consensus of clinical management thought and is aimed at reducing unnecessary variation in clinical practice.

What Happens If a Patient Has Too Many Complications and Does Not Fit the Pathway?

- Depending on how specific the pathway is, there may be a great deal of variance.
- In order to customize a patient's care, the caregiver may change or add statements to the path as required, switch to a more appropriate map, or remove the patient from the map if it no longer fits.
- Some paths include common complications; clinicians can "opt-in" or "opt-out" of the problems as assessment indicates.

In What Patient Situations Would a Path Not Be Appropriate?

For an extremely complex patient or when the actual patterns of care are not yet apparent, case managers, as care evaluators, provide the best opportunity to discover the issues of coordination and care management. Case managers will develop the plan of care accordingly.

How Can Data Be Obtained From a Pathway?

- The pathway itself can serve as a collection tool.

- A separate variance tracking form can be used to preprint indicators, document the variance, and collect and analyze the data.
- Data can be obtained from automated computer systems.

How Do Pathways Fit Into the Practice Guideline Movement?

- Practice guidelines are more extensive descriptors of the care of populations, diagnoses, or conditions.
- Practice guidelines are not day-to-day management tools as pathways are, but they provide the context and data that back up the content within the pathway tool.

When Several Disciplines Function in a Generic Clinician Role, How Can a Pathway Show Differences in Approach to That Role?

- Pathways begin to get all caregivers "on the same page" by focusing on patient-centered outcomes. Caregivers define their special contributions to care, establishing and clarifying ownership of their contributions.
- It is often not a single discipline contribution in mental health care that makes a difference, but rather the cumulative effect of consistent caregiver actions.

Will Pathways in Mental Health Show Cost and Quality Results of Care?

- Pathways describe results in terms of outcomes, which is measurable and objective terminology.
- Even in mental health where a patient's progress is often a subjective measurement, some quality issues can and must be defined. As an example, the National Committee for Quality Assurance developed the Healthplan Employer Data and Information Set (HEDIS) project to collect information from organizations. The HEDIS standards for mental health reflect the following criteria:
  - Ambulatory patient follow-up within 30 days of hospitalization.
  - Standards for triage, treatment approach, case management, alternative treatment settings, outcomes measurement, benefit design, access, quality management, prevention, education, and early intervention.

Can Mental Health Workers Document on a Map?

- Nonprofessional staff and per diem staff rely on pathways for information about the day-to-day management as well as the "big picture."
- Nonprofessional staff will document tasks completed; however, the outcomes of care remain within the realm of professional assessment and are to be signed off only by professional staff.

Is It Possible to Define an Approach in Behavioral or Psychiatric Mental Health In Terms of the Categories Stated on a Pathway?

- The care categories on the pathway can be changed to reflect a facility's environment.
- Many facilities, while they use the classic eight categories of care (e.g., assessments/consults, medications), dedicate separate rows to other disciplines such as psychology and social work or to treatment modalities, such as milieu and group programs.
- Sometimes categories are reduced to assessments, treatments, and discharge planning as the only essential categories of care.

Are Pathways Flexible Enough to Address the Varied Reasons That Patients/Families Seek or Need Care?

- Although patient preparation varies, the rationale for admission to a given level of care is becoming less variable. Managed care requires that facilities develop utilization (level of care) criteria.
- While it seems that scope of care is being reduced in each setting, responsible care across the continuum is increasingly becoming the focus of most organizations and payers.
- The best organizations are affiliating with a number of diverse settings, both public and private, to support the highest level of wellness and prevention for psychiatric patients within their own community.

TAKING ANOTHER LOOK

You are now ready to respond to the questions that were raised in Gaining a Perspective at the beginning of this chapter. After you have written or thought about your responses, you may wish to look at the Suggested Responses on page 337.

44 CASE MANAGEMENT

GAINING A PERSPECTIVE

Think about the questions below, and after you have read the Key Concepts for this chapter respond to the queries in greater detail.

1. Why are nurses in a good position to manage care for psychiatric patients?

2. Why do you think that the community-based psychiatric mental health nurse case manager model is workable?

KEY CONCEPTS

- **AS CARE SHIFTS FROM INSTITUTIONAL TO COMMUNITY-BASED SYSTEMS, PSYCHIATRIC NURSES ARE REQUIRED TO ADAPT TO EXPANCED ROLES** and, at the same time, preserve psychiatric nursing knowledge. Changes in health care delivery systems also suggest that professionals will work less as individual care providers and more as part of multidisciplinary teams focusing on an entire episode of illness, rather than on the most acute piece. The emphasis will be patient-centered care that is coordinated and outcome-focused.

- **CASE MANAGEMENT IN HEALTH CARE,** as a coordinating and evaluation strategy, was first practiced in the 1980s when nursing took the lead in establishing care management programs for patients with certain diagnoses. Those initiatives demonstrated dramatic results in cost stabilization, quality improvement, and understanding the realistic care processes for populations of patients.

- **CASE MANAGEMENT IS DEFINED AS** a clinical system that focuses on the accountability of an identified individual or group for coordinating a patient's or group of patients' continuum of care. Accountability addresses the following:

  - Insuring and facilitating the achievement of quality clinical and cost outcomes

  - Negotiating, procuring, and coordinating services and resources needed by the patient and family

  - Intervening at key points and/or at significant variances for individual patients

  - Addressing and resolving patterns in aggregate variances that have a negative quality or cost impact

  - Creating opportunities and systems to enhance outcomes

  Case management roles assumed by psychiatric nurses present another opportunity, other than primary care, to apply professional skill and clinical reasoning to psychiatric mental health nursing.

- **LOOKING BEYOND THE IMMEDIATE SETTING FOCUS AND INTO THE NEAR FUTURE, THE NURSE CASE MANAGER USES THE NURSING PROCESS** to assist the patient toward identified outcomes. The patient is supported in attaining outcomes beyond the immediate setting. The absence of a practice model that promotes collaborative, outcome-based practice dooms achievement to mere chance.

  Patients and their families want care to be predictable and compatible with their resources. When clinical cases are managed by psychiatric nurses familiar with the patient and the patient's history, the result can be early mobilization of resources and further episodes are more likely to be prevented. Nurses are in an excellent position to coordinate care and manage outcomes.

- **SYSTEMS OF CARE DELIVERY ARE NEEDED THAT PRESERVE QUALITY CLINICAL PRACTICE, EMPHASIZE OUTCOME ATTAINMENT, AND CONTAIN COSTS ACCORDINGLY.** Until recently, clinical care providers have not tracked both cost and quality. Instead, this information was split among care providers, support services, and payer systems, which fragments the picture of cost and quality.

  All care requires managing. Clinical case management, as a strategy for managing care, positions the professional care provider as the source of accountability for coordinated outcome-based care. Care is proactively planned; thereby results are anticipated, and interventions not left to chance.

- **VARIOUS PROGRAMS OF CASE MANAGEMENT HAVE BEEN DESIGNED.**

  A system-wide approach to cost accountability utilizes case management initiatives for the facility.

  Case management initiatives at a unit, or local, level may be a first initiative.

  Goals for case management include:
  - To increase coordination of complex processes and case type needs
  - To link actual costs to care
  - To define and measure outcomes
  - To decrease costs, while stabilizing and improving quality
  - To enhance collaborative practice
  - To improve patient satisfaction
  - To operationalize continuous quality improvement at the care management level
  - To clarify accountability for processes and outcomes.

- **THE CASE MANAGER ROLE MUST BE CLEARLY DEFINED** when psychiatric nurses undertake the responsibilities (see Study Guide Table 44-1).

  A short list of responsibilities includes:
  - Assessment
  - Planning
  - Intervention/coordination
  - Monitoring and evaluation

  The long list of responsibilities includes:
  - Facilitating development of care paths/maps
  - Facilitating collaborative practice
  - Conducting daily utilization reviews
  - Discharge planning
  - Nursing assessment
  - Joining health care team rounds
  - Negotiating with payers/insurers
  - Recording and correcting variances
  - Consulting with staff as variances occur
  - Coaching staff
  - Teaching patients and families
  - Collecting and preparing statistics
  - Giving direct care to assist staff
  - Making shift/home care assignments
  - Following up telephone calls
  - Consulting with peers
  - Keeping financial records

  If all responsibilities are to be undertaken, case management may be shared, with the psychiatric nurse accountable for the clinical aspects of care coordination. Disciplines and departments may share case management

TABLE 44–1.
SAMPLE CASE MANAGEMENT JOB DESCRIPTION

General Role Description

Coordinates, negotiates, procures, and manages the care of complex patients to facilitate achievement of quality and cost outcomes.

Works collaboratively with interdisciplinary staff internal and external to the organization.

Participates in quality improvement and evaluation processes related to the management of care.

Role Functions

Identifies patients for case management services.

Develops a network of the usual services and disciplines required by a typical patient in the case type.

Establishes a coordinating system of care spanning each geographic area of care.

Establishes methods for tracking patient progress across the continuum of care.

Maintains a working knowledge of payer requirements for the case type.

Maintains a working knowledge of community resources available for patients and families.

Demonstrates flexibility and creativity in identifying resources to meet patient and family needs.

Establishes a collaborative communication system with MDs, payers, administrators, and other team members.

Explores, implements, and documents strategies used to decrease length of stay and resource consumption.

Evaluates the effects of case management on the target population.

Introduces self to the patient and family, explains the case manager role, and provides written information.

Tracks and assesses patients within the caseload to identify and confirm care plan.

In collaboration with the patient, team, payer, and available resources forms, implements, evaluates, and revises plan of care.

Manages each patient transition through the system and transfers accountability to appropriate persons or agencies on discharge from case management services.

Maintains appropriate documentation of care and progress.

Coordinates, negotiates, and procures needed services and disciplines.

Communicates with other members of the health care team re: patient needs, plan, and responses to care.

Works collaboratively with team.

Identifies need for health care team meetings when necessary to facilitate coordination of complex services or resources.

Educates health care team colleagues about case management, including the role and unique needs of the case type population.

As a member of a case management practice seeks and provides peer consultation about problem cases, consistently attends meetings of the practice group and participates in them, participates in regular peer review, participates in quality review and case management evaluation processes, and arranges for and participates in coverage during long, short, and unexpected absences of self and other case managers.

Reviews pertinent literature about case types and shares with peers.

Adopted from Zander K, *The New Definition.* South Natick, Mass: The Center for Case Management, 1995.

within complex or inpatient facilities by taking the following actions:

- Merge department staff roles (utilization review/continuous quality improvement, social work, discharge planning, and clinical care roles) based on goals of specific case management programs and population

- Spell out expected role description and behaviors

- Define regular case management planning meetings, peer review, and peer consultation

- Define indicators for health care team meetings and case consultations

- Establish which caregivers to consult when accountability is an issue

- Increase the frequency and quality of meetings in proportion to the need for a daily unit-based management system

- **DEFINING WHICH POPULATIONS WILL BE ASSIGNED CASE MANAGEMENT EFFORTS AND WHEN** is another important responsibility of case managers. Sometimes only the most complex patients require case managers (see Study Guide Table 44-2).

- **A SUCCESSFUL CASE MANAGER IS USUALLY A HIGHLY SKILLED CLINICIAN WITH GOOD CLINICAL JUDGMENT AND HIGHLY REGARDED AND TRUSTED BY COL-**

TABLE 44–2.
MENTAL HEALTH CASE TYPES TARGETED FOR CASE MANAGEMENT INITIATIVES

High Cost	Unpredictable	Significant Variance	Repeat Admits	High Risk	Program Mission	Complex Care: Multiple MDs, Units
Psychosis	Axis II	AWA (Absent Without Authority)	Axis II	Bipolar (rapid cyclers)	Affective disorders	Medical psychiatric patients
Depression	Dual diagnosis	Gesture		Anxiety/panic	Women's program	Chronic schizophrenia
Dual diagnosis	Alcohol/drug abuse	Restraint/seclusion		Males: dysphoric, angry		
Axis II		Major socioeconomic problems				
		Med nonresponsive				
		Medical psych				

Adapted from Andolina K, The Center for Case Management, 1995.

LEAGUES. Case managers know about systems, are creative, and appreciate the culture of patient care. They are good communicators, critical thinkers, evaluators and problem solvers, and skilled negotiators.

- **STANDARDS OF PSYCHIATRIC MENTAL HEALTH NURSING PRACTICE** support case management.

    Standard III, which refers to identification of outcomes and individualizing them for patients, provides direction for continuity of care.

    Standard V (f) presents the rationale and measurement criteria for case management. The psychiatric nurse case manager ensures continuity by maintaining a relationship with agencies and providers within the network of services the patient is using. Jurisdictions of care, however, are defined differently for individual patients, and psychiatric nurse case managers will encounter different continuity situations.

    Standard V (f) emphasizes patient centeredness (e.g., matching resources to needs and respecting the patient's wishes) and extending nursing accountability beyond narrow care settings (e.g., urging negotiation for additional services and maintaining relationships with agencies and individial providers to ensure continuity of care).

- **DEFINING WHEN CASE MANAGEMENT STRATEGIES ARE REQUIRED IS KEY TO TIMELY COORDINATION AND EVALUATION.** If multiple resources are not coordinated, patient outcomes could be at risk. Do you activate services on admission or by the nature of the case? The answer to this depends on established criteria: In some inpatient settings, case management begins when three or more serious complications, variances, or anticipated problems have been identified.

- **CRITICAL PATHWAYS DIRECTLY LINK ACTUAL CARE TO SPECIFIC CARE STANDARDS AND HELP MEASURE THE EXACT COSTS OF CARE.** In the CareMap® tool (See Chapter 43) the entire nursing process can be described in relation to a case management population. A communication system must be designed to support the flow of information acquired from critical pathways or CareMaps® (see Study Guide Table 44-3).

- **PSYCHIATRIC CASE MANAGERS FACE SIMULTANEOUS ACCOUNTABILITY ISSUES FOR COST/QUALITY AND ADVOCACY.** The case manager identifies conflicting agendas (unrealistic outcomes, unrealistic time frames) and then addresses the conflict as early as possible.

- **NURSE THERAPISTS WHO PROVIDE PSYCHOTHERAPY MAY EXPERIENCE ROLE CONFLICT WHEN CASE MANAGEMENT SERVICES ARE REQUIRED.** Because case management and psychotherapy are different services, nurses who are not comfortable switching roles may set up a referral relationship with case managers.

TABLE 44–3. PARTIAL SAMPLE: BIPOLAR AFFECTIVE DISORDER CAREMAP® TOOL (296.44) DRG 430.

Case type: bipolar affective disorder, 296.44. Description: dysphoric manic episode with psychotic features, high safety risk, may be rapid cycler (>4 episodes per year), requires medication evaluation, may present with noncompliance, financial, legal, or family problems. Length of stay: 10 days.

Problem/Focus	Emergency Room to Admission to Unit/Day 1	Day 2	Day 3	Day 4
1. Reason for admission (individualize)				
2. Pathological coping: safety, impulse control, difficulty functioning, maintaining roles	No injury to self/others; self-destructive impulses managed w/assist. Fam/SO has appts, phone #'s of unit and care-givers for contact.	No injury to self/others. Self-destructive impulses managed w/assist.	No injury to self/others. Self-destructive impulses managed w/assist.	No injury to self/others. Self-destructive impulses managed w/assist.
	Cooperates with initial behavioral/ medical management plan. Accepts meds.	Accepts meds.	Accepts meds.	Accepts meds.
3. Physiological: sleep, appetite, weight loss, increased motor activity	Cooperates with sleep, rest, activity plan w/assistance.	Cooperates with sleep, rest, activity plan w/assistance.	Follows sleep, rest, activity plan.	Follows sleep, rest, activity plan. Physical status stabilized.
4. Delusions (grandeur), denial	Shares thoughts, perceptions as appropriate with staff.	Shares thoughts, perceptions as appropriate with staff.	Shares thoughts, perceptions as appropriate with staff.	Stabilized or diminished psychotic features.
1. Assessment/consults	MD: H & P, med hx. RN: VS BID, Ht, Wt, assess health, nutrition, activity patterns, mental status, strengths, coping. Family/support hx. Nutrition consult prn. Medical consult prn. Psychopharm consult prn.	MD: evaluate for ECT.		
2. Specimens/tests	Routine admission labs, toxic screen, med levels.			
3. Treatments: Groups prescribed as appropriate for reasons for hospitalization	Destimulation program; compensatory health, diet, rest interventions.	Destimulation program. Compensatory health, diet, rest interventions. Groups as tol.	Destimulation program. Compensatory health, diet, rest interventions. Groups as tol.	Destimulation program. Compensatory health, diet, rest interventions. Groups as tol.
4. Medications	MD: med hx. RN: Collect meds brought in.	Med hx available, target s/s identified, initial antimanic regimen begun.		
5. Nutrition/diet: push fluids, finger foods unless contraindicated	Diet.	Diet.	Diet.	Diet.
6. Safety/activity	Unit restrict, routine checks, safety and impulse contracts negotiated. Introduce verbal and behavioral strategies.	Assess for level 1 privileges.	Level 1 privileges.	Level 1 privileges.
7. Teaching/support	Orient to room, staff, unit rules, boundaries. Offer support and consistency (avoid excessive verbal interventions until mania subsides).	Review/reinforce information as necessary. Orient to room, staff, unit rules, boundaries, meds. Offer support and consistency (avoid excessive verbal interventions until mania subsides).	Review/reinforce info as necessary: unit rules, boundaries, meds. Offer support and consistency (avoid excessive verbal interventions until mania subsides).	
8. Discharge planning	Contact w/fam/SO, information given	Contact out-patient care-givers.		Collaborative team meeting.

SO = Significant Other, H & P = History and Physical, VS = Vital Signs
Andolina K., Copyright CCM (1994).

Review & Study Guide

- **SOME OF THE MOST THORNY ISSUES IN DEFINING A PSYCHIATRIC NURSE CASE MANAGER ROLE** have to do with determining the parameters of the role. It would not be unusual for the psychiatric nurse to be the primary care nurse for some clients, a group therapist within the treatment community, a psychotherapist for some, and a case manager for others. Keeping roles straight in the nurse's own mind becomes as much a challenge as communicating which role is being enacted at any one time.

- **PSYCHIATRIC NURSE CASE MANAGERS MUST DEFINE THE SCOPE OF THEIR ROLE.** Case management may be a "within the walls" model; it uses different frameworks such as primary nursing, unit-based, clinical-ladder programs, or nurse-technician partnered models. A "beyond the walls" model focuses on the role of the community-based nurse case manager as both care coordinator and provider of preventive and health maintenance services. Case management beyond traditional geographic boundaries incurs costs that must be anticipated in order to provide a case management service that truly spans the continuum.

- **WHEN A PSYCHIATRIC NURSE CASE MANAGER ADDRESSES ISSUES IN PRACTICE THAT INTERFERE WITH PATIENTS ACHIEVING OUTCOMES,** collaborative practices are enhanced.

- **FORMAL REPORTING SYSTEMS,** such as indicator tracking, variance analysis, or outcomes measurements, are used by psychiatric nurse case managers to track the results of care. Once patient outcomes are measured and tracked over time, nurse case managers, as cost-quality leaders, are able to identify strategies that sustain results and consequently support care approaches that consistently succeed.

- **THE IMPACT OF THE PSYCHIATRIC NURSE CASE MANAGER ON PATIENT OUTCOMES AND THE NURSING PROFESSION MUST BE RESEARCHED** in order for the psychiatric nurse to thrive in the manager role. Psychiatric nurse case management requires research to test its scope and cost effectiveness and its application

and limits as a model that bridges population-based care and individual-based care.

TAKING ANOTHER LOOK

You are now ready to respond to the questions raised in Gaining a Perspective at the beginning of this chapter. After you have written or thought about your responses, you may wish to look at the Suggested Responses on page 338.

45 PSYCHIATRIC HOME HEALTH CARE

TERMS TO DEFINE

Carson's Model of Psychiatric Home Care

homebound status

National Alliance for the Mentally Ill (NAMI)

psychiatric home health care

reimbursement policies

supportive home care services

GAINING A PERSPECTIVE

Think about the following two questions, and after you have read the Key Concepts for this chapter present your ideas in greater detail.

1. What questions would you, as a nurse, consider when deciding whether psychiatric home care is appropriate for a particular patient?

2. How does a psychiatric nurse's experience working in home care generally differ from the experience working in a facility?

KEY CONCEPTS

- **AT HOME, SURROUNDED BY FAMILY AND POSSESSIONS, AN INDIVIDUAL MAY RESPOND TO CARE WITH A MORE PEACEFUL SPIRIT AND GREATER WILLINGNESS OF MIND AND BODY.** Yet formalized psychiatric care in the home did not begin until 1979 when Medicare agreed to reimburse home care agencies for providing psychiatric home care. At that time, the deinstitutionalization movement was well under way. As more patients were moved into the community, psychiatric providers became increasingly aware that many communities and families were unprepared. Psychiatric home care emerged as an alternative to facilitate a comprehensive continuum of care.

- **PSYCHIATRIC HOME CARE PROVIDES A BRIDGE TO EASE THE TRANSITION FOR PATIENTS LEAVING THE HOSPITAL AND MOVING BACK HOME.** In addition, home care is an anchor to assist patients to remain at home when stress threatens to destabilize the patient's situation. Generally, psychiatric home care is intermittent and transitional, rather than continuous or long-term.

- **THE OVERALL GOALS OF PSYCHIATRIC HOME CARE** are to shorten and/or prevent hospitalization, improve the patient's quality of life, and maximize the patient's potential to live at home. To achieve those goals, specific interventions will be helpful. Generally, the interventions facilitate the transition of emotionally and psychiatrically impaired individuals from acute and long-term facilities to family care or to other community-based living arrangements.

  - Support the individual and family to help them cope with the symptoms of psychiatric illness.

  - Provide respite to families and caretakers who are responsible for the continuous care of psychiatrically ill persons.

  - Inform the patient, family, and/or significant other about such issues as medication and diet regimens, interpersonal and communication strategies, and individual coping techniques.

- Intervene psychotherapeutically to maintain patients at their maximal functional level and retard further deterioration.

- Assist the patient to develop appropriate diversional activities.

- Assist the patient to develop appropriate social interaction skills.

- Coordinate the necessary follow-up services of other community-based health and social services.

- Assist the homebound patient to achieve a spiritual sense of well-being by finding purpose in his or her present situation and by accessing spiritual resources within the environment.

- Define the mental health needs of patients to the nonpsychiatric medical community.

- Collaborate with nursing schools to provide educational experiences for future mental health professionals.

- **AN APPROPRIATE MODEL FOR PSYCHIATRIC HOME CARE IS CARSON'S MODEL OF PSYCHIATRIC HOME CARE.** A home's architectural structure is used to illustrate this type of care.

  The Foundation of the model is a spiritual one.

  The nurse approaches the patient as a person of worth deserving care and respect. Patients need to relate to an ultimate other, to make sense out of their lives, and to answer questions such as, "Why am I here?"; "What is my purpose?"; "Do I make a difference?"

  The Walls of the model are relationship and assessment skills.

  • A detailed assessment is performed when care begins and continues as long as the nurse is involved in the patient's life.

  • Developing a trusting relationship is a primary goal. The alliance is critical to the patient's compliance with home care instructions.

  The Second Floor of the model consists of medication issues: patient compliance and knowledge about prescribed medications; administering parental medications; and drawing blood samples to determine serum levels of medications, such as Tegretol and lithium.

The Roof of the model is teaching/psychotherapeutic interventions and case management.

  • The patient is helped to establish a regimen of care.

  • The patient is linked with a support system of other people; care is coordinated with other providers.

- **PSYCHIATRIC HOME CARE IS PROVIDED THROUGH STATE-LICENSED AND MEDICARE-CERTIFIED HOME CARE AGENCIES OR SINGLE-SERVICE AGENCIES,** which in some states are not Medicare-certified. Three forces have increased the numbers of psychiatric patients receiving home care:

  - Increased public awareness of benefits

  - A dramatic growth in the population needing home health services, such as the dependent elderly

  - Cost containment pressures resulting in inpatients being discharged "quicker and sicker"

  Because the population using home care services is varied in age and needs, a broad range of services should be available.

  Direct nursing care provided by a psychiatric nurse to patients with primary DSM-IV Axis I psychiatric diagnoses or emotional problems that develop secondary to a medical diagnosis.

  Access to medical and nursing skills; dental care; pharmaceutical services; social services; physical, speech, and occupational therapies; laboratory testing; and nutritional advice.

  Supportive services include those of a homemaker or home health aide. In addition, durable medical equipment and supplies should be available.

- **FOR PATIENTS MEETING CRITERIA, PSYCHIATRIC HOME CARE IS 100% REIMBURSED UNDER MEDICARE AND MEDICAID.** Criteria at this writing are:

  - Patient must be psychiatrically homebound, which does not mean bedbound or physically immobile.

  - Patient must have a DSM-IV psychiatric diagnosis.

  - Patient must require the skills of a psychiatric nurse.

- Patient must be under the care of a psychiatrist.

Funding may also be obtained through the Veteran's Administration, which has its own criteria. Other third-party reimbursement varies, and each private insurance company has its own regulations.

Managed care companies are using psychiatric home care. Their primary criteria are that the patient has failed traditional modes of psychiatric care and uses a significant amount of health care dollars. Psychiatric home care is also available to those who wish to pay for the service.

- **MEDICARE STATES THAT PSYCHIATRIC NURSING CARE MUST BE DELIVERED BY "A PSYCHIATRICALLY TRAINED NURSE WHO HAS SPECIALIZED TRAINING** and/or experience beyond the standard curriculum for a registered nurse (RN)." For Medicare to reimburse an agency the nurse must meet one of the following criteria:
  - Be a licensed RN with a master's degree in psychiatric or community mental health nursing.
  - Be a licensed RN with a BSN degree and 1 year of related work experience in an active treatment program for adult or geriatric patients in a psychiatric health care setting.
  - Be a licensed RN with a diploma or associate degree and 2 years of related work experience in an active treatment program for adult or geriatric patients in a psychiatric health care setting.
  - Possess certification by the American Nurses Association (ANA) in psychiatric or community health nursing.
  - Possess other qualifications that may be considered on an individual basis.

- **PATIENT POPULATIONS THAT ARE APPROPRIATE FOR PSYCHIATRIC HOME CARE** services include the following:

Elderly
Services and support allow the elderly to continue to derive a sense of meaning and purpose from their activities, although their activities may become more restricted.

Patients with Acute Psychiatric Disorders
Patients have been treated in an acute care facility, but no longer require 24-hour supervision. They do, however, require intense monitoring when they go home, perhaps daily visits by a psychiatric nurse who assists them in making the transition from hospital to home.

The Seriously and Persistently Mentally Ill
Many are in and out of institutions, but seem to benefit from home care services and actually require less frequent hospitalization.

AIDS Patients
Patients require medical supervision and psychiatric therapy as they deal with depression, anxiety, grief, and AIDS dementia.

Children
Although few are currently seen in their homes, the number is growing. They may be seen for continued individual therapy and to help families deal with problematic behaviors in the home environment.

- **THE ENTRY-LEVEL PSYCHIATRIC HOME HEALTH NURSE IS GUIDED BY THE STANDARDS OF PSYCHIATRIC PRACTICE,** which encompass the nursing process. Nurses' approaches in the home differ; the nurse is the patient's guest which may influence how a nurse assesses a patient or recommends treatment. Working in different homes, the nurse must be more innovative and flexible.

Assessment of Patient Needs
- A holistic assessment of physical and mental status and functional ability should be done, as the nurse may be the only practitioner to see the patient. Standardized assessment tools may be used to measure depression, anxiety, and psychotic symptoms, movement disorders, and spiritual well-being. A baseline is obtained and the continued use of the tool allows the nurse to trend changes in the patient.
- Family dynamics must be assessed. In the home environment, the relationship with the family is more collaborative.
- Social support systems are assessed to determine who is available to assist with activities of daily living, finances, emotional

support, companionship, and transportation.

Diagnosis

Understanding the DSM-IV and the nursing diagnosis system (NANDA) is important. If patient assessments and DSM-IV diagnoses are not congruent, the referring agency/psychiatrist must be notified to determine what modification is needed. DSM-IV criteria do not shed light on the patient's coping styles, suffering, or other unique problems. NANDA diagnoses, on the other hand, address individuality of the patient and the family and provide direction for care.

Outcomes Identification

Third-party payers want to know what the results of psychiatric interventions will be. Outcomes must be measurable. Psychiatric nurses usually establish outcomes that focus on what the patient and family will learn and what the patient will demonstrate through behavior.

Planning

To establish short-term goals, the nurse works with the patient, other care providers, and the patient's family. Priorities are set and aspects of care delegated.

Interventions

COUNSELING. Supportive intervention, such as teaching problem-solving skills, and relaxation techniques.

MAINTAINING MILIEU. Ensure safety and that the patient will not be victimized.

IMPROVING PATIENT'S SELF-CARE SKILLS. Have other personnel assist patients.

CARRYING OUT MEDICATION AND OTHER PSYCHOBIOLOGICAL INTERVENTIONS. Monitor or administer medications (usually only parenteral administration is reimbursable) or draw bloods to obtain medication serum levels.

HEALTH TEACHING.

CASE MANAGEMENT.

HEALTH PROMOTION AND MAINTENANCE.

Evaluation

Evaluation, an ongoing process, also includes looking at specific outcomes. Were outcomes achieved in a cost-effective manner? Was patient satisfied with care?

Documentation

To meet Medicare standards, several documentation issues in home care must be addressed.

- Every note must stand by itself and include:
  - Current assessment of the patient.
  - Statement of homebound status.
  - Goals for that particular visit.
  - Specific measurable interventions and patient's response to each intervention.
  - Evaluation of goals achievement.
- Notes are written in negative, indicating what deficits the patient still has that justify continued home care.
- Every visit is documented separately.
- All communication is documented; for example, interdisciplinary, nurse to family.
- All verbal orders of the physician are documented as verbal and sent to the physician for review and signature.
- Interventions must be written in concrete language, for example, "teaching regarding medication management."

TAKING ANOTHER LOOK

You are now ready to respond to the questions raised in Gaining a Perspective at the beginning of this chapter. After you have written or thought about your responses, you may wish to look at the Suggested Responses on page 338.

SUGGESTED RESPONSES
for "Gaining a Perspective" Questions

CHAPTER 1

BEGINNING THE PSYCHIATRIC NURSING EXPERIENCE

1. It is impossible for others to describe the type of feelings you will be experiencing as you begin your psychiatric nursing experience, as those feelings are derived from your previous life experiences. Most students, however, feel frightened, anxious, and inadequate before beginning this new venture.

2. Exactly how you plan to prepare for this new experience is your choice; however, it is strongly suggested that you spend time interviewing yourself. Ask yourself questions that give you insight about youself and your feelings about caring for people who are mentally ill or who have emotional problems. When beginning your self-inventory, you will may want to consider the following questions:

   Who am I?

   What have my relationships in school and with my family and others been like?

   What is it about the patients that I am afraid of?

   Answering these and similar questions will help you to begin to focus on what is unique about the patient without projecting your own misconceptions and emotions on the patient.

   In addition to reading and studying textbooks and articles about psychiatric mental health nursing, you may wish to read books about individuals who have had difficulties with interpersonal relationships or a "psychiatric" problem. If you want specific recommendations, ask your instructor or a librarian.

CHAPTER 2

PSYCHIATRIC NURSING

1. It is difficult to say exactly what your purpose may be in learning about psychiatric nursing. It may be that you are only meeting an educational requirement. One hopes, however, that whatever your particular reasons, your expectations of this study should be to gain more understanding of human behavior. In addition to serving as a basis for the practice of psychiatric mental health nursing (should you choose to practice in that specialty), learning about psychiatric nursing will help you in understanding your own behavior, as well as that of your patients. By learning to use neurobiological principles and theories of human behavior, as well as purposeful use of self, your practice of nursing in general should become enriched.

2. One has the feeling that psychiatric nursing will continue broadening its scope, based on the idea that psychiaric nursing has developed over the ages, beginning primarily in in-patient facilities with individuals who had psychiatric problems and emerging later in the community with patients who have emotional problems as well as psychiatric illnesses. As the focus of all health care goes from treatment to prevention, the psychiatric nurse's role will move into all segments of the community. With continuing emphasis on the concepts of multiculturalism and diversity, psychiatric nurses are likely to conduct research to determine effective interventions that will best serve the mental health needs of differing populations.

3. It becomes clear that which qualifications you need depends on the type of nursing practice you intend to have. However, considering statements by the Coalition of Psychiatric Nursing Organizations (COPNO), the trend is toward further education, certification, and perhaps more subspecialization. Functions and roles will continue to be defined, and research, both

clinical and theoretical, will advance the profession and expand its repertoire of activities and knowledge base.

CHAPTER 3

PATTERNS OF PSYCHIATRIC NURSING PRACTICE: INTEGRATING THE ARTS WITH THE SCIENCE

1. Each of us has a different learning style and a different way to approach a new situation. Some would probably like to read all about "how to" do psychiatric mental health nursing; others would like to see films; still others would like to have a "hands on" experience, particularly with mentally ill patients. It is our feeling that to learn about psychiatric mental health nursing you need a framework to approach it—and that is dealt with in Chapter 3. The framework deals with Carper's patterns of knowing, which include empiric personal knowledge, ethics, and esthetics. With that framework in mind, an entire psychiatric mental health nursing curriculum is presented (see Study Guide Table 3-1).

   The experiences you need to help the learning process are manifold and may include:

   - Interacting with patients in community mental health clinics

   - Teaching families about mental illness

   - Working in interdisciplinary settings to determine effective assessment and treatment modalities and critical pathways for patients with minor and major illnesses

   - Assisting parents to deal with their children who have behavior problems

   - Assisting with emotional crises

   - Doing self-inventories.

   Ideally, one would want unlimited time in these areas, as your nursing skills should deepen with each experience. By applying all your patterns of learning and nursing knowledge to the practice setting, you should be better able to understand and deal with human behavior, whether it be a patient's, a community's, a colleague's, or your own.

CHAPTER 4

THE BRAIN AND BEHAVIOR

1. The brain is a complex organ that is involved in controlling many body functions, including those related to human behavior and emotions. Specifically with regard to emotions and behavior, having an understanding of the brain's structure and function enables one to better understand "normal" human reactions, particularly in stressful situations. One should then be able to appreciate the uniqueness of individuals by observing one's patients and even exploring one's own reactions in such situations. By having a beginning understanding of the specific functions of each part of the brain, you, the nurse, can begin to realize what may result from damage to one part (e.g., severe damage to the cerebrum may impair intellectual functioning and the ability to process emotions). The whole idea of neurotransmitter involvement is fascinating. For example, dopamine's involvement in schizophrenia; norepinephrine in depression, mania, and anxiety; and serotonin in regulating eating disorders.

2. Nurses should know how drugs prescribed for "physical" illness can affect patients' behavior. For example, when caring for patients who have psychiatric symptoms, such as hallucinations or disorientation, the nurse who is familiar with the brain's functioning, as well as the effects of the drug the patient is receiving, can make better decisions about appropriate interventions and recognize the need to obtain good psychiatric, behavioral, and/or laboratory data. As one studies the interactions of prescribed and over-the-counter drugs with the body's chemicals (particularly neurotransmitters), one sees that all body systems are affected by the brain's functions.

CHAPTER 5
MENTAL HEALTH LEARNING AND TEACHING

1. Learning theory should assist the nurse in determining what approaches are likely to be appropriate for teaching patients and significant others. By knowing about major approaches to motivation, whether it be the content approach based on Maslow's hierarchy of needs theory or the process approach based on reinforcement theory, the nurse knows that motivation to learn is based on multiple needs, and that the patient's needs for satisfaction can be linked to desired outcomes. These learning theories in conjunction with information processing theories give the nurse a sound foundation for understanding how most people learn. The nurse's task is to operationalize these theories in dealing with individual patients and their significant others. Nurses, particularly those involved in psychiatric nursing, are interested in assisting patients and/or their significant others to change ineffective behaviors to effective behaviors. The more nurses know about how people learn and grow (change and develop), the more effective is the time nurses spend with all their patients.

2. A nurse might deal with this situation in a variety of ways. Some important ideas to consider are presented in the discussion below.

   The nurse would have to be or become knowledgeable about mental illness. In addition, the nurse would have to be knowledgeable about teenagers in general and about these teenagers in particular. Some questions the nurse might want to ask are:

   • How old are these teenagers? What are their educational and sociocultural backgrounds?

   • What are the goals of this program? Why was this program requested? Who is requesting this program? What and why do these teenagers need to know about mental health?

   • What is the time frame?

   • How will the teenagers be evaluated to determine that learning took place?

The nurse wants to present the material in a meaningful and relevant way and, therefore, must consider what will motivate the teenagers. How will learning about mental illness affect their lives? The nurse will also have to consider his or her teaching skills and teaching style. Much will depend on the size of the group and the goal of the program. The nurse must also consider the time available for preparation and presentation, as well as the resources (financial and physical) available for the program. The nurse's own feelings about the program are likely to influence the success of the program.

CHAPTER 6
STRESS, COPING, AND DEFENSIVE FUNCTIONING

1. Because stressors vary from person to person, it is difficult to determine what your stressors may be. Many students experience stressors related to attending school. Some are internal (the need to be number one in the class); some are external (financial strain or family responsibilities).

   High-adaptive defense mechanisms are effective in coping with stress: anticipation, thinking about emotional reactions in advance; affiliation, turning to others for support and talking with them (perhaps individuals in similar situations who are coping well); humor, seeing the amusing or ironic aspects of a situation; and self-assertion, being able to express your feelings about what is happening directly and to the appropriate person.

2. The nurse might first stop and wonder why he or she is not treating the patient especially well. What stressors are causing the nurse to act in this way to a patient? Is the nurse feeling inadequate, or overwhelmed? What is going on in the situation? Is the nurse in any way using devaluation as a defense mechanism?

   Perhaps in some way the patient discerns that the nurse "does not like her"; the nurse's behavior may be acting as a stressor to the patient. If that is so, the patient may be using idealization as a way of coping.

That is one scenario. Perhaps you can think of others. The important factor is that human responses (yours and the patient's) must be viewed in terms of their precipitating factors, in terms of humans' perceptions of themselves and the events within and around them. Stress responses are as complex as they are common.

CHAPTER 7

HUMAN GROWTH AND DEVELOPMENTAL TASKS

1. Fifteen-year-olds are in the process of forming an adult identity. One task that adolescents should accomplish is to renegotiate their role within the family. When a parent dies at this stage, turmoil occurs and this task may be delayed or accelerated depending upon other dynamics within the family. The adolescent, due to his or her age, is already dealing with psychological upheaval leading to disruptions in personality organization, disequilibrium, and disturbance in mood behavior. In addition, one would also need to know a great deal about previous experiences the adolescent has had with loss, the kind of defense mechanisms the adolescent has previously used to deal with severe stress, and the relationship the adolescent had with the parent who died, the remaining parent, and the family in general. Much also depends on the sex of the parent and the adolescent's stage of sexual development. The adolescent continues to learn and model much about sexual roles and identity from both parents.

Intellectually, the adolescent has the capacity to deal with the reality and finality of death. The nurse's knowing what social and cultural factors, including religion, are affecting this adolescent will be important in determining the kind of support that is likely to be available. The adolescent's relationships with peers will be equally important. Does this 15-year-old have peers that will be helpful in a "healthy" way?

The above points are only some of the factors to be considered. Each individual is unique,

and so, too, is his or her response to the death of a parent. Understanding normal developmental tasks, however, helps the nurse come to the situation with some preparation and insight about the effects of this type of loss during adolescence.

2. When an infant is able to successfully form a secure attachment with the caregiver (parent), the infant is learning to trust people and, probably, the world in general. The infant learns that when he or she is in a new situation or afraid, he or she can turn to parents for feelings of safety. This relationship with parents is the infant's first intimate relationship. The infant can take this sense of trust and use it as a basis for forming other relationships, first with other familiar people (family and close friends) and then in beginning to relate to strangers, as in school.

Infants who do not develop secure attachments may have difficulty forming intimate, lasting relationships later in childhood, adolescence, and adulthood. Poor attachment promotes an expectation of rejection, which leads to a defense posture of maintaining emotional distance, avoiding intimacy and commitment.

CHAPTER 8

SYSTEMS THEORY AS A MODEL FOR UNDERSTANDING FAMILIES

1. Numerous examples could be given of what might take place if members of a family used coercion as a mode of transaction. Here is one example. One subsystem (A) might say, "I want you to stop annoying me." The other subsystem (B)'s question in return might be, "Why should I?" Subsystem A would answer, with some sort of intent to use force, "Because I'll beat you up if you don't."

2. The genogram for each family is different. After you have completed yours, review the Flanagan Family Genogram.

3. Without some assistance, a nurse who comes from a family that the nurse feels is not operating normally may have problems dealing with

families who operate in a similar way. The nurse may view these families suspiciously and diagnose them as pathological. In some cases, the nurse cannot be empathetic or objective when dealing with these families.

Nurses with these kinds of problems must decide exactly why they feel their families of origin are abnormal. What kind of structures, interactions, and behaviors were operative in their families? There are many deviations in families, e.g., divorce, which may not match the "ideal" model of family. No single pattern distinguishes well-functioning families from those that are pathological.

4. The changing role of women in our society, for example, working outside the home, may place new stress on men. What will be each family member's role in the future? How will child care be provided? If there continue to be trends such as single-parent families, homosexual partnerships with children, and blended and step families, what will be the model/norm for the "ideal" family? What about the effect of such issues as increased violence, economic plight, and longevity? As the U.S. population becomes more diverse, what effect will it have on the norms for family that professionals have clung to? Further research is needed to understand the effects of culture, class, and minority status on the family? Will systems theory and interactional understanding keep us from needing new norms for understanding the family?

CHAPTER 9

CULTURE, ETHNICITY, AND RACE IN MENTAL HEALTH AND ILLNESS

1. It should not matter whether you, the nurse, are African-American, white, or of any other racial origin or whether the nurse you are working with on the unit is African-American, white, or of any other racial origin. It is probably best to ask the nurse to be totally honest and examine his or her own cultural, ethnic, and racial origins, including beliefs, values, and prejudices. Then it would be helpful for the nurse to assess his or her knowledge about black Americans and their beliefs, values, and experiences in this

country. Reading about black Americans may be the next step. The nurse should know that racism is a reality in the United States.

The nurse should be prepared to come to the psychiatric unit with the idea that each patient, regardless of ethnic and racial background, is a unique individual and that listening to the patient's experience will assist the nurse to gain specific information about how that patient's ethnicity and/or race has affected him or her. The nurse should be prepared to establish a relationship based on mutual respect. The patient's beliefs must be respected and should help in assisting the nurse to provide more culturally sensitive care.

CHAPTER 10

SPIRITUALITY AND PATIENT CARE

1. A way to approach the situation about the patient's perceived loss of faith is to discuss with the patient exactly what "things have gone badly." You, the nurse, might then be able to have the patient deal more constructively with those identified issues.

In addition, depending on how comfortable you, the nurse, are with discussing the topic, it would be important to discuss two other areas with the patient. First, what his or her previous relationship with God was and second, what he or she means by "my life has no meaning."

It is crucial that the nurse be aware of the importance of a patient's spiritual well-being. In order to provide holistic care, the nurse should be able to assess and then intervene in situations where the patient seems to be in spiritual distress. Of course, this presumes that the nurse has dealt with his or her own feelings about spirituality and has some understanding or insight into his or her personal philosophy of life.

CHAPTER 11

LEGAL AND ETHICAL ISSUES IN PSYCHIATRIC NURSING

1. Before discussing with a patient voluntary admission to an inpatient facility, the nurse should clearly understand the legal implications for any patient in the state in which the nurse is working. Then the nurse would probably explain to Mrs. Jones that voluntary admission means that she must consent to treatment and that she will have the right to be released upon request within a specified period of time. Consenting to treatment usually means that the patient will be given treatment choices and be asked to give informed consent; the right to be released depends on the state's law. Mrs. Jones would have to understand that if she refused treatment options or wanted to leave at a time when the staff thought she was a danger to herself or others, the staff, depending on state law, could decide not to release her and initiate a petition for judicial commitment. It would be helpful to explain to Mrs. Jones that none of her rights as a citizen or an individual would be denied because of her inpatient status.

2. First the nurse should assess Mrs. Lawton's understanding and concept of ECT treatments. The nurse might wish to explore questions such as:

   Does she know why ECT is the treatment being advised?

   Does she understand the goals of treatment?

   What are her fears concerning the ECT treatments?

   Have other treatment options been offered to her?

   Has she discussed her feelings or fears with the psychiatrist?

   How did the psychiatrist respond?

   The nurse, in the role of advocate, should be aware of the patient's right to refuse treatment. The nurse should also be aware of the procedure the patient follows in order to refuse treatment. The nurse must know the state laws regarding the rights of mentally ill persons.

In addition, or perhaps initially, the nurse needs to explore his or her own feelings about the use of ECT, or any therapy, as the nurse's feelings will affect nurse-patient interactions.

3. In a therapeutic relationship with a patient, the nurse is bound by the concept of privilege; however, the nurse also has the "duty to protect." In the example given of a patient who threatens to harm her family, the nurse should discuss what the patient said with his or her supervisor and an appropriate course of action should be determined. Perhaps the patient should be seen by another mental health professional (psychiatrist); perhaps voluntary inpatient treatment is possible; or perhaps emergency involuntary commitment would be appropriate. There are many choices depending on further assessments and the availability of resources. The issue here is that there may be potential danger to a third party and the nurse must take some action and, of course, document the findings and actions.

CHAPTER 12

THERAPEUTIC COMMUNICATION

1. You are the only one who knows what influences how you communicate. But, in responding did you consider your culture, your socioeconomic background, your age, and whether you are comfortable with verbal language, and your comfort level in a group and in a one-on-one interaction. Are you shy or outgoing or somewhere in between? Have you been encouraged to verbalize or were you raised to be "seen but not heard"? Do you think what you have to say is important? How well do you feel in general? What about the clothes you wear? What about your body language?

2. As communication takes place between at least two individuals, the misunderstandings between what a person says and what the other person hears may have to do with a problem between these individuals. It may be that the person sending the message is not clear, or does not use proper language; in other words, this person has sent a "wrong" message. It may be

that the words are clear, but because of the intonation or the body language of the sender, the sender is sending mixed messages. Or it may be that the second person (the receiver) just does not understand the message. This misunderstanding may be due to the fact that the receiver thinks the words have a different meaning, due to connotation or not understanding the vocabulary. The receiver may not be listening attentively and may miss important nuances, or even does not "hear" the message at all due to other factors, e.g., his or her own anxiety. The receiver may also have expected, based on past experiences, to receive a different message, and, therefore, that is what the receiver "heard."

These are but a few examples of how communications are "misunderstood." That is why it is so important in therapeutic communication with patients that the nurse to be sure that a feedback mechanism is built into the interactions. Does the nurse hear what the patient is saying and understand what the patient means?

3. Therapeutic communication is a well-planned, goal-directed, patient-focused interaction. You, the nurse, employing therapeutic use of self, interact with the patient to meet the patient's needs, not your own. The nurse needs to structure the environment so that the patient feels safe enough to trust the nurse. The nurse must not only be interested in what the patient is saying but also accepting of the patient's behaviors; empathy is shown by using active listening skills, and respect is shown for the patient. In social communication, some of these elements may or may not apply, but there is usually more of a mutuality in meeting one another's needs.

4. In many situations, silence, a nonverbal technique, can enhance communication. Basically, silence gives the patient, and sometimes the nurse, a time to think, and to gather information, and silence allows the patient or nurse time for responding. Therefore, any situation you described that uses silence in this way is appropriate.

Silence can also convey acceptance. Quite often, when a patient is very upset or afraid, having a nurse sit silently nearby conveys the nurse's acceptance of these feelings. It also shows empathy and genuineness. This use of silence is often the true use of the therapeutic self and sets up an atmosphere of trust, which is essential for therapeutic communication.

CHAPTER 13
SOMATOFORM DISORDERS

1. Patients who have somatization disorders are likely to be seen by a nurse in any setting. Many patients with these disorders frequently visit the emergency room, the urgicare center, and/or the physician's office and are in severe physical distress at the time of the visit. Although the etiology of these disorders is unknown, they are presumed to be psychological in origin. The outcomes are generally to have the patient cope with stress (not be preoccupied with physical symptoms) and to have the patient verbalize an understanding of the relationship between emotional problems and physical symptoms.

2. It is very important for the nurse to assist the parent to understand that regardless of the cause of the pain, the sensation of pain is very real. Psychological pain is as debilitating as physical pain. Explain to the parent that his or her daughter does not do this on a conscious level and needs assistance in expressing her feelings, such as anger or anxiety, in a more productive way.

CHAPTER 14
ANXIETY DISORDERS

1. First the nurse should remain with the patient and maintain as calm an environment as possible. The nurse should attempt to relax the patient by asking the patient to take deep breaths and attempt to "talk the patient down." The nurse should try to break the patient's thought patterns, which are usually focused on the symptoms of the attack — pounding heart, shortness of breath — and have the patient fo-

cus on some external elements, not the attack or the anxiety. The nurse should refrain from asking about the attack or the anxiety as that will only increase the feelings.

2. When responding to a person who says that he has a specific fear or phobia, two main areas of concern. First, does the phobia interfere with the person's ability to function in his roles and interact socially? Second, does the phobia cause the person discomfort (anxiety or panic attacks)? In this case, depending on your friend's job or living environment, it seems unlikely that his fear will interfere with his daily living or make him sufficiently uncomfortable. It is important for you to understand, and perhaps share with this your friend, that many individuals have irrational fears which probably derive from childhood. Of cause, you may want to talk with him further to explore his concern that he is "psychiatrically ill."

CHAPTER 15

DISSOCIATIVE DISORDERS

1. One of the characteristic symptoms of a dissociative identity disorder (DID) is that the patient may experience "voices inside" the head (talking directly to the patient or to another). The voices may tell the patient to harm himself or herself or others in the environment. Therefore, the nurse needs to question the patient about the presence of voices and the content of the "dialogue." The nurse's responsibility is to ensure safety.

   The patient with DID tends to become depressed, have little ability to concentrate, sleep poorly, and feel out of control. All of these occurrences are assessed so that proper interventions can be taken with the goal of guaranteeing the patient's safety.

CHAPTER 16

LOSS, GRIEF, AND BEREAVEMENT

1. It is impossible for anyone but you to answer this question about cultural factors that might help you cope with grief; however, you should consider such questions as those that follow:

   What is your belief about death? Is it part of the life cycle?

   What customs and rituals do you perform when death occurs? Is there a specific mourning period? When are you expected to resume your previous responsibilities?

   How is grief expressed? Are you expected to be emotional or stoic?

2. The nurse in the hospice might intervene to assist the patient, depending on the patient's condition, to do some anticipatory grief work. The nurse would try to provide an environment where the patient could freely express his or her thoughts and feelings. The nurse would encourage the patient to talk about what his or her needs and wishes are concerning death and dying. Does the patient wish to leave written or spoken mementos for family and friends? What are the patient's wishes concerning funeral arrangements, etc.? From a cultural or religious assessment, the nurse would consider how the patient relates to his or her background. The nurse would be an active listener and convey a presence so that the patient will continue to feel connected and have a sense of hope. Time would be spent encouraging the patient to reflect on her life, not only with the nurse but with friends and family. Of course, it is essential that the nurse address the patient's physical needs, as this activity shows a sense of caring.

3. Caregivers of persons with AIDS are in very difficult situations, as by and large their patients tend to be young and face abbreviated life spans. The caregiver may also be a young person and be aware of the deaths of many friends and associates. The nurse may encourage the caregiver to use some of the following coping skills:

- Take some time for self, a respite from caregiving.

- Find a supportive social network.

- Live "one day at a time."

- Learn some stress management strategies.

- Set short-term goals.

- Be aware that you will have feelings of loss and grief.

- Keep informed about the course of the illness.

- Know what is in your control and what is not.

CHAPTER 17

CHILDHOOD DISORDERS

1. Although each individual is different, it is likely that a nurse (especially an inexperienced nurse) is likely to become angry, fearful, and/or frustrated when a child who has a conduct disorder is defiant, shows poor impulse control, and is physically aggressive. The nurse should develop strategies to deal with these feelings.

    - Identify the existence of the feelings.

    - Take an opportunity to express these feelings in supervision (to prevent the nurse from acting them out with patients).

    - Confer with other staff so that there is consistency in dealing with the patient's behavior, e.g., in setting limits.

2. Regardless of the specific childhood disorder, providing support for the family of children with emotional disorders seems to be a universally appropriate nursing intervention. Depending on the disorder, the parent may feel guilty about the illness, as many of the disorders appear to have a genetic or familial etiology. Quite often these emotional conditions are not treated quickly, and the family may need the nurse's assistance in handling difficulties that arise when a chronic illness is present in a family.

The second nursing intervention that seems appropriate when dealing with children with emotional disorders is providing an environment (nurse) that is accepting of the child as a person and that protects the child from self-harm by setting limits and discouraging inappropriate or harmful behaviors. The nurse must be supportive and accepting of the child, but not of inappropriate behaviors.

Above are but two examples of interventions. Those that you see as universal may be equally appropriate.

CHAPTER 18

ISSUES IN ADOLESCENT MENTAL HEALTH

1. Describing your feelings about your adolescence is a personal reflection. For some, adolescence is remembered fondly; for others it is not. For all, adolescence is a time of change. Your ability as a nurse to deal with adolescents requires that you consider your feelings about that time in your life.

2. It is difficult to say how exactly a nurse would handle a teenager who indicates that she wants to commit suicide. One needs to know the context in which the remark was made. However, regardless of the context, the remark must be taken seriously. The nurse should find out more about the teenager's situation. Has anything happened recently to disrupt this teenager's life. Is she depressed? Has she ever felt this way before or considered suicide previously or made an attempt? Depending on the answers to these questions, it may be essential to refer the teenager for treatment, with the real possibility that she be hospitalized. Teenagers who talk about suicide may indeed commit suicide.

3. First during the interview it would be appropriate for the nurse to introduce himself or herself and explain the interview process. It is likely that the adolescent will resent the nurse having to interview his parents. It will be important for the nurse to explain that the purpose of interviewing the parents and the adolescent separately is to have an opportunity to hear each one's view of the situation. It is not

to take sides, but to have a clearer picture of the situation. The nurse should also discuss confidentiality. During each interview, the nurse explains that certain statements will be shared with professional staff; however, what happens during each individual interview will not be shared during the other interview with the family.

When interviewing the patient, in addition to making him comfortable (perhaps by offering him a soft drink or snack), it will be vitally important that the nurse show the adolescent proper respect and acknowledge that this is a very difficult time for him. The nurse should know under what circumstances the young man was admitted. If it was his parents' idea, he is likely to act out and make his parents very uncomfortable, particularly in the nurse's presence. The parents may be experiencing feelings of doubt and guilt and need assurance that the staff is there to assist their son and to support them as well.

CHAPTER 19

AGING AND MENTAL HEALTH

1. The nurse's exact response to an elderly person concerned about forgetting would, of course, depend on the context in which the concern was voiced. The nurse would want to engage the person in a conversation about forgetting to get a clearer picture of the symptom. The nurse may also want to discuss other pertinent events in the individual's life and ask about his or her physical health. It is important for the nurse to understand that in the normal aging process there is occasional forgetfulness, especially of the recent past.

2. Depending on your age, health, outlook, and experience in life and your experience with retired people, your response to the question of what it would be like to retire is likely to differ from someone else's. In general, retirement is usually viewed as a loss. There is a change in role, time structure, and for many financial and societal status. It matters whether retirement is planned or forced. It matters whether the per-

son is alone or has family and friends. One also needs to realize that retirement is an issue to be dealt with and one that may be related to considerations of one's own mortality.

3. The questions a nurse would probably consider in determining the functional status of a mentally and emotionally well elderly patient include:

   - Can the patient take care of her personal needs, that is, bathe, toilet, dress, and feed herself?

   - Can the patient do necessary household chores, that is, shop, cook, and do light housekeeping as well as heavier housekeeping (vacuuming, shoveling snow)?

   - Does the patient have any problems with mobility, that is, managing stairs, and walking unassisted?

   - What transportation is available?

   - Does she have access to health care, and knowledge of available resources?

   - What resources does the patient use now, that is, household help, support persons, and medical services?

   - Is she working or volunteering outside the home and/or retired?

   - How does she spend a typical day? A typical night?

   - What would the patient like the nurse to know?

4. Depression among the elderly often goes unnoticed because the symptoms tend to be more physically oriented than the mood changes that we see among younger adults. The elderly tend to have more physical diseases with symptoms that resemble those of depression, e.g., loss of appetite, or low energy. In addition, many people feel that the aged tend to be "depressed," and consequently, do not think that the complaints warrant attention. If an older adult is not diagnosed as being depressed, he or she may suffer needlessly and even commit suicide.

It is imperative for nurses to listen carefully to what elderly patients are saying. Do not assume that an elderly patient's physical complaints reflect only physical problems, but be aware that complaints may be signs of depression. Nurses must have good assessment abilities to determine if depression is the problem. Nurses must understand the normal aging process and realize that although the reaction to such losses as widowhood or forced retirement may cause some depressive emotions, depression itself is a definite illness. With proper treatment the elderly need not continue to be depressed.

5. It would probably be most appropriate for you, the nurse, to first ask your co-worker why the patient should be restrained. In other words, what behaviors is the confused patient demonstrating? Then the nurse might decide that some of the behaviors were the result of something that could be "fixed." For example, was there anything new happening physiologically with the patient? Was the patient dehydrated? Were the patient's electrolytes in balance? In addition, the nurse might look at the environment. Was there a great deal of noise or confusion on the unit? Had someone recently interacted with the patient?

Prior to considering restraints, a nurse should consider alternatives. Could someone stay with the patient? Would some activity or another environment calm the patient? Had a medication been ordered to use if behavior became uncontrollable? Restraints are always a last resort, as they usually make the patient more agitated and fearful. You, the nurse, and your co-worker need to realize the implications of using restraints.

CHAPTER 20

MOOD DISORDERS

1. The answer to how you feel when you are depressed is personal. Most people have times when they feel "depressed," and the mood is described as despair, gloom, a sense of foreboding, feeling numb. Every person deals with these feelings differently. Some may cry, while others talk to a supportive person, treat themselves to something special, and, in general, find ways to deal with the mood. If depression is related to a loss, then the individual must allow time to process the grief.

2. The nurse should remind the patient that the behavior (persistent telephoning using credit card to order gifts) is inappropriate. If the patient is willing to stop the behavior immediately, what happens next depends on the plan of care that was agreed to by the patient and staff. Frequently, a specific approach has been agreed on; for example, take the patient to a quiet place, see if the patient understands the consequences of the behavior, take the card away from the patient, and remove a privilege. If the patient is not willing to stop the behavior, it may be that the nurse will need to take action to prevent the patient from making further telephone calls — first by verbally insisting that the patient stop, and then by reminding the patient of the limits that have been set regarding this or similar behavior. The nurse may have to summon assistance to remove the patient from the phone area so that the patient understands the behavior is unacceptable and will not be allowed to continue.

3. It is difficult to say how you would feel; however, nurses must be sure that patients and their families fully understand electroconvulsive therapy (ECT). When the patient gives consent, the nurse is expected to support the patient's decision. If a nurse is having difficulty accepting ECT as a viable treatment, the nurse should share those feelings with the treatment team and discuss the subject in supervision. The nurse should understand that the treatment is painless but that memory loss, particularly of recent events, does occur. The patient needs to know the benefits and risks of ECT and other treatment options.

CHAPTER 21

SEXUAL ISSUES, DISORDERS, AND DEVIATIONS

1. Reactions are always personal. One reaction to the woman struggling with the idea that her son is gay would be to show empathy and understanding for the parent's feelings. The nurse would need to have dealt with his or her own feelings about homosexuality and have a clear understanding that all homosexual individuals have the same rights in the health care system as any individual. The nurse must recognize that parents often have difficulty accepting their children's homosexuality.

   After the nurse does the initial intake and identifies the exact problem, he or she may begin a counseling session. The decision will depend on the nurse's skill.

   The nurse should be aware that the etiology of homosexuality has always reflected conflict between nature (biological makeup) and nurture (environment). The nurse should also keep in mind how different religious and cultural groups, and society in general, respond to homosexuality and what effect these attitudes have on this woman. The nurse, depending upon his or her role, may not be the person to deal with the woman directly. Instead, the nurse may do the initial intake, as with other persons coming to the clinic for a first visit, and refer the patient to the appropriate health care provider in the clinic. During the initial intake, the nurse is concerned with the woman's feelings and responses and should be accepting and nonjudgmental when interacting with her. This parent is very likely "blaming" herself for her son's homosexuality.

2. The nurse must have a good understanding of human sexuality, including modes of sexual expression. The nurse should understand and know about common sexual disorders and their etiologies. Then, perhaps, the nurse can help determine the etiology of the problem by interviewing the patient and obtaining answers to the questions following. These questions are not meant to be asked directly, nor are they in any particular order of importance, nor are they the only questions to ask.

   - What does the woman mean by "having sexual problems"?
   - What are the exact problems?
   - Does the woman have adequate knowledge about anatomy, physiology, and the sexual act itself? What are her sexual expectations and past experiences?
   - What stressors are present in the lives of the woman and her partner?
   - Does the woman or her partner have any medical or psychiatric problems? Have they ever had any?
   - Does the woman or her partner use or abuse drugs or alcohol?
   - Has the woman discussed her problem with her partner? Is her partner aware that she has come for help?

   The information obtained from these questions and others you may have thought had priority should allow you to begin to prepare appropriate interventions.

CHAPTER 22

EATING DISORDERS

1. Our society has placed much emphasis on being fit and thin. Women are influenced by the "ideal" models they see on television, in the movies, and in magazines, and may strive to reach that ideal. The women's movement has liberated women in many ways and opened opportunities for women to succeed. For some women, however, the changes have placed them in positions of additional stress. Women must be successful in their work, as wives, as mothers, and socially. These additional stresses may have given some women a need to gain better control of their lives. Some see getting thin as a way to control themselves. (An increase in eating disorders was noted during the 1970s when the women's movement was becoming established.)

   Diets and exercise are big business in the

United States. Many quick-fix solutions are advertised. Thinness is linked to popularity and self-worth. For some who diet and exercise underlying problems need to be assessed. Teenagers have many stresses placed on them. They are experiencing the need to achieve; often they must deal with parental divorce or other losses, dysfunctional families, and developmental issues such as separation from family. They may feel out of control, or unpopular, and, in general, have low self-esteem. All these are risk factors for developing eating disorders.

2. It would be important for the nurse to remind the patient of the rule that she stay in the dayroom following meals. It is advisable to offer the patient an opportunity to tell the nurse why she must return to her room. The patient may want to purge. If, however, she gives another reason for wanting to return to her room, the nurse should remind that patient that someone must accompany her. The patient is likely to challenge the nurse with a statement such as "Don't you trust me?"

It is important for the nurse to indicate that this is not the time to test the nurse's trust. Remind her what the rule is and offer the patient an opportunity to sit and discuss her feelings at this time. If the patient becomes very anxious, other interventions may be required.

CHAPTER 23

SLEEP DISORDERS

1. First, the nurse might ask the colleague with the sleeping problem whether it is a new or ongoing problem. The nurse might want to know if the colleague has recently had a complete physical. Can the colleague think of any reasons for this problem? The nurse might want to know exactly what the colleague means by "having trouble sleeping." If these assessments provide no clues to the colleague's difficulty, the nurse might want to discuss some simple interventions that might promote sleep, such as establishing a regular bedtime and awakening time, avoiding caffeine in the evening, avoiding alcohol prior to sleep, exercising reg-

ularly and moderately, and trying to clear the mind prior to sleep. Advising the colleague not to struggle to fall asleep might be helpful.

2. Patients in hospitals often have difficulty sleeping because their presleep habits and rituals are disrupted. They may be very anxious or in pain. The environment may be noisier than at home. Patients may have to be disturbed during sleep to have certain procedures or assessments done and may not be able to return to sleep. These are but a few reasons why a hospitalized patient may have difficulty sleeping. The nurse should make every effort to minimize sleep disruptions and try to keep the environment conducive to sleep.

3. Sleep disturbances are very frequently seen in patients with psychiatric disorders. It is essential for nurses to determine what kind of problems specific patients have so that sleep-related symptoms, such as insomnia, can be treated. Promoting adequate sleep and rest is always a major nursing concern. When psychiatric patients are sleep deprived, it is likely that their psychotic or abnormal behavior may worsen. Anxiety is likely to become worse, especially if the patient is anxious about not being able to fall asleep or is frightened of having nightmares (may be common in patients with posttraumatic stress disorder). Patients with dementia may tend to wander because of sleep disturbances.

CHAPTER 24

TREATING CHILD SEXUAL TRAUMA

1. The major role for the nurse in caring for a sexually traumatized child is to be sure that the child is in a safe environment. The child needs time to process the abusive experience. The victim ideally will integrate the event into his or her life experience. All attempts are made to give the child enough support so that the child is able to relate to the abuse experience, but not be compelled to dwell on it or avoid it. This action is an attempt to prevent posttraumatic stress disorder.

CHAPTER 25

VICTIMS OF SEXUAL ASSAULT

1. It is difficult to know how you would feel as a nurse interviewing a youngster who has been raped by a man in his thirties. Feelings are personal. In being aware of their values and biases, nurses may anticipate how they are likely to react in a variety of situations. How the nurse feels is also tempered by the nurse's knowledge base and previous similar nursing situations. To recognize and deal with one's feelings when working with individuals who have been sexually traumatized helps ensure that the nurse is respectful and honest. The nurse needs to realize that the victim and the victim's family and significant others are sensitive to the nurse's reactions and particularly to how the nurse conveys information about the event to others.

In addition to dealing with the traumatic event, the victim must disclose what happened. Unless the nurse is able to be supportive and respectful, the victim may be further traumatized by the interview. The victim must be informed of what will be done and the reason for each activity. A young adolescent may need special preparation to relieve the anxiety of having a pelvic examination, perhaps her first pelvic examination. An adolescent's reaction to sexual trauma will, of course, depend on the nature of the assault, the adolescent's life experiences, and the type of care provided to the adolescent following the incident.

CHAPTER 26

PERSONALITY DISORDERS

1. Usually there is someone with whom we interact who seems very inflexible, and when we discuss our perceptions with others they have similar thoughts. If one gets to know this inflexible individual, one will find that this individual is very uncomfortable in interactional situations, whether they be occupational or social. This is not to say that all these individuals have personality disorders. Sometimes, if the environment enhances self-esteem, these people can learn to feel trust and move toward more flexibility.

2. After ensuring that assessment data are complete, the nurse may want to begin by teaching Mrs. Jamison several different ways of self-soothing that she can use when she is alone and anxious. Listening to music, exercising, gardening, doing handicrafts, and reading comforting materials are some self-soothing activities. In addition, the nurse would want to focus Mrs. Jamison on identifying a purpose in her life that enhances self-esteem. Being alone is not as threatening when a person begins to feel more confident and has more self-esteem.

CHAPTER 27

CHILD MALTREATMENT

1. How anyone feels is always a personal experience. The nurse must recognize, however, that personal feelings about child maltreatment must be dealt with or they will interfere with the nurse's ability to assist a parent and child. Nurses working with parents who physically abuse their children should have dealt with their own feelings about their parents, their own childhood experiences, and their moral/value system.

The nurse needs to review the factors in the abusive parent's life that could have led to the behavior; the nurse may, as a result, be able to begin to understand how a parent could behave abusively. Some of the behaviors may be a result of the parent not learning parenting skills or being maltreated as a child.

2. The nurse must be aware of the physical signs of child maltreatment first and foremost because the nurse is a protector of children. It is part of the nurse's function to ensure that patients, children, and adults are in safe environments. In the case of children, if their environment is unsafe, children's protective services must be notified. Children who are abused can be fatally abused if left in an unsafe environment.

A child may be in contact with a nurse when child maltreatment is not the issue at hand; for example, a child is brought to the health care provider for a routine examination.

At that time, the nurse may notice some physical signs of abuse, e.g., bruises, or old burn scars. Unless the nurse has in his or her mind that assessment for abuse is part of any child's evaluation, then many children who are abused will not be identified and proper interventions will not be taken.

In the roles of child advocate and teacher, the nurse is responsible for teaching other individuals, such as day-care workers, the physical signs of child maltreatment.

Early identification and reporting of child abuse not only prevents damage to the child, but will help salvage a dysfunctional family or individual in need of help.

CHAPTER 28

VIOLENCE IN FAMILIES

1. Several factors suggest why women are more likely to be vicitms of family violence. In general in our society, power is not equally distributed between men and women. Men usually have more physical and social power and tend to use it to maintain their dominant position within the family. Some factors linked to women make them particularly vulnerable to violence, e.g., passivity, low self-esteem, and being more educated then their partners. A very important factor is violence within the family of origin. More women are sexually abused as children, a factor that is associated with abuse as an adult.

   In addition, in a patriarchal society children are socialized to the idea of male dominance and aggression.

2. Based on the situation described of the fearful neighbor, the nurse would want to support the woman in her desire to leave the home. It is a crisis situation.

   A quick assessment may reveal that a family member or friend might provide a safe haven. Many abused women, however, are either so ashamed of their circumstances or so isolated from a social support network that they are truly alone. The nurse may suggest a specific shel-

ter or a hotline with information about services for battered women and their children. It may be that a community/social service agency has a program or a social worker who can be immediately contacted.

The important action on the part of the nurse is to assist the neighbor to find safe housing for herself and her children. The woman also needs to be assured that she has done nothing wrong in sharing this information and that the nurse is trustworthy. The woman should also be reassured that she is not to blame for her husband's violence. It is important for her to realize that until her husband is free of alcohol, he is unlikely to change his violent behavior. The issue of police intervention should also be discussed.

CHAPTER 29

SCHIZOPHRENIA

1. Patients with schizophrenia require long-term treatment. The disease drastically alters their ability to experience the environment and other people. Although a patient may be able to control symptoms, the disease does not seem curable. Because the etiology of schizophrenia is so complex, we are not able to pinpoint its causes. The assumptions are that if the stressors and vulnerabilities respond to medication, if the patient is assisted to learn about symptom recognition, and if environmental stressors are somewhat controlled, then the patient is less likely to require intensive treatment, such as hospitalization.

   In all our lives there are daily stresses, but for the patient with schizophrenia, these stresses become intolerable. Patients' symptomatology generally includes impaired cognitive processing during stress. Patients are unable to focus their attention selectively and become overwhelmed by normal stimuli. Because of their bizarre behavior, which many times is a response to hallucinations, they become isolated from a social support system.

   Unless the family and close associates understand the disease process and are accepting of it, the patient may become completely isolated and ridiculed. Many times when patients require brief periods of hospitalization, they and their families feel they have failed with treatment. Schizophrenia needs to be better understood by the general public as well so that patients are able to function to their maximum potential when their symptomatology is in check.

2. The first thing the nurse wants to know is if the voices are frightening or telling the patient to harm self or others. As always, the safety of the patient is first and foremost. If the voices are telling him to kill himself or harm others, immediate interventions must be taken. It is also important for the nurse to acknowledge that the voices may seem real to the patient, but the nurse can not hear the voices.

CHAPTER 30

THE SERIOUSLY MENTALLY ILL, HOMELESS POPULATION

1. When deinstitutionalization was conceived, the idea was to provide services to individuals in their own community, keeping them part of the community. It would also save taxpayer monies. When individuals, many of them schizophrenics who had been hospitalized for long periods of time, were released into the community and their homes, neither the community nor families were ready. Many of these people no longer had families or their families were unable to cope with the patient's behaviors. In the institutions, the patients had been constantly supervised; their medication and activities of daily living were taken care of. Now, they were, in effect, turned loose into a new world. They had no skills to earn a living; they were unaccustomed to managing their own lives. Similarly, community mental health centers were not totally prepared. Many times, the patients' symptomatology returned and they were unable to access services, such as hotlines. Seriously ill patients became homeless.

2. Whether you think you could or could not work with seriously mentally ill persons who are homeless depends on what you see as your

strengths and weaknesses. Working with this population requires that the nurse clearly understand that progress, if any is to occur, will be made very slowly. The patient will have to trust the caregivers enough to comply with the treatment plan. Often the only way the patient will relate to the nurse is for the nurse to connect with the patient on some emotional level. These patients are likely to be very isolated and alienated individuals with very little ability to communicate their needs. They may also be substance abusers. The nurse must find a positive feature of the patient and use this feature to begin a relationship.

The reality of the situation is that these individuals are not the most appealing people to work with. The nurse must deal with personal feelings. Support and supervision will be required. The rewards of the work are likely to be on a very personal level.

CHAPTER 31

SUBSTANCE ABUSE

1. Prior to dealing with any individual who is involved with alcohol, it is critical for the nurse to assess his or her own beliefs, values, and attitudes about alcohol. It is vital that the nurse not have a punitive attitude. The nurse must realize that denial, an ego defense, is frequently used by individuals who abuse alcohol. If the nurse becomes impatient with the denial and thinks that the patient is lying, the patient may become anxious and more defensive, even hostile. A therapeutic relationship will be blocked.

How you feel in the situation described (the man's denying that he is an alcoholic) depends on the outcome of your assessment of yourself.

2. The nurse's first concern is the safety of the patient; therefore, the nurse would want to know, if possible, the name of the drug or the kind of drug that the patient abused, and when the patient last took the drug. This would make the nurse aware of the potential for withdrawal symptoms and what those symptoms are likely to be. The nurse would have to keep the addiction in mind when considering the patient's

postoperative anxiety and pain level and the doses of medication that would be required to manage them. The nurse would also be concerned about the physical effects the drug abuse has had: Is the patient malnourished, or more susceptible to infection? The nurse might begin to think about what the patient's view of his addiction is: Does the patient deny the problem? Does the patient want to be treated for the addiction? These are but a few concerns; you may have thought of many others.

CHAPTER 32

MANAGEMENT OF SUICIDAL PATIENTS

1. The first action that a nurse would take when suspecting that a patient is suicidal is to use therapeutic communication skills to introduce the topic of suicide and then ask direct questions about it. The nurse who suspects suicide must have gotten some clues from the patient. Is it that the patient sounds depressed? Does the patient demonstrate risk factors; e.g., does he have an "incurable" or painful disease? The nurse must determine if the patient is having suicidal thoughts and take actions to protect the patient from harm.

   The nurse also needs to discuss his or her suspicions with the other team members so that they can have input and assist with a plan of care. Patient safety is always a first priority.

2. The nurse should be aware that adolescents tend to do "copy cat" suicides. This places other students in the high school at risk for suicide. The teachers and staff should be made aware that other students are at risk.

   The students in this high school need specific counseling. An appropriate educational program might include how emotional problems can be treated and specific information about community organizations and other resources that are available, such as hotlines.

3. Suicide is considered an occupational risk for nurses who work on psychiatric units. Unless there is a collaborative team effort to assist team members to deal with the stress, individual nurses are likely to experience undue emotional suffering.

   How a particular nurse feels when a patient commits suicide depends, of course, on the individual nurse and the nurse's feelings toward the patient. Before working on the unit the psychiatric nurse should have assessed and dealt with his or her morals, beliefs, and values about suicide. A suicide on the unit is always a devastating event, and it is important that the nurse not blame himself or herself. The suicide should be dealt with by the team, so that methods of prevention can be reviewed and feelings addressed.

CHAPTER 33

MANAGING ASSAULTIVE PATIENTS

1. Nurses differ in their responses to violent threats, although most would be frightened. If the nurse had not dealt previously with his or her own feelings about violent and aggressive behavior and how to act when that behavior occurred, it would be hard to predict what other responses might occur. What is important for the nurse to realize is that all threats are serious and the nurse must act immediately by reporting the threat, getting assistance, and setting limits on the patient's verbal, as well as nonverbal, aggressive actions. The patient must understand that verbal threats cannot be tolerated in this, or any, environment and be taught acceptable ways to deal with aggression. The patient must also understand the consequences of making these remarks. The nurse must not be punitive toward the patient, but understand that the statements may be a symptom of mental illness. An effective way to talk with an aggressive patient is to project a calm, soothing manner.

2. The patient should participate in the development of a contract and agree to specific response patterns and expected behavior changes. The contract should describe staff interventions that evolve from the least restrictive to more restrictive, contingent on the patient's response. Contracting may be successful in patients who have some impulse control.

CHAPTER 34

HIV-POSITIVE PERSONS AND THEIR FAMILIES

1. Patients react in many different ways when they are told that they are HIV-positive. For some, there is almost a sense of relief; the time of uncertainty is over. Some become extremely depressed and distraught and focus on their hopelessness and helplessness. Others react by changing their behaviors; they may start to engage in no-risk sex or, conversely, take great risks during sexual activities. Still others may, with help, begin to deal with the reality of the situation.

   The patients' past coping experiences will all affect how they deal with the news that they are HIV-positive: e.g., whether they have dealt with their sexual orientation or the reasons for their are intravenous drug abuse.

   The nurse's role is to assess the patient's ability to deal with the HIV infection and to be supportive and assist the patient to deal with the problem constructively. The nurse must examine how he or she might react on learning of HIV infection in oneself or a significant other.

2. The problem of pain in patients who are HIV-positive and have neuropsychiatric problems is difficult to deal with. Generally, the patient with HIV disease is debilitated and does not tolerate analgesics well; therefore, the problems of respiratory depression and other side effects loom large. Opiates may confuse the patient who has organic mental problems or AIDS dementia. Patients may be unable to take tricyclic antidepressants at their therapeutic level, due to the anticholinergic side effects which tend to appear more frequently in patients with AIDS.

   If the patient has been a drug abuser, a physician may hesitate to prescribe narcotics for pain. These patients, however, do not tend to need large doses of drugs to relieve the pain, and they do not seem to complain of pain if there is none. The general rule is to give medication for pain on a regularly scheduled basis, rather than PRN. In that way, pain and anxiety about pain is kept at a lower level.

   In addition, it may be helpful to use non-pharmacologic methods to assist the patient. If the patient can be taught relaxation, imaging, or biofeedback techniques, they may be helpful used alone or in combination with pain medication.

CHAPTER 35

CONCEPTUAL MODELS AS GUIDES FOR PSYCHIATRIC NURSING PRACTICE

1. A conceptual model gives a clear focus from which we can delineate goals. The model allows us to approach the process of nursing and the events that are occurring using a particular framework that others can understand. Nurses can talk in the same language; we know "where we are coming from." Having a conceptual model helps nurses to know how to observe and interpret phenomena for their particular practice specialty. Actually, having a framework tells both nursing and society what the mission and boundaries of the profession are. A nursing model articulates a nursing process format that encompasses parameters for assessment, labels for patient problems, a strategy for planning care, a set of nursing interventions, and criteria for evaluating outcomes of nursing practice.

2. The three conceptual models are applicable to nursing and present the individual as a complicated system. Although they use different terminology, physiological and psychosocial components run through all the models and all deal with internal and external environments as having an effect on the person. Each model defines nursing as separate and apart, a unique profession, implying a distinct body of knowledge. Each model's goal is to have a therapeutic effect on the patient, but each one suggests a different way to approach the person. All models can be used in conjunction with the nursing process.

CHAPTER 36

THE THERAPEUTIC NURSE-PATIENT RELATIONSHIP

1. The idea that each person is a unique individual is an important one for the psychiatric nurse. Understanding this gives the nurse an awareness that each individual has had different life experiences, has a different biological make-up, and has different strengths and weaknesses. Hopefully, this knowledge will encourage the nurse to realize that each person must be cared for differently. Early in the development of a therapeutic nurse-patient relationship, the nurse and the patient must get to know each other's feelings. Hopefully, the nurse is projecting feelings of empathy and unconditional positive regard. The nurse helps patients to learn about their uniqueness — those defining aspects of self that will help or hinder an individual in moving toward a productive life. These identifying characteristics may be used to help the patient not feel so helpless and may begin to assist the patient to learn about how he or she can address present problems.

2. The patient's desire to show gratitude to the nurse is normal and natural. The nurse, however, will want to explain to the patient that a gift is not appropriate because their relationship is a professional one. The nurse may assist the patient to find more appropriate ways of expressing his or her feelings, such as talking or writing about the feelings. The nurse needs to be sure that the patient understands that the feelings of gratitude are accepted, and that it is only the method (the gift) that is in question.

CHAPTER 37

THERAPEUTIC MILIEU MANAGEMENT

1. If one views the milieu as an environment in which responsibility and decision-making power are distributed, then one must understand that decision making is usually a group process. The group, whether it be through its daily community meetings or the rules of behavior it establishes, has a great deal of power. The milieu, or environment, is structured, usually with staff input and approval, in such a way that norms underlie what is acceptable and unacceptable behavior. In addition, the consequences of displaying behavior that is not tolerated are stated. It is always important, however, that an individual's needs not be subordinated to the group by coercion.

CHAPTER 38

CLINICAL ASSESSMENT AND NURSING DIAGNOSIS

1. As a nurse it is important to first consider the purpose of any action you are asked to take. Conducting an initial assessment interview, the nurse's purpose is to find out what brought the patient to the clinic, what the patient expects from the clinic, and what in the patient's history might have contributed to the need for help. As the first professional person in the clinic with whom the patient interacts, the nurse must be sure to introduce himself or herself and explain what the goals of that day's meeting are. The nurse will also want to explain the purpose and need for collecting assessment data.

2. Making a nursing diagnosis assists the nurse in systematically analyzing the assessment data. The process helps the nurse to identify a patient's patterns of response, or potential or actual mental health problems. Nursing diagnoses themselves provide the nurse and patient with ideas for appropriate expected outcomes and interventions. Nursing diagnoses communicate to other nurses what the identifiable problems are and, in general, what the problems are related to.

CHAPTER 39

CRISIS INTERVENTION

1. The first priority in assisting anyone who is in crisis is to assess the lethality of the situation and the safety needs of the individual. A crisis might be precipitated when a patient who was threatened or battered by a spouse is now afraid

to return to the company of that individual, or when a patient who lost a loved one is so overwhelmed that suicidal ideation is present. Unless a patient is safe, it is impossible to move forward.

2. Crisis by definition means that even when using the coping mechanisms that the individual is familiar with, the individual is in a state of disequilibrium. If during crisis the individual is not helped, maladaptive coping generally results. The individual is likely to continue to be uncomfortable. The immediate crisis situation will eventually be diffused, but then the person usually functions at a lower adaptive level. The person is usually more vulnerable in problematic situations and may come into crisis more easily; that is, more or similar situations may be emotionally hazardous. It is possible that without treatment the person in crisis may become self-destructive. Crises may also trigger — immediately or in the future — such mental disorders as depression and post-traumatic stress syndrome. Crisis intervention not only helps the person with that crisis but also assists the individual to learn new and more adaptive coping responses. Consequently, in the future, the person will function at a more mature and stable level.

CHAPTER 40

TREATMENT MODALITIES: CRISIS, BEHAVIORAL, RELATIONSHIP, AND INSIGHT

1. In deciding what kind of treatment modality to use with a patient, the nurse would have to consider his or her own skills. Although one modality may be preferable, if the nurse is unable to do the "tasks" required, then the nurse has two options: to learn how to use that therapy, or to refer the patient to someone with the necessary skills. The nurse must consider the patient and the context in which the therapy is to be given. A part of considering the context is to determine what resources are available; patients differ in the severity of their problems, the amount of dysfunction that they have, and the amount of time they have available.

2. In discussing insight therapy with a colleague,

the nurse would explain that the therapy focuses on assisting people to increase self-awareness and self-control, and thereby decreases their need to use defensive patterns that may interfere with self-actualization. This type of therapy is really for those who have subtle problems, who want to be more in touch with their feelings. Sometimes, the person has some unrealistic expectations or some difficulties in relationships that may have to do with past experiences.

CHAPTER 41

THERAPEUTIC GROUPS

1. In preparing a patient for therapy in a group that uses the interpersonal model, the nurse should explain that by interacting in the group the patient will begin to understand more about herself. The nurse should inform the patient that she will need to be open and honest in the group, and that there may be group members she does not like or who do not like her. Most important, however, is that by learning about oneself in this guided experience, the patient will develop more adaptive ways of thinking, feeling, and behaving.

2. Adolescents often have problems dealing with authority. Therefore, a one-to-one relationship may make adolescents feel that they are being scrutinized. Consequently, they may become blocked or unwilling to verbalize their feelings or thoughts in the individual setting. The peer group experience should be part of a normal adolescent's developmental experience. If the adolescent is isolated, withdrawn, and has no exposure to peers, the group experience may also be indicated.

3. Numerous factors might lead to difficulty within a multiethnic therapy group. Perhaps the nurse has not dealt with his or her own biases and prejudices. In addition, everyone might not speak the same language, or expressions used in speech might mean different things to different ethnic groups, or silence may be honored by a particular ethnic group or person.

It also could be that the nurse never prepared

the group properly for therapy. The group must deal with its own biases and prejudices. The larger society may devalue cultural difference, and this devaluation may have been internalized by minority groups within the society. The minority groups, or individuals from these groups, may have a negative sense of self.

Many factors may be problematic within a multiethnic or, for that matter, any group. The leader must recognize the problem. Then, with the group, the leader will try to identify the problematic factors and work on methods to deal with the problems that are identified.

CHAPTER 42
PHARMACOTHERAPY

1. In addition to obtaining baseline psychological data, functional and behavioral assessments provide the nurse with a great deal of data about the patient's beliefs about drug therapy. The patient's misunderstandings can be addressed. The patient will have to give informed consent regarding the use of drugs and, in order to make a reasonable decision, the patient must have adequate knowledge. During the assessment period, the nurse and the patient are forming a therapeutic alliance through the thoughts they are sharing. In addition, the nurse can observe the patient's behavior. Does the patient have any hallucinations or illusions that may interfere with the therapy or that one needs to be aware of, as they may be the symptoms for which the therapy is prescribed?

Having all the baseline data is most helpful when monitoring the patient once the drug is started. Then, the nurse is better able to judge whether the changes that occur are due to the drug's action.

2. Nurses need to empathize with patients who become noncompliant with psychopharmacological interventions because many of the drugs have very uncomfortable effects. For example, antipsychotic drugs can cause parkinsonian-like symptoms; tricyclic drugs, such as lithium, may slow one's thinking processes. Gaining weight and sexual dysfunction are side effects

of other drugs. Effects may be therapeutic or side effects, but in either case, patients may not feel comfortable because of them.

Patients may also be using drugs to stabilize a chronic condition and those patients may be, albeit an unrealistic expectation, looking for a cure. Patients may say, "This drug is not making me any better," and stop using it.

In addition, patients may have restrictions placed on them when they are taking medication. They may have to stay out of the sun, avoid drinking any alcoholic beverage, or be unable to drive an automobile because of a drug's sedative effect. Some drugs require that blood tests be done periodically, and patients may find the tests painful and inconvenient. Money for purchase of drugs may also be an issue.

For these, and many other reasons, the nurse should be able to empathize with a patient who becomes noncompliant. The nurse needs to counsel these patients in terms of the therapy's benefits and what the patient sees as risks (downside).

CHAPTER 43
CRITICAL PATHWAYS FOR MENTAL HEALTH AND PLANNING CARE

1. For the first time, there is a single multidisciplinary plan of care. It is beneficial that all disciplines involved in caring for a psychiatric patient must now be aware of what the goals and outcomes of care are and how these goals can be achieved in a specific time frame. One hopes that pathways will be somewhat individualized when dealing with specific patients so that they do not become useless professional tools.

Pathways are used to document variance. If used properly, pathways may make all of those involved in psychiatric mental health aware of improvements that are needed in patient care delivery.

2. One problem that might be foreseen in using critical pathways is the possibility of their standardizing care too much. Because the pathway is based on current standards of care, one

also wonders how experimentation and creativity are going to be built in. One can imagine, that in this era of cost containment, if one finds a creative approach that is also a cost saver, no problems in implementation will arise. In dealing with behavior, however, one sometimes learns through own's mistakes, and it is hoped that by standardizing care this approach will not be totally lost.

CHAPTER 44
CASE MANAGEMENT

1. Nurses, particularly those in mental health care, have good access to patients and information about their wants and needs. Psychiatric nurses are, or should be, excellent communicators; therefore, they should be able to take on the multidisciplinary collaborative role that is part of case management. By using an outcomes approach, the nurse, whether in an inpatient or community-based setting, can use the nursing process to determine patients' care needs across the health-illness spectrum. The nurse should be aware of community resources so that the best cost-effective care can be provided to the patient. Then, through the relationship that is generally set up when a psychiatric nurse works with a patient, the nurse can easily act as case manager and ensure that the outcomes that are achieved in one setting are not lost in a transfer to another care setting.

2. The patient who has psychiatric mental health problems needs to be viewed on a continuum. It is usually the goal to keep the patient in the least restrictive environment and use inpatient services only when they are essential. Most psychiatric patients, therefore, are in the community where they may need preventive and health maintenance services, in addition to more intensive treatment during crises. The community-based psychiatric nurse will probably spend more time with the mentally ill patient and the family and get to know them, and their desires and needs better then would a case manager who is hospital based. Moreover, the community-based nurse is part of the patient's community — aware of its culture, and, on a day-to-day basis, knowledgeable about its resources and deficiencies.

CHAPTER 45
PSYCHIATRIC HOME HEALTH CARE

1. Some of the questions a nurse may consider in deciding whether home care is appropriate for a patient are listed below. They are not in priority order.

   - Is the patient ready to go to an environment without 24-hour supervision?

   - Can the patient's psychiatric needs be met at home? What are those needs?

   - Is the patient considered psychiatric homebound? On what basis?

   - How will the patient's home care be funded? Is the patient eligible for Medicare or does the patient's insurance pay for these services?

   - Will the patient require supportive services, e.g., a homemaker in addition to psychiatric nursing care?

   - If the patient has a family or significant others, how do they feel about the option of the patient staying with them?

2. In a patient's home, the nurse is a guest. The patient permits the nurse to come in. Usually no peers or supervisors are present; the nurse, therefore, functions more independently in the home and needs to have very well honed assessment, evaluation, and intervention skills. The nurse may need to be more flexible and innovative, as the nurse may not be able to change many situations in the home environment, such as messiness or noise, but, instead, will have to work around them. The family and significant others may be present, and establishing collaborative relationships with them may become critical.

NCLEX-TYPE QUESTIONS
for reviewing the text

1. A patient is to be discharged from a psychiatric inpatient unit to his home. The patient's wife is to receive instruction regarding the patient's medication regime and his care at home. Prior to beginning the teaching, the nurse assesses the wife's level of anxiety. For which of these reasons is the nurse's assessment appropriate?

   A. Learning usually does not take place when the level of anxiety is too high.

   B. Unless there is at least a moderate level of anxiety, learning is unlikely to take place.

   C. If a high level of anxiety is present, audio-visual materials should not be used.

   D. The level of anxiety indicates how great is the need for the information.

2. The nurse informs a patient that a privilege he was to have had if he kept an agreement to participate in a unit activity has been removed because he did not participate in the activity. The patient does not respond to the nurse at the time the nurse informs him of the loss of the privilege. A little while later, however, when his wife visits, the patient shouts at her and shows other signs of anger inappropriate to the situation.

   The nurse interprets correctly that the patient is using which of these defense mechanisms?

   A. Reaction formation

   B. Displacement

   C. Projection

   D. Sublimation

3. A mother of a 26-month-old boy says to the nurse, " I'm really concerned. Lately my son has become afraid of the dark and seems so scared of loud noises." In order to respond appropriately, the nurse should know that at this age this behavior is

   A. a sign of abuse.

   B. an indication of faulty attachment.

   C. commonly seen in overprotected children.

   D. a part of normal growth and development.

4. A patient is admitted to an impatient facility. The nurse does a careful assessment of the patient's cultural background. The purpose of the assessment is to

   A. plan appropriate patient care.

   B. compare the patient's experience with external norms.

   C. encourage the patient to talk about a nonthreatening area.

   D. identify experiences that are similar to those of the interviewer.

5. In a mental health clinic a patient says to the nurse, "Please don't tell anyone, but I've been thinking about driving my car into a wall." The nurse's intervention will be based on which of these understandings?

   A. Patients often threaten destructive acts as a way of getting more attention.

   B. When a patient threatens a destructive act, it is the duty of the nurse to protect the person.

   C. When a patient discusses a destructive act with a nurse, it is a sign that the patient does not intend to commit the act.

   D. Patients who allow time to elapse after they have considered a destructive act do not commit the act.

6. Over the past 10 years a 27-year-old woman has repeatedly been treated both medically and surgically for abdominal discomfort. Recently she was diagnosed as having a somatization disorder. Which of these nursing diagnoses is most appropriate?

   A. Ineffective individual coping

   B. Sensory-perceptual alteration

   C. Alterations in pain

   D. Self-care deficit

7. A patient says to the nurse, "Why do I have to have electroshock treatments?" Which of these responses by the nurse is most appropriate?

   A. "Can you be specific about what you would like to know?"

   B. "Did you understand what the doctor told you?"

   C. "You are fearful about the treatments."

   D. "The treatments will hasten your recovery."

8. A nurse is interviewing a newly admitted patient and says, " Tell me what brought you to the hospital." The patient does not answer immediately. Which of these actions should the nurse take initially?

   A. Find out if the patient heard the question.

   B. Rephrase the question.

   C. Touch the patient's arm gently.

   D. Wait for a while in silence.

9. A patient tells the nurse that she feels a panic attack coming on. Which of these nursing interventions is appropriate?

   A. Find out from the patient what she thinks is triggering the attack.

   B. Ask the patient to describe what she is feeling

   C. Try to focus the patient on another issue.

   D. Find out when the patient had similar feelings.

10. A male patient is admitted to the psychiatric unit and diagnosed as having obsessive compulsive disorder. He has rituals concerning bathing, dressing, and eating that prevent him from functioning. Which of these treatment goals is appropriate for the time of discharge?

    A. Is able to demonstrate some flexibility in activities of daily living

    B. Is able to maintain focus on immediate surroundings

    C. Can begin to verbalize thoughts while conducting activities of daily living

    D. Can encourage others to assist him with unaccomplished chores

11. To assist a patient who is terminally ill effectively prepare for her death, it is appropriate for the nurse to include which of the following measures in the patient's care?

    A. Limit the time the patient spends with her family.

    B. Provide opportunities for the patient to face the shortness of her life constructively.

    C. Avoid situations that are likely to evoke painful memories.

    D. Suggest that the patient see a member of the clergy on a daily basis.

12. The daughter of a male patient who is terminally ill says to the nurse, "My father and mother, although they have been married for a long time, disagree about so many things. Now things seem to be worse than ever. You'd think that now that my father is going to die my mother would just let him have his way."

    The nurse's response should be based on the understanding that

    A. this is an unexpected reaction at this time.

    B. family members tend to exaggerate difficulties.

    C. a family member may tend to project his or her own feelings about the terminally ill member as death approaches.

    D. terminal illness may exacerbate difficulties in family relationships.

13. An elderly patient who has suffered a severe heart attack says to the nurse, "I have a living will and my children do not agree with what I have decided. I hope the doctors will abide by my wishes." Which of these responses by the nurse is most appropriate?

    A. "Your wishes are the most important."

    B. "Do you expect your children to be here when these decisions have to be made?"

    C. "You and your children should really decide together."

    D. "Don't you think you should reconsider your decisions?"

14. A child has been diagnosed as having attention deficit hyperactivity disorder. The nurse should anticipate that the child will have which of these symptoms?

   A. Difficulty sleeping at night

   B. Poor appetite

   C. Impulsiveness

   D. Intention tremor

15. A child diagnosed as having a conduct disorder becomes physically abusive to another child. The nurse's actions should be based on the understanding that

   A. punishment for aggressive acts needs to be of the same nature as the act.

   B. children need to feel that staff can limit their inappropriate behaviors.

   C. impulse control cannot be learned in an environment where the aggressor is physically stronger then the other people in the environment.

   D. children who are physically attacked should be involved in deciding what discipline should be used for those who attacked them.

16. In discussing the care of a 9-year-old boy who has enuresis with the child's mother, it is appropriate for the nurse to include which of these suggestions?

   A. "Do not give your son any liquids after 4 in the afternoon."

   B. "Place a plastic sheet on top of the regular sheet on your son's bed."

   C. "Remind you son that he won't be able to sleep away at friends' houses if he continues to wet his bed."

   D. "Have your son change the sheets on his bed when he wets the bed."

17. An adolescent patient is admitted to the inpatient psychiatric unit because she is very depressed. The nurse should understand that which of these factors, if present in the adolescent's history, places her at risk for suicide?

   A. Her grandmother committed suicide.

   B. She is chronologically the middle child in her family.

   C. She is the only female child in her family.

   D. Her mother smoked when she was pregnant with her.

18. The nurse is talking to an elderly woman who complains that she seems to be sleeping for shorter periods of time than when she was younger. In order to respond to this woman, which of these understandings should the nurse have?

   A. Shortened sleep periods are the first sign of depression in the elderly.

   B. Shortened sleep periods are a normal part of the aging process.

   C. The elderly have distortions of time regarding sleep.

   D. The elderly who complain of problems with sleep are generally not dealing well with the finality of life.

19. The daughter of an elderly patient who has suffered a cerebral accident says to the nurse, "I think I'm going to begin to make plans to have my mother come and live with us instead of having her return to her own apartment." Which of these responses by the nurse is most appropriate initially?

   A. "You might want to talk to the social worker before you decide."

   B. "Have you considered the alterations that would be required in your home?"

   C. "It might be easier to have someone live with your mother in her own home."

   D. "Have you asked your mother what she would prefer?"

20. A 68-year-old patient seems depressed. The nurse should assess the patient for which of these symptoms that is frequently seen in elderly patients who are depressed?

A. Increase in time spent reminiscing

B. Loss of visual acuity

C. Loss of appetite

D. Ringing in the ears

21. Because of the side effects of the tricyclic antidepressant drug that is being used to treat a depressed elderly patient, the nurse should include which of these measures in the patient's care?

A. Increase his fluid intake.

B. Monitor his cardiac rhythms.

C. Question him about his bowel function.

D. Observe him for bleeding tendencies.

22. A newly admitted 85-year-old patient is suspected of having delirium. Which of these factors, if present in the patient's history, is common in patients with delirium?

A. He has an elevated blood sugar.

B. He is of Mediterranean origin.

C. He was a coal miner for 34 years.

D. He is dehydrated.

23. A resident who is newly admitted to a nursing home seems slightly confused. Which of these measures is likely to assist the resident?

A. Encourage friends or family to bring in objects from the resident's home.

B. Provide the resident with few choices regarding meals.

C. Keep stimuli in the environment to a minimum.

D. Remind staff not to answer the same questions repeatedly, but to ask the resident to give the answers.

24. A patient is admitted to the psychiatric unit with a diagnosis of major depression. A nursing diagnosis of dysfunctional grieving has also been made. Which of these interventions should have priority?

A. Encourage the patient to learn the normal stages of grieving.

B. Have the patient identify behaviors associated with grieving.

C. Determine what stage of grieving the patient is in.

D. Teach the patient adaptive skills to use to cope with grieving.

25. In the dayroom of a psychiatric unit, a patient is talking loudly, pacing, telling other patients what to do, and changing the channels on the television while others are watching a program. In view of this patient's behaviors, which of these actions should the nurse take first?

A. Check to see what medications the patient is receiving.

B. With assistance, place the patient in seclusion.

C. Escort the patient from the dayroom.

D. Find out if the other patients in the dayroom object to the patient's behavior.

26. Because a patient is receiving lithium therapy, the nurse should observe the patient for side effects which include

A. thirst.

B. orange-colored urine.

C. nystagmus.

D. tetany.

27. A patient who is very depressed and scheduled for electroconvulsive therapy (ECT) treatment says to the nurse, "I'm so frightened about having these treatments." Which of these responses is it appropriate for the nurse to make initially?

A. "Would you like to talk to someone who has had the treatments?"

B. "Would you like me to explain what happens during the treatments?"

C. "People usually forget their fright after the first treatment."

D. "Tell me what about the treatment frightens you."

28. A patient who was admitted to the hospital with a diagnosis of anorexia is now permitted out of bed. She is to eat her meals in the dining room. Which of these measures should be included in the patient's care?

    A. Have the patient weigh herself after eating.

    B. Have the patient remain in a public area for at least an hour after meals.

    C. Place the food on the patient's plate so that the proteins are directly in the middle.

    D. Provide child-size utensils for the patient to eat with.

29. A patient who is diagnosed as having bulimia nervosa is to keep a food-intake diary. Which of these statements, if made by the patient, indicates that a goal of using the diary has been achieved?

    A. "I notice that I am eating foods that are high in Vitamin C."

    B. "I notice that I tend to eat the most after I talk to my mother."

    C. "When I eat in a restaurant, I'm likely to overestimate the calories I'm eating."

    D. "When I drink water with my meal, I'm not so likely to have a second cup of coffee."

30. A mother complains that her 6-year-old son occasionally walks in his sleep. Which of these suggestions is it essential for the nurse to give to the mother?

    A. "Make sure that the windows are closed."

    B. "Use a restraint to keep the child in bed."

    C. "Do not allow the child to eat foods containing stimulants, such as caffeine before bedtime."

    D. "Leave a light on in the bedroom."

31. An adolescent is known to have been a victim of child abuse and currently is in treatment. The mother of this adolescent reports that the adolescent is constantly fighting with her peers and family members. In order for the nurse to assist this mother, which of these understandings should the nurse have?

    A. Aggressive behaviors may indicate that the person was not a victim of abuse but the abuser.

    B. This type of behavior is part of the normal development of an adolescent and is not related to the abuse.

    C. This type of interpersonal behavior indicates that the adolescent is also a substance abuser.

    D. Interpersonal disruptions including aggressive behavior are commonly seen in victims of abuse.

32. A 15-year-old girl who has been raped tells the nurse that she feels a sense of total helplessness. In planning care for this girl, it is important for the nurse to be sure that the girl be given opportunities to

    A. evaluate how she could have handled the assault more effectively.

    B. blame herself for the assault.

    C. separate herself from her social network.

    D. make decisions about her care.

33. A patient is diagnosed as having a schizoid personality disorder. The nurse can expect this patient to have a pattern of

    A. excessive emotionality.

    B. attention seeking.

    C. violating the rights of others.

    D. detachment from social relationships.

34. As well as assessing a patient, a nurse has read the patient's chart and learned that the patient is a college professor who has not kept current in his field. The professor has graduate students do his work, particularly preparing material for publication. The professor never acknowledges their work and takes credit for the student's achievements in other areas as well. The professor sees himself as entitled to promotions and raises.

    Based on the information provided, which of these nursing diagnoses is most appropriate?

    A. Defensive coping related to unrealistic expectations of self and others

    B. Self-esteem disturbance related to repeated negative feedback

    C. Risk for violence: self-directed related to perceived threat of self-concept

    D. Altered thought process related to inability to trust

35. The nurse is to care for an infant who has been diagnosed as neglected. In light of this diagnosis, which of these behaviors should the nurse expect?

    A. Hyperactive response to stimuli

    B. Excessive passivity

    C. Continuous crying

    D. Constantly in movement

36. In planning care for a 6-year-old child who is admitted to the hospital because he has been neglected and maltreated, the nurse should give a high priority to which of these measures?

    A. Provide an educationally stimulating environment.

    B. Encourage interaction with other children.

    C. Assign a primary nurse to care for him.

    D. Have him talk with others who have been abused.

37. The nurse in the emergency room suspects that a 10-year-old child, who was brought in by her mother, is being maltreated. After a careful assessment and physical examination, it is decided that the case be reported to the appropriate child protective services agency. Before the mother leaves, the nurse should be sure that

    A. the child has an opportunity to call a friend.

    B. the close relatives of the child have been notified that a report has been filed.

    C. the hospital's clergy have been informed.

    D. the mother has been told that a report has been made.

38. A child is suspected of having been maltreated by his mother. Which of the following findings in the mother's history is considered a risk factor for child maltreatment?

    A. She is the eldest in her family of origin.

    B. She is the only girl in her family of origin.

    C. She is left-handed.

    D. She is physically abused by her husband.

39. A woman comes to the emergency room. She tells the nurse that she is being battered by her husband. Which of the following factors in her history is closely associated with family violence?

    A. She is the youngest child in her family of origin.

    B. She is the same age as her husband.

    C. She was physically abused as a child.

    D. She was married when she was in her mid-twenties.

40. A patient who has been diagnosed as having schizophrenia is readmitted to the hospital. It is the patient's third admission in 3 years. The patient's mother says to the nurse, "I don't understand what my son is doing wrong. Every year he has to be hospitalized." It is appropriate for the nurse's response to be based on which of these understandings?

    A. Hospitalization should not be viewed as a treatment failure.

    B. When hospitalization is needed on a yearly basis, the patient is not being compliant.

    C. Patients with this diagnosis are usually hospitalized every 6 to 8 months.

    D. Hospitalization is often used to reevaluate treatment options.

41. On the psychiatric unit, the nurse is talking to a patient who consistently claims that his food is being poisoned. The nurse should recognize this symptom as

    A. a delusion.

    B. a hallucination.

    C. projection.

    D. dissociation.

42. The nurse is talking with an adolescent suspected of abusing alcohol. The adolescent says, "I really don't have a problem, I just drink for fun." The nurse's response is based on the understanding that the patient's denial is used to

    A. increase the nurse's anxiety level.

    B. encourage the nurse to become hostile.

    C. protect the patient's ego.

    D. gain sympathy for the patient.

43. When the nurse begins to give the patient a prescribed medication, the patient says, "You are poisoning me with the pills you are giving me." Which of these responses by the nurse is most appropriate?

    A. "Tell me why you think I am doing that with the pills."

    B. "This isn't the first dose I've given you."

    C. "I'll get a fresh package of pills so you can see me open the sealed package."

    D. "Are the other nurses giving you these pills?"

44. A patient is brought to the emergency room with symptoms of alcohol withdrawal. It is approximately 24 hours since the patient's last drink. Symptoms of alcohol withdrawal at this time usually include

    A. runny nose.

    B. hypotension.

    C. bradycardia.

    D. nausea.

45. A patient who is known to be a narcotic abuser is involved in an automobile accident and has extensive surgery. In planning for analgesia post-surgery, the nurse should be aware that this patient is likely to

    A. tolerate more pain than a patient who is not a drug user.

    B. require greater doses of medication before pain is relieved.

    C. refuse medication to prove addiction is not a problem.

    D. tolerate oral medication better than intravenous doses.

46. A patient who abuses narcotics tells the nurse he wants to go "cold turkey." The nurse discusses what usually occurs during opiate withdrawal. Which of these statements if made by the patient would indicate a need for further instruction?

    A. "In the beginning my eyes are likely to tear."

    B. "My symptoms will last about 1 to 2 days."

    C. "It's likely that I'll get diarrhea."

    D. "It'll be really hard for me to tolerate any pain."

47. A 78-year-old patient says to the nurse, "I think I've lived long enough. None of my friends are around anymore." Based on the patient's statement, which of these actions is it appropriate for the nurse to take initially?

    A. Refer the patient to a member of the clergy.

    B. Find out how the patient has handled depression in the past.

    C. Remind the patient that all older people have these kinds of feelings.

    D. Call a family member to alert her to the possibility of suicide.

48. A patient is being assessed for suicidal risk. Which of these factors in the patient's history places the patient at risk for suicide?

    A. The patient will be 30 years old this week.

    B. The patient has just completed a food service training program.

    C. The patient is in the sixth month of her pregnancy.

    D. The patient's mother overdosed on sleeping pills.

49. A patient with a history of aggressive behavior comes to the mental health clinic and demands to see the nurse immediately. The nurse is summoned. Was this action appropriate?
    A. Yes. If the patient is kept waiting, the patient is likely to interpret it as a sign that he did not need immediate treatment.
    B. Yes. If the patient is not seen immediately, he will not return again.
    C. No. Other patients may use this type of behavior when they see that it works.
    D. No. Patients need to be seen in turn.

50. A patient on a psychiatric unit says to the nurse, "If you try to keep me from getting a pass this weekend, I'll kill you." The nurse's response should be based on which of these understandings?
    A. Threats of violence must be reported immediately.
    B. Verbal threats of violence are usually a call for attention.
    C. Whether a threat becomes an action is solely dependent on the nurse's emotional response.
    D. An assessment of the patient's impulse control mechanisms needs to be performed prior to taking any action.

51. An 82-year-old patient says to the nurse who has been providing care to her for a long time, "I'd like you to have this necklace that my husband gave me when we were married." In order to respond appropriately to the patient, it is essential for the nurse to consider which of these questions?
    A. Does the patient feel the care she is receiving is adequate?
    B. What does the patient hope to gain from giving the gift?
    C. Does the patient have any suicidal ideation?
    D. What was the patient's relationship with her spouse?

52. The nurse is preparing medication at the nurses' station when a male stranger comes up behind the nurse and says," Unless I get the keys to the narcotics cabinet, I'm going to kill you." The stranger has no visible weapon. Which of these actions should the nurse take initially?
    A. Call for help.
    B. Explain the consequences of this behavior to the man.
    C. Quickly assess the stranger's level of anxiety.
    D. Comply with the stranger's request.

53. A female nursing assistant tells the nurse that she is not comfortable about a young adolescent's behavior and will not provide care to him. The adolescent has poor impulse control, but has never "acted out" or assaulted the assistant. Which of these goals should have priority in the nurse's dealing with the nursing assistant?
    A. To have the assistant care for the patient
    B. To have the assistant identify her feelings about aggressive and violent behavior
    C. To have the assistant confront the patient about his behavior
    D. To have the assistant admit the need for a referral for counseling services

54. The nurse and a patient who resides on a psychiatric unit are discussing the idea of contracting. The patient has a history of violent behavior. The nurse will know that the patient needs further instruction about the concept of contracting if the patient makes which of these statements?
    A. "The patient is responsible for using appropriate methods for dealing with aggressive behaviors."
    B. "The staff alone will determine what the consequences of the patient's behavior will be."
    C. "The contract indicates how nonaggressive behavior will be rewarded."
    D. "The patient is the one who knows what aggressive behavior is unacceptable."

55. Which of these factors in a patient's history places the patient at the greatest risk for HIV infection?

A. Her brother is a drug abuser.

B. Her lymph nodes were repeatedly infected when she was a child.

C. She was abused by an uncle as a teenager.

D. She gets weekly injections for allergies.

56. The nurse suggests to a patient who is in counseling because he has AIDS that it might be helpful for him to either write or tape his life story. The nurse knows that the therapeutic goals for the use of this tool are to give the patient an opportunity to review his life and provide

A. a way to document his care.

B. an aid in the continuing assessment of his psychological status.

C. a method for legally defending his need for financial assistance.

D. a substitute for interpersonal contacts.

57. Because a patient has AIDS dementia complex, the nurse can expect the patient to have which of these symptoms?

A. Seizures

B. Hyperactivity

C. Memory loss

D. Paralysis

58. The nurse is about to give the first dose of a tricyclic antidepressant drug to a patient who is severely depressed and has AIDS. The nurse notes that the dose is extremely small. Which of these actions should the nurse take initially?

A. Give the dose as prescribed.

B. Call the physician to have the dose increased.

C. Assess the patient's T-helper cell count.

D. Check the patient's reflexes.

59. The nurse is interviewing a patient who has been addicted to opiates. The patient tells the nurse that he cannot understand why his drug screening test was positive for opiates, as he is not using the drugs now. The answer to which of these questions should the nurse consider as a basis for explaining why the patient's urine test was positive for opiates?

A. "Is he taking any medications that contain ibuprofen?"

B. "Has he eaten any aged cheese?"

C. "Is he dehydrated?"

D. "Has he increased his salt intake suddenly?"

60. If a patient who is addicted to a benzodiazepine, such as diazepam (Valium), were to withdraw abruptly from the drug, the nurse should expect the patient to have

A. cardiac arhthymias.

B. visual difficulties.

C. respiratory distress.

D. seizures.

61. The patient and nurse are setting up a therapeutic relationship. In the orientation phase, a goal is for the patient to

A. assess her failures in coping.

B. identify the process of seeking help as a learning experience.

C. accept mental illness as a failure of self.

D. make the nurse trust her.

62. In the first interview with a patient, the nurse and the patient are discussing how angry the patient feels about her mother-in-law's attitude toward her children. During this first encounter, it will be vital for the nurse to take which of the following actions?

A. Advise the patient how to avoid these feelings.

B. Reassure the patient that these feelings are normal.

C. Encourage the patient to express her feelings further.

D. Suggest to the patient that she focus on more positive feelings.

63. A nurse has noticed that a colleague, another nurse on the psychiatric unit, seems unable to leave the unit on time at the end of the shift. A young female patient always seems to ask the nurse in question to assist her with something just as the nurse is ready to go.

    Prior to discussing this situation with the nurse in question, the nurse who has observed the situation should understand that the nurse in question may

    A. need help in organizing her work.

    B. be having difficulty setting effective boundaries.

    C. not be aware of the unit rules.

    D. be a dedicated individual.

64. A patient complains to a nurse that the nurse on the evening shift seems so formal and refuses to "chat" with him. The nurse should understand that the patient's complaint reflects which of these feelings?

    A. Projection

    B. Introjection

    C. Delusional thinking

    D. Depersonalization

65. A patient is about to be discharged from the psychiatric inpatient unit to a neighborhood clinic that has its own treatment team. The patient says to the nurse with whom the patient has been working, "I'd like to come back and see you from time to time." The nurse's response is based on which of these understandings?

    A. Maintaining contact with the patient after the patient is discharged to another facility conveys a message of lack of confidence in the patient's ability to move on.

    B. Patients often say they want to maintain contact as a way of testing a nurse's professionalism.

    C. Unless a certain amount of contact is maintained, the accomplishments made in the relationship are likely to be lost.

    D. Maintaining contact conveys to the patient the nurse's interest in the patient as a unique individual.

66. At a community meeting on a psychiatric unit, the nurse notes that one of the patients is interrupting the meeting frequently and the group leader is allowing this behavior. Which of these actions is it appropriate for the nurse to take?

    A. Tell the patient to discontinue this behavior.

    B. Encourage another member of the group to censure the patient.

    C. Ask the patient if he would like to talk privately with the nurse.

    D. Discuss this observation during the postmeeting process.

67. A nurse is to assess a psychiatric patient's response to medication. Prior to the assessment, which of these questions should the nurse consider?

    A. What is the purpose of the medication?

    B. What is the cost of the medication?

    C. When does the patient take the medication?

    D. When was the patient's last appointment?

68. A unit has just begun to use a critical pathway system. A nurse notes that a patient is not making progress according to the prescribed pathway. Which of these actions should the nurse take?

    A. Determine who from the nursing staff decided that this was a proper goal.

    B. Find out if the physician is aware of this problem.

    C. Determine what is interfering with the patient's ability to meet goal.

    D. Try to find out what other team members have done when a problem like this occurred.

69. A patient's family is talking with the nurse about their daughter who has just come to the clinic for crisis management. The nurse explains to the family that the purpose of this therapy is to

    A. cure her illness.

    B. focus her on past events that led to this crisis.

    C. assist her to learn new coping strategies.

    D. encourage her to learn operant techniques.

70. A 36-year-old female patient who comes to the nurse for crisis intervention after the loss of her spouse says,"I know I am going to die of a heart attack just like my husband did." Which of these responses by the nurse is most appropriate?

A. "Many people are fearful of having heart attacks."

B. "Did your husband have heart problems before he died?"

C. "Have you asked your doctor what your actual risk of having a heart attack is?"

D. " Your husband's life experiences may have led to his heart problems."

71. A patient is being prepared by the nurse to start pharmacotherapy. The patient talks about his fear of drugs; however, after the discussion with the nurse about the specific medication, the patient decides to begin the therapy. The nurse's reason for discussing the medication with the patient was based on the knowledge that shared decision-making leads to empowerment and can prevent

A. regression.

B. delusions.

C. illusions.

D. ideas of reference.

72. After a patient has been on a specific medication for a while, the patient says to the nurse, "I feel lots better, and I'd like to try taking smaller doses of the medication and see how that works." The nurse's response should be based on the understanding that the patient's request indicates the patient

A. is in the beginning stages of noncompliance.

B. does not understand that the responsibility for drug adjustment lies with the physician.

C. is testing staff regulations.

D. has a desire to self-monitor his drugs.

73. A patient who is diagnosed as having schizophrenia is to receive long-term antipsychotic drug therapy. Because one of the side effects of the drug is sedation, the nurse should understand that a goal of therapy is for the patient to

A. learn methods to prevent drowsiness.

B. schedule events so that a daytime nap can be taken.

C. drink small amounts of stimulant liquids, such as coffee, throughout the day.

D. take one bedtime dose of the drug.

74. A patient who has been on long-term antipsychotic drug therapy has beginning signs of tardive dyskinesia. The nurse's action is based on the understanding that

A. anti-parkinsonian drugs are used for treatment.

B. the drug will be discontinued.

C. increasing the dosage of the drug slightly will retard the progression of symptoms.

D. this is an expected effect of the drug.

75. A patient who is taking an antipsychotic drug complains of beginning symptoms of dystonia. Which of these actions should the nurse take?

A. Remind the patient that the side effects are expected.

B. Obtain an order for benztropine mesylate (Cogentin).

C. Teach the patient relaxation techniques to lessen the side effects.

D. Discontinue the drug immediately.

76. A patient is to start clozapine therapy. Because of the risk for agranulocytosis, the patient will have periodic blood counts and should be observed for symptoms of agranulocytosis, which include

A. muscle rigidity.

B. pill rolling movements.

C. tremors.

D. sore throat.

77. A female patient is started on chlorpromazine (Thorazine) therapy. The patient has received instructions regarding the drug's side effects. Which of these comments if stated by the patient indicates that she understood the instructions?

   A. "I'm likely to have a decrease in my desire to have sex."

   B. "I'm likely to lose weight while I'm taking the drug."

   C. "I should wear protective clothing so I'm not in the direct sun."

   D. "I should feel more energetic now."

78. The nurse and the patient on a psychiatric unit are talking about the patient's experiences in group therapy. Which of these statements if made by the patient indicates that a goal of therapy has been reached?

   A. "I've learned how to change the direction of the conversation in the group."

   B. "I feel like I'm not so isolated from everyone when I go to group."

   C. "It's nice to watch the leader try to get everyone involved in the group."

   D. "I know now that I don't have to go to group when I'm feeling low."

79. A patient, who talks easily with his family and friends and with all the nurses on the unit, is attending group therapy with six other patients. The nurse notes that the patient is silent and withdrawn in the group. Prior to talking with the patient about his behavior, the nurse should initially consider which of these questions?

   A. Does he have difficulty hearing?

   B. Does he have difficulty being in a group where a staff member is present?

   C. Is this a bad time of day for the patient?

   D. What are his cultural values about sharing problems?

80. A patient is being discharged from an inpatient facility to a psychiatrist in an outpatient clinic. Prior to discharge, which of these questions is it essential for the nurse to ask the patient?

   A. Has anyone the patient knows ever attended the clinic?

   B. What type of transportation services does the patient have available?

   C. Can someone remain in the clinic while the patient is seeing the doctor?

   D. Will the patient be remaining in contact with any of the patients in the inpatient facility?

81. A nurse is talking with a 78-year-old male patient on a psychiatric unit who is to be discharged. Because of the patient's condition, he is considered psychiatrically homebound. Plans are being made for psychiatric home care services. The patient is very concerned about payment for the services.

   The nurse's response should be based on which of these understandings?

   A. If the patient is unable to pay, the patient will be referred to social services.

   B. The home care providers use a sliding scale to determine appropriate rates of payment.

   C. Medicare will reimburse for qualified home care services.

   D. Other resources, such as outpatient clinics, are used when reimbursement for home care is a problem.

82. A nurse is reviewing the work of a nursing student. The student has listed an outcome for a patient as: The patient will improve his ability to express his feelings.

   The nurse should recognize that this statement is

   A. properly stated because it is an appropriate outcome.

   B. properly stated because it deals with a psychiatric concern.

   C. improperly stated because it is not stated in measurable terms.

   D. improperly stated because it does not address the means of assessment.

83. A patient who is taking an antipsychotic drug tells the nurse that she finds it difficult to concentrate and feels restless. To determine if this complaint is akathisia, a side effect of the drug, the nurse should determine if the patient

    A. has pain when urinating.

    B. feels better when walking around.

    C. can count backward by sevens.

    D. can drink a glass of water without swallowing difficulties.

84. When a patient begins taking chlorpromazine (Thorazine), which of the following statements is appropriate for the nurse to make because of one of the drug's adrenolytic effects?

    A. "You may perspire a great deal."

    B. "You may have some ringing in your ears."

    C. "Be sure you have tissues or a handkerchief with you at all times. You are likely to have a runny nose."

    D. "Take your time getting out of bed in the morning. You may feel a little dizzy on arising."

85. A male patient is being treated with an anti-parkinsonian agent. Which of these statements if made by the patient indicates that he is experiencing a side effect of the drug?

    A. "My wife says my heart rate is very rapid."

    B. "I seem to be going to the bathroom to urinate more frequently."

    C. "I sometimes feel sleepy."

    D. "My wife says that I don't hear her when she speaks."

86. A patient who is taking chlorpromazine (Thorazine) says to the nurse, "The doctor told me not to take any antacids that have magnesium in them. Why is that?" The nurse's response is based on the understanding that concurrent administration of Thorazine and this type of antacid

    A. causes bowel impaction.

    B. increases the side effects of Thorazine.

    C. significantly lowers the serum levels of Thorazine.

    D. tends to increase absorption of Thorazine in the stomach.

87. A patient is started on antipsychotic drugs. His family wants to know when the drug will begin to have some effect on the patient's symptoms. The nurse's response is based on the understanding that symptoms usually are in control within

    A. 24 hours.

    B. 48 hours.

    C. 3 to 4 days.

    D. 5 to 10 days.

88. A patient on the psychiatric unit refuses drug therapy as a treatment option. After much discussion, the patent continues to refuse. What information does the nurse need in order to proceed?

    A. The state's ruling about the rights of hospitalized psychiatric patients

    B. The American Nurses Association's position on patient's rights

    C. The protocols for the drug that was to be administered

    D. The length of time the patient has been in the facility

89. A patient was admitted to the psychiatric unit with a diagnosis of bipolar affective disorder — manic type. The patient is overactive, grandiose, and talks and walks about constantly. Because of the patient's behaviors, which of these measures should the nurse include in the patient's care?

    A. Encourage the patient to go to the bathroom every 2 hours.

    B. Take the patient's vital signs around the clock.

    C. Provide the patient with a high-calorie diet.

    D. Test the patient's reflexes regularly.

90. A patient who has a bipolar disorder and is slightly manic is to start on lithium therapy. The patient and the nurse have discussed its actions. Which of these statements if made by the patient indicates the patient understood the discussion?

    A. "If I get diarrhea, I know the drug is reaching its effective dose."

    B. "I can expect my thought processes to slow down."

    C. "Within a few days I will feel generally terrible, and that will last for at least 3 to 4 months."

    D. "I can expect my stomach to hurt as long as I am taking the drug."

91. A patient who attends a community-based clinic is to be started on lithium therapy. Which of these instructions should the nurse give the patient?

    A. "I will teach you to test your urine for the presence of lithium."

    B. "You will need to learn how to take your own pulse."

    C. "You will need to have someone you can rely on be taught to take your blood pressure."

    D. "I will give you a schedule as to when you have to have blood drawn so lithium serum levels can be determined."

92. When a patient who is taking lithium has a fever, it is extremely important for the nurse to be sure that the patient

    A. does not have food high in sodium.

    B. stays away from direct exposure to sunlight.

    C. does not become dehydrated.

    D. is in an nonstimulating environment.

93. If a patient's lithium level is 4.5 mEq/L, the nurse should expect that the patient might be prepared for

    A. a blood transfusion.

    B. dialysis.

    C. a liver biopsy.

    D. a brain scan.

94. A nurse is in a group therapy session with patients who are all on drug therapy. One of the patients says, "I'm sick and tired of taking these drugs." Many group members express similar feelings. In addition to discussing the patients' feelings and the importance of and reasons for drug therapy as a treatment modality, which of these goals should the nurse have?

    A. Patients will work closely with staff when they discontinue medications.

    B. Patients will understand that their taking the drugs shows a trust in the nurse.

    C. Patients will understand that once they start a drug, they are not permitted to discontinue it.

    D. Patients will find other outlets for their feelings.

95. Prior to a patient's starting on carbamazepine (Tegretol), the nurse should prepare the patient for the fact that he must have

    A. a bone scan.

    B. a T-helper cell count.

    C. an intravenous pyelogram (IVP).

    D. an electrocardiogram (ECG).

96. A patient who attends a community-based mental health clinic is to start on tricyclic drug therapy. The nurse should instruct the patient that the patient will have to have routine

    A. white blood cell counts (WBCs).

    B. electroencephalograms (EEGs).

    C. blood pressure checks.

    D. blood sugar values.

97. A patient who is depressed and taking tricyclic antidepressant medication complains of headaches. Which of these actions should the nurse take first?

    A. Assess to see if the complaint is part of the patient's depressive symptomatology.

    B. Ask the patient if she has been eating cheese.

    C. Determine if the patient is dehydrated.

    D. Check the patient's abdominal girth.

98. A depressed patient, who attends a mental health outpatient clinic and who has admitted suicidal ideation in the past, is started on tricylic antidepressant drug therapy. Which of the following actions is it appropriate for the nurse to take?

    A. Explain to the patient that the drug should be taken before eating.

    B. Tell the patient that weight loss is a common side effect.

    C. Instruct the patient to keep a diary where recurring thoughts should be recorded.

    D. Give the patient only a week's supply of the medication.

99. A 25-year-old woman, married 3 months ago, comes to the crisis center. She is feeling depressed and overwhelmed. The nurse obtains a complete history. Which of these factors is a likely precipitant for her crisis?

    A. She was sent to a boarding school as a child.

    B. She has a new job.

    C. She went to college with her husband.

    D. She was her father's favorite child.

100. When a patient is taking an antianxiety drug such as alprazolam (Xanax), the nurse should instruct the patient to

    A. avoid alcoholic beverages.

    B. increase potassium intake.

    C. discontinue use of such drugs as Tylenol.

    D. check for signs of edema.

Answers and Rationales for
NCLEX-TYPE QUESTIONS

1. A A mild level of anxiety generally helps to motivate learning. In that state, the person's sensory field increases. When a higher level than mild anxiety is present, learning is not usually possible. By assessing a person's anxiety level, the nurse tries to ascertain if the person can comprehend the materials which are to be discussed.

2. B Displacement is the reduction of an emotion (anger) from one area or person to another area or person (wife).

3. D Fears are part of the normal growth and development of children between the ages of 24 and 30 months. Common fears are of loud noises, dark, animals, and separation from parents.

4. A Broad knowledge of the patient's culture, racial identity, and ethnicity can be used to make care delivery more culturally sensitive.

5. B When a patient indicates that he or she is going to do harm to self, it is always the duty of the nurse to protect that person and inform others regarding the intention to harm.

6. A Patients with somatization disorder usually have a diagnosis of ineffective individual coping, as they tend to handle their emotional problems by having physical symptoms.

7. A In order to provide information to help patients understand their treatments, nurses should use clarifying statements as a way to attempt to find out what it is that patients want to know.

8. D Silence allows a patient time to gather his or her thoughts. The patient, particularly a newly admitted patient, may need time to think. It also conveys a sense that the nurse is interested in what the patient is thinking and has time to listen.

9. C When a patient begins to have a panic attack, it is important for the nurse to have the patient put his or her mind on another issue in order to draw the patient out of self, rather than going into the anxiety. If the patient begins to respond to the panic by focusing on the feelings, the feelings of anxiety escalate.

10. A The goal of treatment for a patient who is not able to function due to his ritualistic behavior is to limit and perhaps even eliminate that behavior so that the patient can function. The patient can be taught how to avoid the behaviors or circumvent the rituals so that he can participate more normally in the activities of daily living.

11. B Patients who are terminally ill need a time to contemplate their lives. It is appropriate for the nurse to encourage patients to engage in anticipatory grieving activities to deal with the shortness of their lives.

12. D Due to the stress of terminal illness, it is not unusual for unresolved conflicts and difficulties in relationships and communication patterns among family members to continue or even become worse.

13. A The living will offers competent individuals a mechanism to document what medical intervention they do and do not want should they become mentally incompetent and require medical technology to keep them alive. It is the responsibility, and legal duty, of the health care team to respect the wishes of the individual who has a living will.

14. C Children with attention deficit hyperactivity disorder are described as impulsive, restless, inattentive, distractable, and fidgety.

15. B Therapeutically, it is essential that children who have conduct disorders feel and believe that staff can limit their inappropriate behaviors, in this case aggression.

16. D The child should be allowed to assume some control over the condition. Having the child change the soiled sheets may give some sense of control.

17. A Clinical risk factors for suicide include a major psychiatric disorder and a family history of suicide or psychiatric illness.

18. B A change that is normal during aging is that the elderly are likely to sleep shorter periods; many older people normally complain of insomnia.

19. D The elderly feel a loss of control when they are not included in decision making. Relocation is a stressful event, and the elderly should have their preferences and choices considered.

20. C The depressed older adult may experience loss of appetite and disturbances in sleep as symptoms. These manifestations may be more evident than other symptoms found in younger adults who are depressed.

21. B Tricyclic antidepressants may increase the risk of cardiac rhythm irregularities, cause a drop in blood pressure, and cause urinary hesitancy and retention.

22. D The list of potential physiological causes of delirium is long. Significant attention must be paid to maintenance of hydration, nutrition, and electrolyte balance as any deviations from the norm may cause symptomatology.

23. A The best environment for a resident is a familiar one that provides many orienting clues. Having family and friends bring familiar objects from home is one way to help the resident in a new and confusing environment from becoming more confused.

24. C In order for the patient to be assisted in the grieving process, the nurse must first determine what stage of the grieving process the patient is in. Then the nurse can talk with the patient about the normal process and abnormal responses and teach the patient appropriate coping skills.

25. C The nurse should attempt to encourage the patient to leave the dayroom and either find a less stimulating environment or provide him with activities that allow him to release some of his energies — perhaps use a punching bag.

26. A Common side effects of lithium include thirst, nausea, fine hand tremors, polyuria, fatigue, and mild muscle weakness.

27. D The thought of having ECT treatments can be frightening. It is important to determine if the patient has any misconceptions regarding the therapy. One way to determine this in this situation is to ask what the patient is afraid of.

28. B Patients who have anorexia nervosa may vomit after eating. It is best to be able to observe the patient for at least 1 hour after the patient has eaten a meal.

29. B The purpose of a food diary is to keep track of what has been eaten and what feelings or activities were present before, during, and after eating.

30. A Sleepwalking can cause injury. Make sure that windows are closed, doors locked, and stairways blocked.

31. D After abuse, post-traumatic syndrome disorder (PTSD) may occur and interpersonal performance may be disrupted. An aggressive pattern of PTSD is common and characterized by fighting with peers and family.

32. D A sense of helplessness divorces the victim from her ability to be self-assertive and take charge of her life. Self-blame leads to a fragmented sense of self, separating the victim from sexual and aggressive capacities essential for living and relating to others.

33. D Schizoid personality disorder is a pattern of detachment from social relationships and a restricted range of emotional expression (DSM-IV-1994).

34. A The nursing diagnosis that is made is defensive coping because the patient is denying he has obvious problems (lack of current knowledge, projection of responsibility, and a superior attitude toward others).

35. B Neglected infants and toddlers may appear dull, inactive, and excessively passive.

36. C A primary nurse is assigned to the neglected child as a way to establish a beginning therapeutic alliance and decrease the number of strangers that the child would need to interact with.

37. D Parents should always be informed that a report is being made and what the purpose of the report is: It is a referral to an agency that will visit the child's residence to ensure that the child's environment is safe.

38. D Parental risk factors for child abuse include spouse/partner abuse; the other factors are not considered risks.

39. C Most studies have shown that a risk factor for being a victim of physical abuse is having been a victim of parental abuse as a child.

40. A Schizophrenia is a chronic disease and various factors may lead to intermittent hospitalization for acute exacerbation of symptoms. These occasions should not be viewed as a treatment failure.

41. A Delusions are fixed beliefs maintained despite experience and evidence to the contrary.

42. C In the early development of the addiction, it is very threatening to the ego to allow the possibility of addiction into one's awareness. Thus, the individual tends to deny the problem.

43. C Patients who are having delusions, such as thinking that their medications are being poisoned, need to be given an appropriate degree of choice, e.g., seeing a closed medication packet and watching the nurse open the packet.

44. D Nausea or nausea and vomiting, visible tremors, increased anxiety, tachycardia, or mild systolic hypertension are usual symptoms in the early stages of alcohol withdrawal.

45. B As addicting drugs, narcotics produce tolerance in the individual; therefore the patient will probably require more pain medication than a patient who has not abused drugs.

46. B Symptoms of withdrawal usually last 4 to 7 days. The symptoms are extremely unpleasant (increased pain and anxiety perception from low serotonin levels). Tearing usually begins first; then diarrhea is likely.

47. B When a patient expresses feelings of distress about life and indicates loneliness, suicide is possible. It would be most helpful to determine the patient's past coping behavior.

48. D Suicide tends to run in families. It may be that because one family member committed suicide, suicide can be viewed by other family members as an "appropriate" coping mechanism.

49. A Aggressive patients should not be kept waiting, as they interpret the wait as a sign they are not important or do not require immediate treatment. The patient's behavior is viewed as a symptom of an illness and must be taken seriously.

50. A The nurse must immediately report threats of violence. To prevent violence, it is vital to set limits on a patient's aggressive behavior — verbal and physical.

51. C Giving away possessions may often be a clue that an elderly person is considering suicide; an assessment of suicidal ideation is essential.

52. D The nurse should not place himself or herself in jeopardy of being killed, especially when no one else's life is at risk. Therefore, if the stranger is threatening to kill the nurse, the nurse should take the threat seriously and comply with the demand.

53. B Prior to caring for patients, staff need to deal with their own feelings toward violence and aggression. Then, the staff can learn techniques to deal with their own and the patients' feelings and behaviors.

54. B Contracting is a system whereby the nurse, staff, and patient together decide how aggressive behavior will be handled. The patient is responsible for using methods that work for him, selecting from a variety of suggestions. Aggressive/violent behavior is always unacceptable.

55. C Child abuse, particularly sexual abuse, may be a factor in the transmission of HIV infection.

56. B The continuous recording of the patient's life story aids in the continuing assessment of the patient's psychological status. It is not a substitute but rather an adjunct to the interactions of the nurse, other health care providers, and others in the patient's social network.

57. C Cognitive symptoms include memory loss, mental slowing, poor concentration, and confusion. Motor symptoms include unsteady gait, leg weakness, tremor, spasticity, and hyperflexia.

58. A The rule to follow in giving psychotropic drugs to patients with AIDS is "Start low and go slow." Because of the anticholinergic effects of the drug, the patient must be assessed for side effects before more therapeutic doses can be given.

59. A Ingestion of ibuprofen may cause a false positive on a urine screen for opiates.

60. D When a patient becomes addicted and develops a tolerance to Valium, the seizure threshold of the brain is raised. Abrupt cessation lowers the threshold and causes seizures.

61. B In the orientation phase, the goal is for the patient and nurse to become acquainted with each other and for the patient to identify the process of seeking help as a learning experience. The patient's problem is a learning deficit rather than a personal deficit in coping.

62. C In the orientation phase, the focus is on encouraging the patient to identify and express feelings. Advice, reassurance, and suggestions are of little value when offered about dealing with feelings.

63. B Ineffective boundaries are demonstrated when nurses stay with patients beyond working hours serving the patient's needs rather than theirs or those of the treatment setting.

64. D Feelings of depersonalization can a occur when the nurse refuses to "chat." The patient feels that he is not being treated as an individual, but rather as a diagnosis or bed number.

65. A Maintaining contact with the patient after termination conveys a subtle message of lack of confidence in the patient's independence.

66. D The nurse is a part of the community and must use discretion about when to intervene. The nurse does not want to usurp the leader role and may choose to discuss what occurred after the meeting as a part of the postmeeting discussion. There may have been reasons for the leader allowing the behavior or it may be that the leader needs some assistance in curbing this type of behavior.

67. A In order to know if a patient is responding appropriately to a medication, the nurse needs to know the purpose of the medication. If the purpose is to slow the patient's thinking, then finding that the patient is complaining that his or her thinking has been slowed has an entirely different meaning.

68. C A critical pathway is a multidisciplinary plan of care. If there is a variance between what has been planned and what has occurred, the first step is to determine why the variance has occurred.

69. C The goal of crisis management as a therapeutic modality is to strengthen the patient's coping processes.

70. C During crisis intervention, the nurse should help the patient recognize irrational beliefs. Sometimes a carefully worded question to challenge the belief is most appropriate.

71. A The discussion of the patient's fears about drugs often strengthens the therapeutic alliance between the patient and the nurse because of the thoughts shared and the decisions that the patient must make. This empowerment can prevent regression.

72. D Patients should learn self-monitoring procedures and be taught to communicate and negotiate drug dosage.

73. D Antipsychotic drugs are long-acting. Once a dose level to control symptoms has been achieved, a single dose can be given at bedtime to overcome problems with daytime sedation.

74. B At this time, the only known treatment for tardive dyskinesia is discontinuance of the antipsychotic drug causing the symptoms.

75. B Dystonia requires immediate treatment. It is easily treated with an anti-parkinsonian drug, such as Cogentin.

76. D Agranulocytosis is initially recognized by a sore throat, fever, and general malaise.

77. C Photosensitivity may occur with Thorazine therapy; staying out of the sun and wearing protective clothing are the best ways to deal with this problem.

78. B A goal on the inpatient unit is that the patient will overcome feelings of isolation. Therefore, one of the goals of the group is for a patient to feel less isolated.

79. D Some ethnic group members remain quiet and withdrawn even when language proficiency is not an issue.

80. B Prior to discharge, if a patient is expected to attend a facility for follow-up care, it is vital to know if the patient can get to the facility or if some means of transportation is required.

81. C For patients who meet eligibility criteria, psychiatric home care is 100% reimbursed by Medicare.

82. C Outcome must be stated in concrete measurable terms. This outcome could be stated (if the feelings in question were negative), "The patient will state three reasons for expressing negative feelings."

83. B For patients taking antipsychotic medications, akathisia, which usually is manifested by feelings of restlessness and agitation, must be differentiated from increasing anxiety. If the akathisia is due to drug side effects, the patient will report that she feels better when walking about.

84. D One example of an adrenolytic side effect of Thorazine is postural hypotension, which may be manifested by dizziness upon arising.

85. A Peripheral anticholinergic side effects (the side effects from anti-parkinsonian agents) include tachycardia and urinary retention.

86. C Studies indicate that the concurrent administration of Thorazine and alum or magnesium gel-type antacids results in significantly lower serum levels of Thorazine.

87. D When a patient is receiving antipsychotic drug therapy, symptoms are usually in control within 5 to 10 days, and a positive drug response should occur within 3 to 6 weeks.

88. A In many states, patients can refuse drug treatment when they are hospitalized.

89. C A patient in a manic state is using a tremendous amount of energy and needs a greater caloric intake than usual.

90. B When lithium is used to treat mania, the patient may be aware of a slowing down of the thought process. Symptoms of toxicity include abdominal pain, diarrhea, and general malaise. If any of these symptoms occur, the drug should be withheld.

91. D A major nursing responsibility is to monitor lithium blood levels. It is necessitated by lithium's very narrow therapeutic index and the consequences of the drug's buildup as a result of its pattern of excretion.

92. C Dehydration caused by excessive heat or fever can cause a buildup of lithium due to sodium loss, and toxicity may then occur.

93. B Severe lithium toxicity is a medical emergency. Some physicians believe that for patients with a serum level of 3.0 mEq/L or more, hemodialysis or peritoneal dialysis may be started.

94. A The nurse must make it clear to all patients that they have the right to refuse treatment; however, once a drug treatment regimen is started, patients must work closely with nursing and medical staffs if they wish to discontinue the medication.

95. D Incidents of heart block have been noted during treatment with Tegretol; therefore, a baseline ECG should be done.

96. C Cardiovascular side effects, including hypotension, are common when using tricyclic drug therapy. Blood pressure should be checked weekly.

97. A When patients who are taking tricyclic antidepressants complain of headaches, it is important for the nurse to assess the frequency, quality, and severity of the headaches. Frequently, depressed patients have somatic complaints as part of their symptom presentation.

98. D Outpatients need to be monitored carefully and frequently to decrease the chances of lethal overdosage, particularly with tricyclics. Sometimes it is best to give only a week's supply of the drug.

99. B A crisis can occur with too many changes in one's life. The stress of a new job and a new marriage concurrently can precipitate a crisis.

100. A Xanax is a benzodiazepine, and alcohol or another central nervous system depressant should not be used when the patient is taking this class of drug.